Concise Clinical Pharmacology

Concise Clinical Pharmacology

Ben Greenstein

BA(Hons), BSc(Hons), DHPh, PhD, FBIH, MRPharmS

Senior Visiting Research Fellow
Pain Management Team, Royal Free Hospital,
London, UK

Adam Greenstein

BSc(Hons), MBBCh, MRCP

Specialist Registrar in Elderly Medicine
Leeds General Infirmary, UK

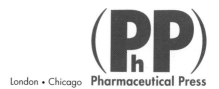

London • Chicago **Pharmaceutical Press**

Published by the Pharmaceutical Press
An imprint of RPS Publishing

1 Lambeth High Street, London SE1 7JN, UK
100 South Atkinson Road, Suite 200, Grayslake, IL 60030-7820, USA

© Pharmaceutical Press 2007

(**PP**) is a trade mark of RPS Publishing

RPS Publishing is the publishing organisation of the Royal Pharmaceutical
Society of Great Britain

First published 2007

Typeset by Photoprint, Torquay, Devon
Printed in Slovenia by Compass Press Ltd, Ljubljana

ISBN-10 0 85369 576 8
ISBN-13 978 0 85369 576 9   OCT   2007

A catalogue record for this book is available from the British Library

Contents

Preface

Clinical pharmacology is one of the most important subjects of the medical curriculum, especially in view of the central position of drug prescribing in general and specialist medicine. Now that other health professionals, notably nurses and pharmacists, are poised to take an expanded role in the prescribing of drugs, particularly licensed medicines, the need for a readily accessible and user-friendly textbook and reference guide for prescribers becomes imperative. Many clinical pharmacology curricula will need revising and updating and this book has been designed with those needs in mind.

Medical students have an especially onerous task in the assimilation of knowledge about a vast range of medicines and their uses, and in the experience of the authors a common complaint among students has been the lack of a clinical pharmacology textbook that presents concisely the information needed for note preparation, revision and reference. There are undoubtedly several worthy clinical pharmacology textbooks available, but none as far as we know that tackles the needs of the embattled student head on. It is hoped that this book will come to be regarded by all students who use it as a valued friend.

It may be helpful for the student to approach the study of medicines with the attitude that drugs are not mainly about mechanisms, receptors, enzymes and chemical structures but about patients who need help to prevent and cure diseases, reduce or remove unpleasant symptoms, and allow them to get on with a normal life as far as possible. This book therefore attempts to relate all aspects of drug study to the patient and to motivate the student who wants to know about drugs for the sake of the patient, and not just for academic study needs.

Ben Greenstein
Adam Greenstein
August 2006

Acknowledgements

It remains only to thank all those kind colleagues who have scrutinised the manuscript critically; their corrections, suggestions and revisions are gratefully acknowledged. We should also like to thank Louise McIndoe and Victoria Brown of the Pharmaceutical Press for their superb editorial patience and support.

About the authors

Ben Greenstein originally qualified as a pharmacist in South Africa, where he worked mainly in rural areas before immigrating to the UK to work for 3 years as a community pharmacist. He obtained a PhD in Pharmacology at the University of London in 1975 and lectured in pharmacology at the University of London for 18 years, after which he decided to devote himself to the writing of textbooks in his areas of expertise. He is currently an Honorary Visiting Senior Research Fellow in the Pain Management Service at the Royal Free Hospital, Hampstead, London and is also a Fellow of the British Institute of Homeopathy.

Adam Greenstein obtained his degree in medicine at the University of Manchester and is a member of the Royal College of Physicians. He is a specialist registrar in general medicine and elderly care medicine in Yorkshire.

1 Introduction to pharmacology

Pharmacology is the scientific study of the properties of drugs and their interaction with living organisms, including viruses.[1] The term 'drug' is in common usage for any chemical used to treat disease or for recreational purposes. Strictly speaking, the term describes any chemical that is used to change the activity of a living cell.

Pharmacology has two main branches: **pharmacodynamics** and **pharmacokinetics**. Pharmacodynamics is the study of the interaction of drugs with cells. It can be thought of as how the drug affects the body. Pharmacokinetics is the study of how the body handles the drug, including how it is absorbed and distributed among the various compartments of the body, how long it remains in the body in a therapeutically effective form, and how it is metabolised and excreted. Pharmacology also embraces the study of adverse reactions to drugs, drug–drug interactions and the consequences of drug overdose. Pharmacology also covers toxicity of chemicals.

Clinical pharmacology is devoted mainly to the choice and use of drugs to prevent and treat disease and to the consequences of drug misuse. Clinical pharmacology is nowadays becoming more and more involved in the socio-economic implications of clinical drug use. An example of this is the relatively new science of **pharmacovigilance**, which is concerned with the follow-up of drug use, and **pharmacoeconomics**, which examines the economic implications of prescribing and dispensing increasingly more expensive treatments.

Drugs may originate from natural sources or be synthesised. Digoxin, for example, was originally extracted from the foxglove, *Digitalis purpurea*, but is now synthesised. Once a drug is identified as a possible treatment for a specific condition, it undergoes an intensive battery of tests to determine its mechanism of action, its potency, its specificity of action and its safety for the patient. The drug's fate in the body is studied, as well as its effects on the tissues and organs. Its possible teratogenicity (ability to harm the unborn embryo or fetus) is also investigated. Once a suitable dose and formulation are decided upon, the drug undergoes rigorously controlled clinical trials, and if it passes all tests it may be licensed for use in patients. Clinical pharmacology encompasses all aspects of the drug's use in patients, both before and after licensing.

Modern clinical pharmacology involves the expertise not only of doctors, but also of nurses and pharmacists, who are involved in the choice of drug, and dosage and administration, especially in hospitals. In outlying districts and in developing countries, the pharmacist and nurse are often the only immediate resource for patients, both for advice and for the monitoring of, for example, adverse drug reactions and patient compliance. Pharmacists have prescribed some remedies for hundreds of years. Nurses, both in hospital and in the community, are now prescribing certain drugs and need pharmacological knowledge to underpin their use of drugs for patients and to treat, for example, adverse reactions and overdose.

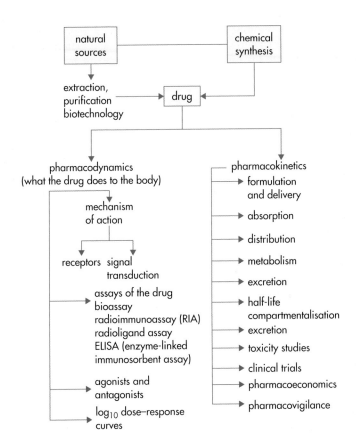

2 Sources of modern drugs

One of the first, and still arguably the most widely used, of all drugs is aspirin, a synthetic derivative of salicylic acid, which was used for centuries as an extract of willow bark for the treatment of what used to be called ague (rheumatism). Natural products are, however, still very much in circulation, because of the huge resurgence of interest in their use (**A**). In more developed countries, e.g. the USA, it has been estimated that approximately 40% of annual expenditure by the public on medicines and treatment can be attributed to the use of herbal, homoeopathic and other alternative remedies and treatments, including acupuncture. This amounts to several billions of dollars. The phenomenon has been recognised by government and other research-funding agencies in the UK and other countries, and treatments such as glucosamine sulphate for osteoarthritis are the subject of intensive scientific research.

In conventional pharmacology, the discovery of drug structures and the characterisation of the active sites of their receptors and receptor subtypes in tissues have led to the synthesis of a whole battery of new drugs (**B**). Examples include the synthetic morphine analogues such as pethidine and methadone. The discovery of the body's own opioids, the endorphins and enkephalins, and their various receptors, resulted in the synthesis of novel short-acting general anaesthetics and analgesics such as fentanyl and alfentanil. The structure of antihistamines was altered until a drug was found that selectively blocked histamine H_2-receptors, and the introduction of the anti-ulcer drugs cimetidine and ranitidine. The characterisation of the different norepinephrine and epinephrine receptor subtypes (α_1, α_2, β_1, β_2 and β_3) has produced the selective receptor-blocking drugs, e.g. the selective β_1-blockers for cardiovascular diseases, such as atenolol (page 40). The elucidation of the body's means of terminating neurotransmitter action through metabolism of the neurotransmitter or through the neurotransmitter's re-uptake into the nerve terminal after it has done its work has generated a powerful group of drugs for psychiatric use, notably antidepressants such as monoamine oxidase inhibitors (MAOIs), the tricyclic antidepressants and the selective serotonin re-uptake inhibitors (SSRIs). Nevertheless, work needs to be done to reduce or eliminate adverse effects. SSRIs, for example, are proving to be problematic because of the development of drug dependence.

Pharmacological research, e.g. into the mediation of inflammation by the immune system, together with powerful techniques in recombinant DNA technology, has produced new and important drugs. The discovery that the peptide tumour necrosis factor-α (TNF-α) is an early mediator of the immune system has led to the introduction of proteins designed to combine with circulating TNF-α and neutralise it. An example is **infliximab**, an **antibody** that binds to circulating TNF-α, thus inactivating it. These drugs are large foreign peptides or proteins and may cause an anaphylactic (allergic) reaction; the same immune response by the body also serves to inactivate the medicine itself. Nevertheless, these drugs are proving dramatically effective in reducing the inflammation of rheumatoid and psoriatic arthritis. There is no doubt that many of these so-called 'biologic' drugs are on the way.

A. Sources of modern drugs

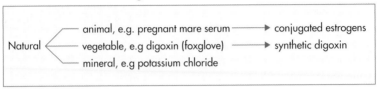

Natural
- animal, e.g. pregnant mare serum ⟶ conjugated estrogens
- vegetable, e.g digoxin (foxglove) ⟶ synthetic digoxin
- mineral, e.g potassium chloride

B. Modern methods of drug discovery

Modern methods

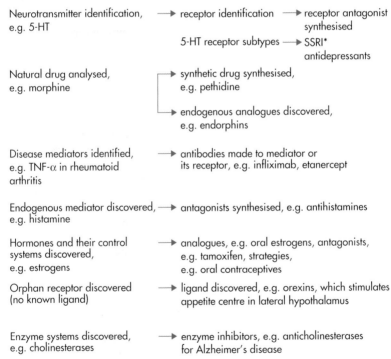

Neurotransmitter identification, e.g. 5-HT ⟶ receptor identification ⟶ receptor antagonist synthesised

5-HT receptor subtypes ⟶ SSRI* antidepressants

Natural drug analysed, e.g. morphine
- ⟶ synthetic drug synthesised, e.g. pethidine
- ⟶ endogenous analogues discovered, e.g. endorphins

Disease mediators identified, e.g. TNF-α in rheumatoid arthritis ⟶ antibodies made to mediator or its receptor, e.g. infliximab, etanercept

Endogenous mediator discovered, e.g. histamine ⟶ antagonists synthesised, e.g. antihistamines

Hormones and their control systems discovered, e.g. estrogens ⟶ analogues, e.g. oral estrogens, antagonists, e.g. tamoxifen, strategies, e.g. oral contraceptives

Orphan receptor discovered (no known ligand) ⟶ ligand discovered, e.g. orexins, which stimulates appetite centre in lateral hypothalamus

Enzyme systems discovered, e.g. cholinesterases ⟶ enzyme inhibitors, e.g. anticholinesterases for Alzheimer's disease

SSRI: Selective serotonin re-uptake inhibitors

3 The use of drugs in medicine

Drugs form a major part of the treatment of disease. They may be used to cure a disease, e.g. the use of antibiotics to clear an infection, and they alleviate symptoms, e.g. the use of aspirin or morphine to reduce pain. Drugs may prevent disease, e.g. the use of quinine for malaria or the use of vaccines. They are also used as aids to other forms of medical treatment, when their use is not necessarily directed towards the treatment of a disease. For example, drugs are used as general anaesthetics during surgery, or when organs are being investigated, e.g. opticians using atropine-like drugs to dilate the pupil when examining the interior of the eye. Drugs are also very widely used by healthy people. Millions of women world-wide take drugs to prevent conception, and travellers take antispasmodics to prevent or treat travel sickness.

Important aims with drug use are to use a drug that is easy and safe to administer, and that acts with high specificity and appropriate duration in order to gain the maximum advantage with minimum damage to the body. (Much of clinical pharmacology is concerned with these considerations when prescribing.) This is an ideal scenario – which at present is seldom, if ever, achieved. Drugs are by definition foreign chemicals that are often toxic, and the body tries to eliminate them as soon as possible, by metabolising them and rendering them easier to excrete. Drugs are most easily administered orally, and have to resist the digestive processes, be easily absorbed and survive their passage through the liver after absorption (page 18). Some drugs actually damage the digestive tract, aspirin being a commonly quoted example, because it is corrosive and can cause stomach ulceration. Drugs may have to be given by injection, and some patients fear injections. Some injectable drugs, particularly some of the anticancer drugs, can damage the tissues into which they are injected.

Drugs have to reach the target tissue, and this can be a problem, particularly if they have to cross the blood–brain barrier. It is worth mentioning that drugs travel not only to the intended site of action, but everywhere in the body, and this to a great extent is responsible for the unwanted, so-called **side-effects** of drugs (see opposite). One of the most notorious examples of this is the drug thalidomide, which was introduced to treat the nausea of pregnancy. It crossed the placenta and caused fetal malformation. Modern pharmaceutical formulation includes attempts to target selectively the tissue where the drug is intended to act.

Another important consideration is the cost of medicines. Medicines are becoming far more sophisticated and expensive to develop, which results in a more expensive drug for the patient, the medical insurance companies and governmental health systems such as the National Health Service (NHS) in the UK. Patients quite reasonably have every right to the drug that will improve or cure their condition, and prescribers are increasingly caught in the middle between the patient and the bodies that pay for the drug. This is pharmacoeconomics.

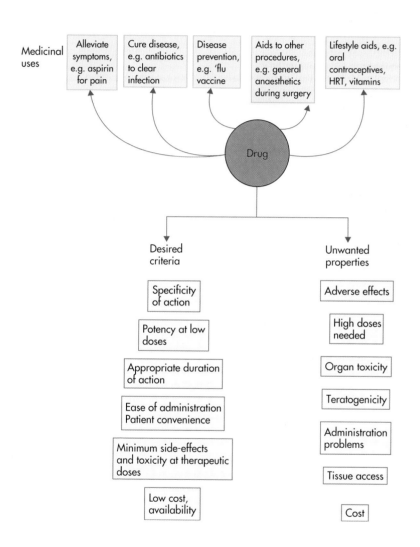

4 The receptor concept

Through their receptors, all tissues can distinguish between different chemical messengers such as hormones and neurotransmitters. These receptors are proteins on the surface of the cell, or within it, that selectively bind these chemicals and transduce the binding reaction into a signal to the cell, which responds appropriately (**A**). Thus, acetylcholine (ACh) receptors on the surface of salivary gland cells bind ACh, and the cell secretes saliva (see also page 39). Implicit in the binding reaction are the receptor properties of **selectivity** and **affinity**. A chemical that binds to a receptor and elicits the appropriate response is called an **agonist**.

Selectivity is the property whereby the ACh receptor recognises only certain chemical structures but not others. Thus the ACh receptor binds chemicals that possess certain chemical groups, but not others. **Affinity** is the degree of attraction between the binding site on the receptor and the chemical groups that bind to it. For example, ACh in relatively low concentrations at its receptor sites in a tissue will be picked up by the receptors sufficiently to elicit a cellular response. Selectivity and affinity underpin most of pharmacology and the design of drugs.

Antagonists: Another extremely important feature of the receptor–chemical interaction is that some chemicals produce a cellular response, whereas others bind to the receptor but elicit no response, and in addition block access to the receptor by an agonist (**B**), (**C**). The property of some drugs to block receptors has been successfully exploited to produce many useful drugs, e.g. the β-blockers for hypertension (page 72) and the H_2-receptor blockers to treat gastric ulcers (page 200). Any chemical that binds to a receptor is also called a **ligand**.

The **structure of the receptor** is dictated to a large extent by its cellular location and function. Thus, receptors on the cell membrane have an extracellular ligand-binding domain, a transmembrane domain and an intracellular domain, all with specific functions. The extracellular domain binds the ligand and possibly identifies it as either an agonist or antagonist; the transmembrane domain conducts the message and also interacts with other membrane proteins that transduce the binding message into the appropriate cellular response, a duty also performed by the intracellular domain, which initiates the intracellular cascade of reactions (**D**). The transmembrane domain may also give the receptor mobility within the membrane. The above is a generalisation, because different membrane receptors may have very different properties and mechanisms of action. Examples of cell membrane receptors are the insulin receptor (page 8), the ACh receptor and the β-**receptor**.

Intracellular receptors occur inside the cell, and examples of these are the steroid hormone receptors (**E**) such as the estrogen receptor. The main receptor families are described in the next spread.

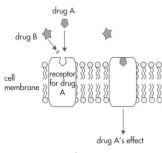

A. Receptor selectivity

B. Receptor antagonist

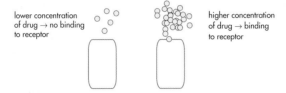

C. Drug affinity for receptor: effect of drug concentration

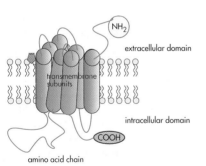

D. Membrane receptor structure

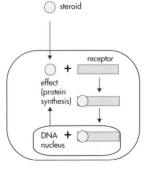

E. Intracellular steroid receptor

5 Signal transduction and the receptor families

Receptor families: Four receptor families are defined in terms of receptor structure and the transduction mechanism. These are: (i) membrane channel-linked receptors (ionotropic) coupled directly to ion channels; (ii) G-protein-coupled (metabotropic) receptors; (iii) kinase-linked receptors, which incorporate domains for protein kinase enzymes; and (iv) intracellular receptor proteins linked to nuclear transcription. The steroids exert their effects mainly through (iv).

Signal transduction: Drugs interact with cells through a primary interaction with receptors. Charged molecules such as peptides and neurotransmitters bind to receptors on the cell membrane, causing a conformational change in other membrane proteins, which may activate ion channels (receptor family (i), or activate enzymes inside the cell, resulting in the synthesis of 'second messengers', which activate phosphorylating enzymes (receptor families (ii) and (iii)).

Second messengers: The first second messenger to be identified was cyclic AMP, the intracellular chemical activated after activation of the membrane β-receptor by, for example, epinephrine, which in turn activates the membrane enzyme adenylyl cyclase through membrane G proteins. Adenylyl cyclase, when activated, converts intracellular ATP to cyclic AMP.

G proteins: There are a number of G proteins in the cell membrane, which mediate the activation or inhibition of membrane-bound enzymes after a receptor has been bound by its ligand. For example, after epinephrine binds to its receptor, the Ga protein moves away from the Gb/g complex to the enzyme adenylyl cyclase and activates it (receptor family (ii)).

PLCb system: Another important second messenger system is the PLCb system. This membrane enzyme is activated when a hormone, e.g. angiotensin II, binds to the receptor and phosphoinositol-4,5-bisphosphate (PIP_2) is cleaved to form diacylglycerol (DAG) and inositol-1,4,5-trisphosphate (IP_3). IP_3 releases Ca^{2+} from the endoplasmic reticulum (ER). Released Ca^{2+} activates several intracellular enzymes, including protein kinases, or it may activate muscle contractility or secretions. DAG together with Ca^{2+} also activates intracellular protein kinases. As a result of the activation of the PLC systems, the activated protein kinases also promote nuclear transcription and subsequent protein synthesis through activation of both intranuclear response elements for various genes and the nuclear cyclic AMP response element-binding protein (CREB).

Kinase-linked receptors (receptor family (iii)) include the insulin receptor. This receptor incorporates a protein kinase on its intracellular domain, and so it can be said to serve as its own second messenger. In the case of insulin, after the hormone has bound to the receptor, it is internalised. Insulin is an example where down-regulation of the receptor serves to limit the action of insulin, and up-regulation of the receptor is induced in order to maximise the effects of insulin.

Intracellular receptors: Uncharged molecules, such as the steroid hormones, thyroid hormone and vitamin D, diffuse into the cell and bind to receptor proteins which may be in the cytoplasm or nucleus or both (receptor family iv). The hormone receptor complex binds to specific hormone response elements (HREs) on the DNA and mRNA, and protein synthesis is altered as a result. These intracellular receptors are often, therefore, nuclear transcription activators, so their full effects are delayed for several hours. Examples of the hormones are cortisol, androgens, estrogens and progesterone.

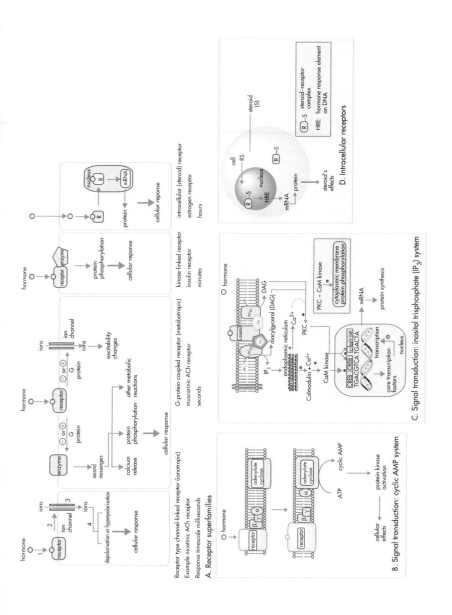

A. Receptor superfamilies

hormone

1 → receptor → 2 → ion channel → 3 → ions

4 → ions

depolarisation or hyperpolarisation

cellular response

Receptor type channel-linked receptor (ionotropic)
Example nicotinic ACh receptor
Response timescale milliseconds

hormone

enzyme ⊕ or ⊕ G protein → receptor ⊕ or ⊕ G protein → ion channel → ions

second messengers

calcium release

protein phosphorylation

other metabolic reactions

excitability changes

cellular response

G-protein-coupled receptor (metabotropic)
muscarinic ACh receptor
seconds

hormone

receptor / enzyme

protein phosphorylation

cellular reponse

kinase-linked receptor
insulin receptor
minutes

nucleus R → mRNA

R → protein

cellular reponse

intracellular (steroid) receptor
estrogen receptor
hours

B. Signal transduction: cyclic AMP system

hormone

receptor | β γ | α

receptor | β γ | α | adenylate cyclase

ATP → cyclic AMP

cellular effects

protein kinase activation

C. Signal transduction: inositol trisphosphate (IP₃) system

hormone

DAG

diacylglycerol (DAG)

IP₃

endoplasmic reticulum

Ca²⁺

PKC

Calmodulin + Ca²⁺

CaM kinase

PKC + CaM kinase

cytoplasmic membrane protein phosphorylation

CREB CREB c-fos/c-jun
TGACGTCA TGACTCA

core transcription factors

transcription

nucleus

mRNA

protein synthesis

D. Intracellular receptors

steroid (S)

cell

R–S

R–S
nucleus
HRE

mRNA → protein

steroid's effects

R–S : steroid–receptor complex

HRE: hormone response element on DNA

6 The measurement of drug activity I: Bioassay

Drugs cannot be used in patients until they have been tested for potency, toxicity and specificity of effect. **Bioassay** is a term used to describe and measure the activity of drugs in biological systems. Historically, bioassay was used to measure the plasma concentration of substances such as the body's own hormones, but it has now been replaced by techniques such as enzyme-linked immunosorbent assay. Bioassay is now used mainly: (i) to identify and measure the pharmacological activity of drugs under development; (ii) to compare the potency of a new drug with drugs already in clinical use; (iii) to investigate the activity of the body's own chemical mediators; and (iv) to study adverse and toxic actions of drugs under investigation.

Bioassay is used *in vitro* on, for example, bacteria, cells, isolated tissues and organs (e.g. nerves, heart or lungs), or *in vivo* in the intact organism (e.g. mice, humans). Clinical trials are bioassays of drugs in human participants. Ideally, a bioassay should be specific for the biological activity being targeted. For example, if a drug is sought to treat hypertension by blocking calcium channels, its clinical potency often correlates well with its ability to block calcium channels *in vitro*. On the other hand, there are few if any bioassay systems (other than treatment of the patient) that will reliably identify a potential treatment for certain psychiatric disorders, e.g. schizophrenia.

An important principle in bioassay is that a drug of unknown potency or efficacy is compared with a drug or standard of known potency. For example, a batch of human insulin prepared by genetic engineering must (among other tests) be tested for its ability to lower blood sugar in comparison with a standard batch of known potency, before it can be packaged and sold. A test may be **quantal** or **graded**. A graded test may involve the use of the $\log_{10}$ dose–response curve (**A**) to measure the degree of lowering of blood glucose. A quantal test (**B**) is a test for an all-or-nothing event such as loss of a reflex.

Problems associated with bioassay include the occurrence of **biological variation**. Tests can become unreliable through factors as unexpected as the variation in water hardness in different areas where a test is done, to variations in responsiveness to a given drug as a result of strain differences within a species such as the mouse or, even more notoriously, to response variability in humans. Ethnicity plays a large part in the variability of response to drugs. For example, certain drugs, such as hydralazine, are inactivated by acetylation, a process involving enzyme action. In the UK about 40% of the population are fast acetylators and 60% are slow acetylators. This characteristic is inherited and the ratio of slow:fast acetylators varies in different societies. Eighty per cent of Egyptians are slow acetylators, whereas the Inuit of Canada and North America are without exception rapid acetylators. In principle, this will affect the outcome of the bioassay of drugs that are acetylators in any clinical trial, and factors such as acetylation rate have to be controlled for.

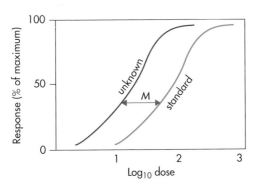

A. A graded test: the parallel line assay. Log_{10} dose–response curves are obtained for a standard preparation and the preparation of unknown potency. The unknown is more potent than the standard because its curve lies to the left of the other. The antilog of M is the potency ratio.

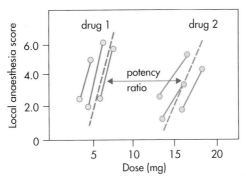

B. A quantal test. Two doses, one high and one low, of a local anaesthetic drug are tested in six patients in two groups of three, and a subjective score calculated for each. A regression line is calculated for each group and a dose ratio obtained.

7 The measurement of drug activity II: Dose–response relationship

Before drugs can be used therapeutically, an effective range of doses has to be determined. A dose–response relationship has to be established *in vivo*, and studied by testing a range of doses on *in vitro* and/or *in vivo* systems. For example, a drug being developed to treat hypertension by slowing the heart might first be tested on an isolated perfused heart. In practice, it is advisable to find a dose that lies on a linear range of responses and, in many cases, a linear relationship between the dose and the response is found when the response is plotted against $\log_{10}$ dose. A dose that produces 50% of the maximal response is usually considered a good starting point for investigation in living systems.

Potency: The $\log_{10}$ dose–response curve can be used to determine the potency of the drug being tested. In practice, the more potent the drug, the further to the left it will lie on a dose–response curve (**A**), and the steeper it will be. This property of a drug should not be confused with its **efficacy**. In pharmacological terms, efficacy is an indication of how much of a dose actually exerts the wanted effect on the problem being treated. A drug may produce a powerful effect *in vitro*, but when used *in vivo* it may not produce the powerful response for a given dose because it may, for example, be attacked by metabolising enzymes in the liver or blood during first-pass metabolism before it can get to its site of action. It may be potent *in vitro*, but not **effective** *in vivo*. This is reflected in the $\log_{10}$ dose–response curve by a lower maximum response to the drug (**B**). **Partial agonists** are drugs that act on the same receptor as an agonist, but they cannot produce the greatest response that the tissue or organ is capable of (as happens in response to a full agonist), and these produce $\log_{10}$ dose–response curves of a drug with less efficacy than that of a full agonist. An example of a partial agonist is the opiate nalorphine, which at higher doses may, for example, precipitate withdrawal reactions in heroin addicts.

Antagonists: The $\log_{10}$ dose–response curve can also be used to test for drugs that block the action of the body's chemicals on their receptors. Histamine contracts gut muscle and causes acid release in the stomach. A putative antihistamine may be tested for its ability to increase the dose of histamine that must be used to achieve a given contraction of gut or acid release. In the presence of a histamine receptor antagonist, the $\log_{10}$ dose–response curves for the action of histamine will be shifted to the right; the more potent the antagonist is, the more the curve will be shifted. Similarly, increasing the dose of the antagonist will cause graded degrees of curve shift for a given dose of histamine.

The 2 + 2 assay: This is an example of the **parallel line assay**, where two doses of an unknown and a standard preparation of a drug that should produce a response lying on the linear portion of a $\log_{10}$ dose–response curve are chosen are chosen and the distance between the two parallel lines obtained gives a measure of relative potencies (see opposite).

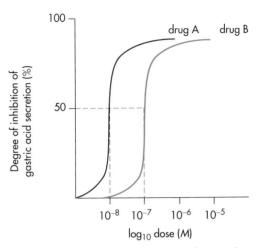

A. Log$_{10}$ dose–response curves for two drugs A and B that block gastric acid secretion. Drug A is more potent than drug B although they have the same efficacy. The similiar shapes of the two curves suggest that they have the same mechanism of action.

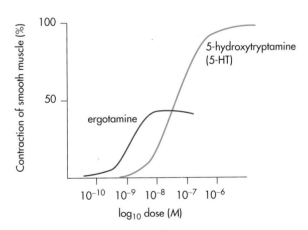

B. Contraction of smooth muscle: ergotamine is more potent than 5-HT (curve shift to the left), but has less efficacy, since its maximum effect is lower.

Log$_{10}$ dose–response curves

8 The measurement of drug activity III: Clinical and human pharmacology and clinical trials

Clinical pharmacology involves the experimental testing of drugs in patients and in healthy volunteers. Clinical trials may involve new drugs and biological agents, or the use of existing drugs for other medical conditions, and can range for anything from weeks to several years. The use of drugs in humans is subject to ethical and safety regulations, usually administered in hospitals or clinics, analogous to the stringent regulations governing the use of animals for scientific research. There are different phases of drug development (see opposite), and clinical trials for new drugs are done during phase III.

The aim is to compare, as objectively as possible, in randomised controlled clinical trials, the results obtained after applying therapeutic procedures to patients in a prospective study. No drug can be introduced for general medical use until it has undergone these trials and been licensed for treating the condition specified in the trial. The trial is designed so that patients are recruited and screened before acceptance into the trial for variables such as age, weight, sex and previous medical history. Patients are separated randomly into at least two groups. One group receives the test drug while the other receives another drug, a placebo or nothing at all. To minimise bias in the minds of those running the trial or taking the drug, the trial should ideally be planned as a double-blind, randomised controlled trial, when neither the doctors and nurses running it nor the patients taking the treatment know which group is receiving one of the treatments (double-blind) and, at some point, the patients switch treatments (crossover). This ideal is not always feasible, possible or ethically acceptable. No patient with a life-threatening disease, e.g. cancer or AIDS, should be asked to take a placebo treatment for any length of time. Ideally, and from an ethical and legal standpoint, patients recruited into a clinical trial should be admitted only after they have given informed consent to take part; this can be difficult to adhere to if patients with diseases such as Alzheimer's disease, which impairs cognition, are being recruited for a clinical trial. In brain degenerative disease, however, permission may be obtained by proxy.

Trial design and data analysis: It is not possible here to give more than an introduction to the problems facing the designers of a clinical trial. Major problems include deciding on the size of each sample, i.e. number of patients in a group (and sometimes even obtaining a desired number), and knowing whether the sample is representative of the population that the trial is designed to test. Other significant problems occur when analysing the results and drawing conclusions. Unintentional error can occur through pure wishful thinking or choosing the wrong method of data analysis. A more recent and popular technique for data analysis of clinical trials is meta-analysis, when data are combined with those from previous trials.

Rarely do clinical trials provide unequivocal differences between groups and appropriate statistical methods should always be applied to results. Even with rigorous planning, errors can occur. The two errors possible are type I (false positive) and type II (false negative).[2] Clinical trials are very costly in terms of effort, time and money, and neither the patients nor the organisers would wish to miss the opportunity of introducing a better drug. Conversely, there is little point in introducing a drug that offers no benefit over existing treatments.

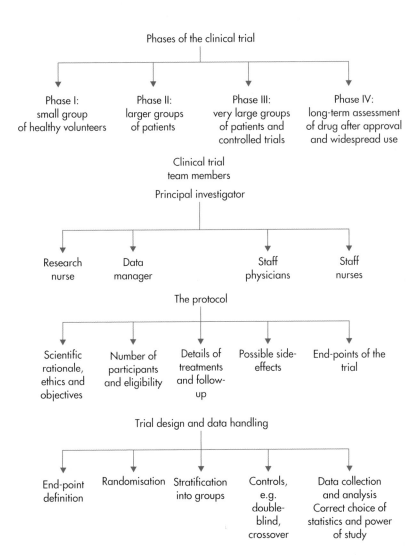

Phases of the clinical trial

- **Phase I:** small group of healthy volunteers
- **Phase II:** larger groups of patients
- **Phase III:** very large groups of patients and controlled trials
- **Phase IV:** long-term assessment of drug after approval and widespread use

Clinical trial team members

Principal investigator

- Research nurse
- Data manager
- Staff physicians
- Staff nurses

The protocol

- Scientific rationale, ethics and objectives
- Number of participants and eligibility
- Details of treatments and follow-up
- Possible side-effects
- End-points of the trial

Trial design and data handling

- End-point definition
- Randomisation
- Stratification into groups
- Controls, e.g. double-blind, crossover
- Data collection and analysis Correct choice of statistics and power of study

9 Principles of drug absorption I: Basic principles

Ideally, a route of administration is chosen to deliver the desired dose of drug selectively to the site of action (**A**). However, this ideal is seldom achieved. Before routes of administration are described, it is necessary to explain the internal and external environments, and bioavailability.

The **external environment** is everything outside of the body. Drugs remain in the external environment until they cross a membrane and enter any of the body's compartments, whether it is, for example, the interstitial fluid, a cell, the circulation or the cerebrospinal fluid (CSF). A grape seed may pass from the mouth through the entire gastrointestinal tract (GIT) until it is expelled, but it will not have entered the **internal environment** of the body.

Bioavailability refers to the proportion of a drug that can be presented to its site of action, and generally refers to the drug in the circulation after it has escaped the liver during first-pass metabolism (page 14).

The **route of administration** will affect the onset of action, the plasma concentration achieved, and the length of time that the drug remains in the circulation (**B**). The ideal route ensures that an effective concentration of a drug is delivered to its desired site of action, and that this concentration is maintained steadily until the condition is cured. The routes available are oral, parenteral and topical (**C**). **Oral** administration means that the drug is put into the mouth and swallowed. **Parenteral** administration[3] is the introduction of the drug into the internal environment by application to or through any membrane (excluding those of the GIT), e.g. the skin or a mucous membrane. Examples include sublingual, rectal, inhalation or vaginal, or by injection. **Topical** means the application of a medicinal preparation directly to a site at which the drug is meant to act. This site could be the skin (e.g. hydrocortisone cream) or a mucous membrane (e.g. a local anaesthetic).

The **choice of route** depends on: (i) patient convenience; (ii) desired speed of onset of effect; (iii) required site of action; (iv) physicochemical, pharmacological and toxicological properties of the drug; (v) duration of drug action; and (vi) organ exclusion.

The oral route is the most convenient for the patient. Some drugs, e.g. insulin, which is digested in the GIT, cannot be absorbed orally and have to be injected. Some patients, however, fear needles. Emergencies and surgical procedures require rapid onset of drug action, so inhalation or intravenous injection is used. Patients with kidney failure should not take drugs eliminated through the kidney. A drug may be applied directly to its site of action, e.g. hydrocortisone cream to the skin or an epidural injection during labour. If a drug's action is to be of short duration, its **half-life** in the circulation (page 18) should be relatively short. If a long duration of action is desired, e.g. months, a slow-release preparation (e.g. a steroid) may be implanted subcutaneously. If a continuous form of administration is required, the drug may be given directly into the vein by infusion.

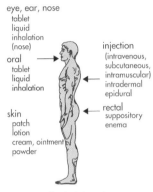

eye, ear, nose
   tablet
   liquid
   inhalation
   (nose)

oral
   tablet
   liquid
   inhalation

skin
   patch
   lotion
   cream, ointment
   powder

injection
(intravenous,
subcutaneous,
intramuscular)
intradermal
epidural

rectal
suppository
enema

A. Routes of administration

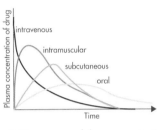

B. Time course of drug concentration

intravenous
intramuscular
subcutaneous
oral

Plasma concentration of drug

Time

intravenous, e.g. general anaesthetic
intramuscular, e.g. antibiotic
subdural, e.g local anaesthetic
intradermal, e.g. local anaesthetic
subcutaneous, e.g. insulin

oral, e.g. aspirin, antibiotics
sublingual, e.g. glyceryl trinitrate
inhalational, e.g. asthma nebulisers

topical, e.g. hydrocortisone cream,
zinc ointment, calamine lotion,
Lassar's paste, powders
oral contraceptive patch
antifungal pessaries
haemorrhoidal suppositories

C. Drugs and routes of administration

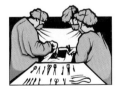

general anaesthesia for surgery

10 Basic principles of drug absorption II: Membrane penetration

Many drugs need to cross biological membranes in order to reach their sites of action in the body. Drugs taken orally have to cross from the lumen of the GIT into the bloodstream, unless, like glyceryl trinitrate for anginal pain, they are absorbed through the mucous membranes of the mouth (**A**). The efficiency with which drugs are absorbed from the GIT depends to a large extent on the nature of the drug and on its solubility in water. Drugs have to dissolve in order to be absorbed. The membrane is a bimolecular lipid, and lipophilic drugs will cross these membranes relatively easily. These drugs, which include alcohol, certain antibiotics and steroids, pass easily through the GIT membranes into the bloodstream through a process of passive diffusion, the rate of which is determined by the concentration gradient of the drug.

Charged molecules such as aspirin, which is a weak acid, can also cross lipophilic GIT membranes, although the efficiency of transfer is much reduced (**B**). Being a weak acid, aspirin is mostly uncharged in the highly acidic environment of the stomach, which enhances its absorption. In the small intestine, which is strongly alkaline, aspirin is mostly charged, and absorption is not as rapid, although the large surface area of the small intestine makes up for this. The pK_a is a useful measure of drug absorption; it is the pH at which the drug is 50% ionised (**C**).

Some drugs and dietary chemicals, e.g. amino acids and pyrimidines, are transported by carriers across GIT membranes into the bloodstream (**D**). For example, the same carrier that transports the dietary amino acid phenylalanine also carries the drug levodopa, which is used to treat Parkinson's disease. The same carrier that transports the natural pyrimidines thymine and uracil, which are used in nucleic acid synthesis, also transports the cytotoxic drug fluorouracil.

Drug absorption from the gut can be affected by patient health, foods, drug action and drug formulation (**E**). For example, tetracycline absorption is impaired if the drugs are taken together with milk or other calcium-containing substances, because calcium salts adsorb the drug. Migraine produces stasis of the GIT and this delays absorption of food and drugs. The absorption of drugs with a site of absorption in the small intestine is delayed if they are taken at mealtimes. Tablets and capsules may be formulated to enhance or delay absorption. For example, nifedipine, a calcium antagonist used to treat angina, has been formulated in delayed-release form that allows once daily administration.

After absorption, drugs may have to cross other barriers to reach their site of action, e.g. the blood–brain barrier. This barrier is extremely resistant to drug penetration because of the absence of pores in the capillary endothelial system. Lipophilic substances such as alcohol and the inhalational anaesthetics pass easily into the neural cells of the brain while other substances, e.g. levodopa, are transported by carrier proteins in the cell membrane.

Mucous membranes of the rectum and vagina are also used as sites for drug transfer into the bloodstream, through the use of suppositories and pessaries, respectively. Aspirin, for example, has been formulated in suppositories to avoid its corrosive effect on the stomach.

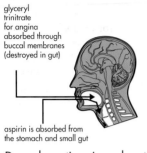

glyceryl
trinitrate
for angina
absorbed through
buccal membranes
(destroyed in gut)

aspirin is absorbed from
the stomach and small gut

A. Drug absorption via oral route

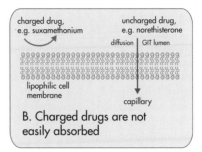

charged drug,
e.g. suxamethonium

uncharged drug,
e.g. norethisterone

diffusion | GIT lumen

lipophilic cell
membrane

capillary

B. Charged drugs are not easily absorbed

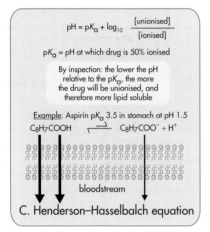

$$pH = pK_a + \log_{10} \frac{[\text{unionised}]}{[\text{ionised}]}$$

pK_a = pH at which drug is 50% ionised

By inspection: the lower the pH relative to the pK_a, the more the drug will be unionised, and therefore more lipid soluble

Example: Aspirin pK_a 3.5 in stomach at pH 1.5

$$C_8H_7COOH \rightleftharpoons C_8H_7COO^- + H^+$$

bloodstream

C. Henderson–Hasselbalch equation

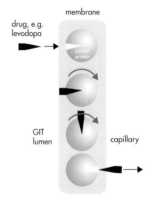

membrane

drug, e.g.
levodopa

carrier
protein

GIT
lumen

capillary

D. Carrier proteins transport drugs across membranes

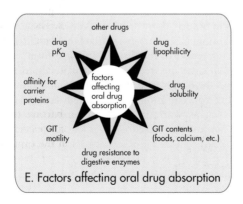

other drugs

drug
pK_a

drug
lipophilicity

affinity for
carrier
proteins

factors
affecting
oral drug
absorption

drug
solubility

GIT
motility

GIT contents
(foods, calcium, etc.)

drug resistance to
digestive enzymes

E. Factors affecting oral drug absorption

11 Drug distribution

Manufacturers of drugs need to know where and how they are distributed in the body. For example: does the drug reach its intended target, e.g. the brain? How is it carried to the target? For how long is a given dose maintained at effective concentrations? Considerations such as these dictate the design of drugs, the route of administration and the dose. Virtually all administered drugs are water soluble, carried to their targets in the blood, and need to cross membranes to get to their site of action. In the blood, drugs may be bound to plasma proteins (A), and this will affect the rate at which extravascular concentrations of the drug build up. In addition, the degree of ionisation, and relative solubility of a drug in water and fat, play a large part in determining its rate and pattern of distribution in the body ([B] and [C]).

For the purposes of drug distribution, several different **body compartments** can be defined (D): total body water (~0.5 l/kg),[4] extracellular water (~0.2 l/kg), plasma (0.04 l/kg), fat (~0.2–0.4 l/kg) and bone (0.07 l/kg). Attempts have been made to measure the distribution of a drug in the body, and the parameters used include the **volume of distribution** (V_D) and the **partition coefficient**. The volume of distribution may be defined as the volume of water that the body would have to have in order to keep the entire amount of drug in the body at the same concentration as in the plasma. The formula used to calculate V_D is given opposite (D). The higher the figure, the more likely it is that the drug is concentrated in extravascular compartments. Salicylate, for example, has a V_D of 12 l/70 kg, while chloroquine, which is highly concentrated in all the tissues, has a V_D of 13 000 l/70 kg. The practical implication of this is that a very large loading dose of chloroquine must be given in cases where rapid onset is needed in order to build up effective plasma concentrations, because it is rapidly removed from the blood and only slowly released back into the circulation. The partition coefficient is a measure of the distribution of a drug between two different types of compartment and has important implications for the disposition of the drug in the body. General anaesthetics, for example, dissolve rapidly into fat, leaving relatively little in aqueous compartments. The value of V_D will reflect this physical property of the drug.

Protein binding in blood: Many drugs become reversibly bound to proteins in the blood. Equilibrium is set up between the bound and free fractions of the drug. Only the free fraction of the drug can escape from the blood into the tissues, and in certain cases the free fraction is relatively small (< 5% of total drug). This prolongs the drug's time in the circulation and delays the build-up of an effective drug concentration at its desired site of action. Potentially dangerous drugs such as warfarin and barbiturates are bound to plasma proteins, and this can cause serious drug interactions (page 54).

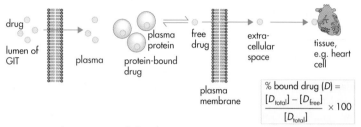

$$\% \text{ bound drug } (D) = \frac{[D_{\text{total}}] - [D_{\text{free}}]}{[D_{\text{total}}]} \times 100$$

A. Drug absorption and distribution

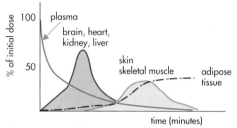

B. Time course of drug distribution in tissues

lipid solubility	degree of ionisation
molecular weight	blood flow

C. Factors affecting the rate of drug distribution

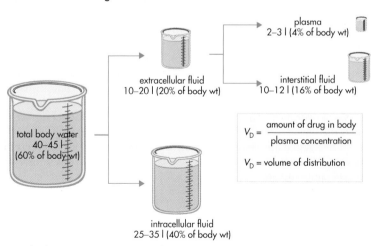

$$V_D = \frac{\text{amount of drug in body}}{\text{plasma concentration}}$$

V_D = volume of distribution

D. Fluid compartments in a 70-kg man

12 Drug metabolism

The body transforms ingested drugs to detoxify them and render them easier to excrete. Drugs may be metabolised to more toxic products, or to substances that are more powerful treatments. Drugs may be excreted unchanged (**A**). Metabolic transformations are called phase I and phase II reactions. Phase I reactions alter the drug's structure (usually) to produce a more easily excreted polar compound, through reactions such as oxidation–reduction, oxygenation or hydrolysis. Phase II reactions conjugate the altered drug by, for example, methylation or glucuronidation to facilitate the drug's excretion.

One important liver enzyme system catalysing **phase I** reactions is the microsomal cytochrome P450 mono-oxygenase, which utilises molecular oxygen and NADPH as a co-factor. Metabolised drugs include propranolol, phenylbutazone, barbiturates and warfarin. These substrates can increase enzyme activity by a process called **enzyme induction**, which results in increased drug breakdown, thus diminishing its potency. This can be serious. For example, if a patient on warfarin is given barbiturates, this will increase the breakdown of warfarin and clotting times will shorten and more warfarin may be prescribed. If the patient is then taken off barbiturates, the enzyme is no longer induced and the increased dose of warfarin may cause haemorrhage (**B**).

Phase II reactions involve the coupling of the phase-I-transformed polar drug to **conjugates** such as glucuronic acid (e.g. digoxin), glutathione (e.g. paracetamol), glycine (e.g. salicylic acid), acetyl-CoA (e.g. clonazepam) or water (e.g. carbamazepine epoxide). Conjugated metabolites are generally inactive and easily excreted. Some of these transformations are potentially dangerous, e.g. the conjugation of paracetamol (**D**). Paracetamol is normally 95% glucuronated and sulphated, with about 5% being coupled to glutathione. If the therapeutic dose is exceeded the glutathione pathway becomes quickly used up and hepatotoxic metabolites are formed. The antidote is glutathione, and some paracetamol formulations do contain glutathione. Some drugs, called pro-drugs, may be metabolised to more powerful agents. A pro-drug may be defined as a chemical that is ineffective, but that is metabolised to an effective chemical, e.g. the antidepressant imipramine loses a methyl group to become the active metabolite desipramine.

The **first-pass effect**: The liver is the principal drug-metabolising organ, although the lungs, GIT, kidneys and skin also metabolise certain drugs. All drugs orally ingested are absorbed by the mesenteric veins, which drain via the portal vein directly into the liver sinusoids. In many cases, e.g. morphine, meperidine and isoprenaline (isoproterenol), a significant proportion of the drug is metabolised by hepatocytes, which reduces the effective dose of the drug, and alternative routes need to be used (**E**).

Many factors affect drug metabolism, including age, sex, state of health, liver function, genetic make-up and other drugs. Genetic factors include variations in acetylation of drugs such as the amine isoniazid caused by an autosomal recessive trait, resulting in reduced synthesis of the metabolising enzyme. There are several other examples of autosomal recessive traits causing altered drug metabolism. Reduced metabolism of drugs may occur in very young or old patients. Cigarette smoking may induce the microsomal enzymes and speed up drug metabolism.

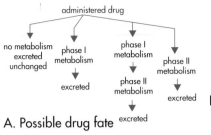

A. Possible drug fate

administered drug

- no metabolism excreted unchanged
- phase I metabolism → excreted
- phase I metabolism → phase II metabolism → excreted
- phase II metabolism → excreted

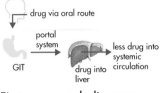

drug via oral route

portal system

GIT → drug into liver → less drug into systemic circulation

E. First-pass metabolism can reduce the efficacy of the drug

phenobarbital
⊕
warfarin ——→ inactive metabolite

more warfarin needed
(potentially dangerous if phenobarbital stopped)

B. Enzyme induction by drugs

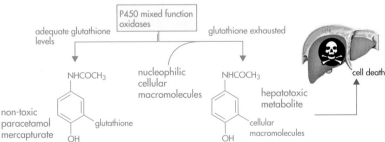

liver microsomes

liver microsomes are induced after phenobarbital

Phase I dealkylation

Phase II conjugation

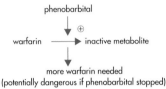

acetylsalicylic acid (aspirin)

$\xrightarrow[\text{P450}]{\text{NADPH, O}_2}$

salicylic acid

glucuronide (excreted)

C. Phases of aspirin metabolism

lower doses of paracetamol

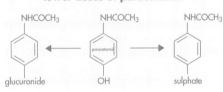

NHCOCH₃ glucuronide ← paracetamol (OH) → NHCOCH₃ sulphate

at higher does of paracetamol

P450 mixed function oxidases

adequate glutathione levels

glutathione exhausted

nucleophilic cellular macromolecules

cell death

non-toxic paracetamol mercapturate — NHCOCH₃ glutathione OH

hepatotoxic metabolite

NHCOCH₃ cellular macromolecules OH

D. Paracetamol hepatotoxicity

13 Drug excretion

Drugs may be excreted in urine, faeces, sweat, milk or saliva, or by the lungs (A). Most drugs in use are excreted mainly in the urine. The body usually (but not always) facilitates the excretion of drugs by making them more water soluble. Drugs may be excreted metabolised or unchanged. The rates of metabolism and excretion largely determine the dose frequency, whereas the route may dictate the drug used. Patients with kidney failure should not, as a rule, be prescribed drugs excreted via the kidney, whereas patients with liver failure should not be prescribed drugs metabolised and excreted via the liver. The rate of excretion depends on both the properties of the drug and the body's handling of it. Excretion rate will depend on whether the drug is a weak acid or a weak base, on the pH of the urine and on whether the drug circulates bound to plasma proteins, because only the free, unbound drug can be excreted (B). The rate may also depend on the size of the drug. Small molecules are more easily filtered than large ones.

Attempts are made to measure the rate of excretion by measuring drug concentrations in plasma or urine at various times after administration. Various parameters are used, namely, the **glomerular filtration rate** (GFR in ml/min), the **volume of distribution** (V_D; page 22), the **clearance**, the **half-life** ($t_{1/2}$) and the **plasma and urine concentration** (mg/ml). The GFR is the rate at which substances are filtered through the kidney glomeruli in the Bowman's capsules of the nephrons. Kidney blood flow in healthy people is around 650 ml/min, and is lower in the newborn, the elderly, and patients with heart or kidney disease. V_D is a theoretical number defined as the volume of fluid necessary for all the drug in the body to be at the same concentration as that in the plasma. The clearance is the volume of plasma cleared of the drug per minute or hour. The $t_{1/2}$ is the time taken to clear 50% of the drug from the plasma.

The half-life is found by administering the drug, measuring how much is left in plasma at different times and plotting a graph of the result (C). With some drugs, the more there is in the circulation, the faster it is eliminated, i.e. the rate depends on the concentration. Mathematically, this is called a first-order process, and the graph gives a straight line on semi-logarithmic paper. This means that (i) the higher the concentration in plasma, the faster the drug is eliminated and (ii) at the end of five half-lives, 97% of the drug has been eliminated. Overall, this makes the drug relatively safe. Furthermore, the drug designer knows at what intervals to administer the drug and, if continuously higher blood levels are aimed at, may aim to repeat the dose at intervals of less than four or five half-lives, and usually less than one half-life.

Drugs that are excreted at a fixed rate regardless of plasma concentration are potentially more dangerous because large amounts are cleared at the same rate as smaller amounts. This is called a zero-order process and, if a patient has overdosed, dialysis may be needed to speed up drug elimination. Examples are phenytoin for epilepsy and ethanol.

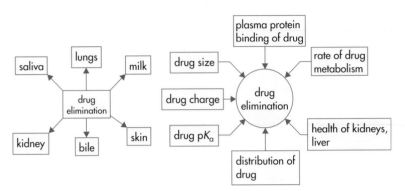

A. Routes of drug elimination   B. Factors affecting drug excretion

First-order kinetics

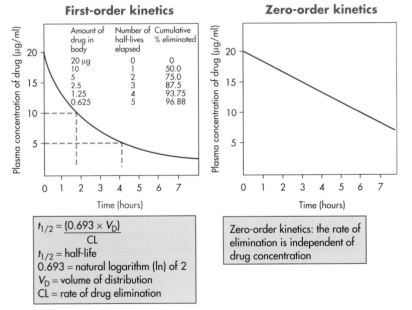

Amount of drug in body	Number of half-lives elapsed	Cumulative % eliminated
20 µg	0	0
10	1	50.0
5	2	75.0
2.5	3	87.5
1.25	4	93.75
0.625	5	96.88

Zero-order kinetics

$$t_{1/2} = \frac{(0.693 \times V_D)}{CL}$$

$t_{1/2}$ = half-life
0.693 = natural logarithm (ln) of 2
V_D = volume of distribution
CL = rate of drug elimination

Zero-order kinetics: the rate of elimination is independent of drug concentration

C. Drug half-life ($t_{1/2}$)

14 Renal drug excretion

The nephron is the functional excretory unit of the kidney. Renal arterial blood is filtered in the glomerulus, which is a knot of capillaries, and the filtrate enters Bowman's capsule. Filtration is driven by a hydrostatic pressure gradient highly sensitive to the blood pressure. The filtrate, which contains water, ions and substances below a molecular weight of about 5000 Da, passes into the renal tubule, where most is reabsorbed and returned to the venous blood. The remaining fluid, called urine, passes through the collecting ducts and drains into the ureter. About 20% of the renal plasma flow is filtered in the glomerulus and the remaining 80% of any drug is delivered to the peritubular capillaries that surround the proximal tubule (A). Most of the filtered water (± 99%) is reabsorbed from the tubules.

Tubular secretion and reabsorption: The tubule and collecting ducts have walls that are highly specialised for the excretion and re-uptake of water and salts, and these re-uptake and excretory mechanisms are targets for the action of drugs, especially the diuretics (page 24). **Active tubular secretion** is the active transport of drugs and other substances from the plasma across the renal tubule epithelial cell wall to the tubular fluid by one of two independent ATP-dependent systems: the anionic and cationic systems. The **anionic system** transports organic acids such as salicylic acid, the penicillins, sulphonic acids and acidic metabolites, e.g. the glucuronide and sulphate conjugates. It also secretes endogenous acids, e.g. uric acid. The **cationic system** transports organic bases such as amiloride, histamine, morphine, pethidine and serotonin (5-HT). Both systems are extremely powerful since they pump substances against a concentration gradient and reduce plasma concentrations of drugs to virtually zero, even if they are bound to plasma proteins, because they promote dissociation of drug from its plasma protein-binding sites (B). The pumps are not absolutely specific and drugs can compete at the anionic pump, e.g. penicillin and probenecid.

Passive reabsorption from the tubules into plasma is by diffusion down a concentration gradient, and the urine:plasma gradient usually favours solute reabsorption, since the active reabsorption of water from the tubules concentrates solutes in the tubular fluid. Nevertheless, the rate of passive reabsorption will also depend on the pH in the tubule and on the lipophilicity of the drug. Uncharged molecules will be rapidly reabsorbed and their rate of excretion is therefore relatively slow. The pH changes from about 4.5 in the proximal tubule to about 8 in the distal tubule. Since only the unionised (more lipophilic) drug crosses biological membranes freely, weak acids such as aspirin will be reabsorbed more readily in the proximal tubule, whereas a weak base, e.g. morphine, will be more readily reabsorbed in the distal tubule. Thus, if rapid excretion of a drug is needed, e.g. through overdose, acidification or alkalinisation of urine is done in order to speed up excretion of weak bases or acids respectively. For example, alkalinisation of urine by administering bicarbonate to the patient will speed up the excretion of aspirin (C).

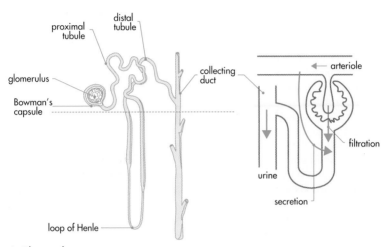

A. The nephron

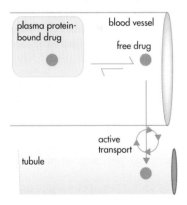

B. Plasma protein binding and drug clearance

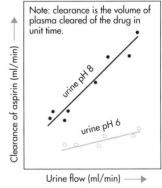

C. Urine pH and aspirin clearance

15 Biliary drug excretion

The liver is an important site for drug metabolism and excretion and is potentially under threat from drug-induced toxicity. It consists of two main lobes, constructed mainly of hepatocyte cells, arranged into functional units called lobules. The lobules are composed of cell plates (A) consisting of hepatocytes that lie adjacent to the bile canaliculi, in which the bile forms and drains into ductules. From here bile, which contains drug metabolites, will ultimately be drained into the gallbladder, and then into the duodenum. Many toxic metabolites, cholesterol and lipid waste products are excreted in the bile (B).

The liver is rich in enzymes that metabolise many different drugs, including alcohol. The liver detoxifies many substances that arrive from the GIT, thus preventing their entry into the general circulation. This places it in the firing line, so to speak, so that it is very vulnerable to drug-induced injury.

All drugs absorbed from the GIT are taken to the liver via the hepatic portal vein, where extensive metabolism of the drug may occur through **first-pass metabolism** by the liver. Furthermore, all circulating drugs also pass through the liver, where they may be metabolised and made more soluble by phase I and II reactions. Drugs such as lidocaine (lignocaine), morphine and propranolol are readily cleared by the first-pass effect (a high extraction ratio – C), whereas drugs such as phenobarbital, tolbutamide and warfarin, which are mainly bound to plasma proteins (D), are less readily metabolised in the liver (low extraction ratio) because only the relatively small free fraction of drug is available for metabolism. Larger and more lipophilic (fat-soluble) drug molecules are usually metabolised and excreted via the hepatic system, whereas smaller molecules are excreted via the urine. The liver renders drugs more water soluble (e.g. as glucuronides), more polar and increases their molecular size, all of which enhance rates of excretion. Metabolised drugs are secreted into the bile ducts, which drain into the gallbladder, and are delivered to the intestine in the bile (E).

Once in the intestine, the glucuronated drug (for example) may be excreted in the faeces or hydrolysed to release the free drug, which is then re-absorbed and the cycle repeated through the hepatic portal cycle, in a process called **enterohepatic cycling**. This process (A) creates a 'reservoir' of recycled drug that can constitute about 20–25% of the total drug and thus prolongs the effect of a given dose. Ethinylestradiol, a synthetic estrogen, and morphine are both recycled this way.

Drug-induced hepatotoxicity can be produced by, for example: paracetamol and carbon tetrachloride, which cause a toxic necrosis; chlorpromazine, which is inflammatory to the liver; or drugs that cause hepatitis-like symptoms, e.g. methylodopa and isoniazid.

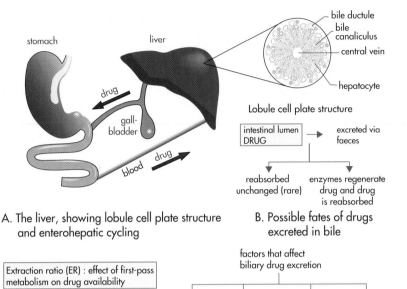

Lobule cell plate structure

A. The liver, showing lobule cell plate structure and enterohepatic cycling

| intestinal lumen DRUG | → | excreted via faeces |

reabsorbed unchanged (rare)   enzymes regenerate drug and drug is reabsorbed

B. Possible fates of drugs excreted in bile

Extraction ratio (ER) : effect of first-pass metabolism on drug availability

$$ER = \frac{CL_{liver}}{Q}$$

CL = clearance
Q = hepatic blood flow (l/h)

C. Extraction ratio

factors that affect biliary drug excretion

age   drug size (larger > smaller)   hydrophobic > hydrophilic   disease

E. Factors that affect biliary drug excretion

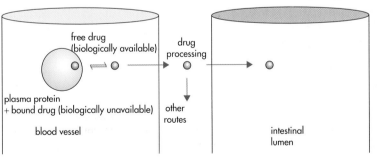

D. Plasma binding and drug availability

16 Determination of drug dosage regimen

The main aim of dosage determination is to achieve a concentration of drug at its site of action in order to produce an effective therapeutic effect for the patient. It is generally not feasible to individualise dosages for each patient and generalisations have to be made, with adjustments for patient age, weight and state of health. It is not yet possible always to measure drug concentrations at their site of action and dosage regimens are adjusted to achieve plasma concentrations that are therapeutically effective and non-toxic where possible. This is called the **target concentration** (TC) and it depends on knowledge obtained from studies of drug administration, absorption, metabolism, excretion and evaluation of effect. For a particular drug, the TC may vary depending on the use. For example, a higher dose of digoxin is needed for treating atrial fibrillation than for heart failure. At least two types of dosages are used, depending on the aim: the **loading dose** and the **maintenance dose**. For example, for an infection, a single loading dose of 500 mg amoxicillin may be prescribed followed by a maintenance dose of 250 mg three times a day for 7 days. The loading dose is used when a rapid achievement of the TC is required or when a drug normally achieves the TC relatively slowly. The loading dose may be given by intravenous injection if feasible, e.g. in the case of aminophylline, followed by oral maintenance administration.

The maintenance dose is calculated to achieve a steady state of drug presence. Ideally, doses should simply replace the amount of drug eliminated and thus maintain the steady state. Therefore the mean clearance (CL) must be determined first. Other parameters that need to be known are F, the fractional systemic bioavailability, and the TC. The dosing interval (DI) to keep the circulating concentration at effective levels also has to be determined. With all these parameters known it is then possible to calculate the dosage regimen (**A**). Calculation of the maintenance dose usually assumes that a single compartment system is being dealt with and this is very seldom, if ever, the case. Examples of calculations used are given opposite.

The loading dose can also be calculated from the data obtained by measuring drug concentrations and clearance (see opposite). In order to calculate the loading dose, the volume of distribution (V_D; page 22) must be known.[5]

The rate at which the drug accumulates in different body compartments needs to be taken into account when determining the loading dose. Failure to do so can result in dangerous toxic effects. An example is the administration of a loading dose of a cardioactive drug such as theophylline.

Maximum and minimum concentrations may be measured in relation to the frequency of dosing (**B**). Intravenous infusion of a drug (where possible) and measurement of plasma concentrations give a value of the plasma concentration of the effective dose to be aimed at. Maximum and minimum concentrations may cycle about this value.

A. Calculation of dosing rate

Aim: To produce a target concentration (TC) of theophylline of 8 mg/l by intravenous infusion to treat acute bronchial asthma in a 70-kg patient.

Parameters needed:

Mean clearance (CL; l/h)

Target concentration (TC; 8 mg/l)

CL: For theophylline this is 2.8 l/h/70 kg[1]

The dosing rate (DR) for this patient will be:

$$DR = CL \times TC$$

$$= 2.8 \text{ l/h/70 kg} \times 8 \text{ mg/l}$$

$$= 22.4 \text{ mg/h/70 kg}$$

1. Data from: Katzung BG, Basic and Clinical Pharmacology, 7th edn. Stamford, CT: Appleton & Lange, 1998, p.37.

Aim: To calculate the oral dose in order to maintain the plasma concentration in the patient using oral slow-release theophylline to be taken every 8 hours.

Parameters needed:

Dosing rate (DR) = 22.4 mg/h

Dosing interval = 8 h

Oral availability (F; 0.96 for theophylline[1])

The maintenance dose =

$$\boxed{\dfrac{\text{dosing rate}}{\text{oral availability}} \times \text{dosing interval}}$$

$$= \dfrac{22.4 \text{ mg/h}}{0.96} \times 8 \text{ h}$$

$$= 187 \text{ mg}$$

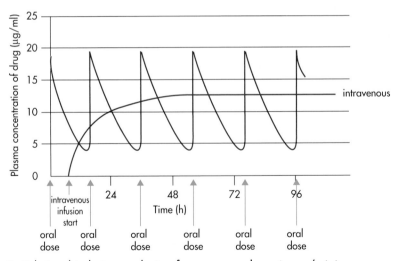

B. Relationship between dosing frequency and maximum/minimum plasma concentrations of a drug

17 The autonomic nervous system I: Introduction

The **autonomic nervous system** (**ANS**) controls involuntary systems, e.g. the cardiovascular system, GIT, hypothalamic temperature regulation, endocrine and exocrine hormonal function, and the genitourinary tract. It also mediates aspects of immune function, although this is poorly understood. It consists of two main components, the **sympathetic** and **parasympathetic** divisions (**A**). These divisions work together to maintain appropriate and adequate function of the various systems (**B**). The ANS is therefore a major target for many drugs.

Structurally, the ANS has virtually all of its main control centres in the brain, from which all efferent nerve fibres run to the rest of the body. Afferent sensory fibres carry information from organs to the brain in the same nerve bundles. In both systems, in general, efferent **pre-ganglionic** fibres run from the brain to ganglia, where they synapse with **post-ganglionic** fibres that run to the target organs. In all cases the ganglionic synapses are **cholinergic**, i.e. **acetylcholine** (ACh) is the neurotransmitter released by the pre-ganglionic fibre, and its post-ganglionic receptors are called **nicotinic**, because they were originally discovered using nicotine. **Post-ganglionic sympathetic** efferent fibres in general release the neurotransmitter **norepinephrine** (noradrenaline), which acts on specific post-synaptic **adrenergic** receptors (page 36) to produce its effects. **Post-ganglionic parasympathetic** efferents release the neurotransmitter ACh, which acts on specific cholinergic muscarinic receptors – known as muscarinic because muscarine, a toadstool poison, was used to discover them.

In both divisions, there are subtypes of the different receptors. In the sympathetic division, α- and β-adrenoceptors are recognised and, within these groups, yet further subdivision occurs. Thus there are α_1- and α_2-adrenoceptors, and β_1-, β_2- and β_3-adrenoceptors which mediate different functions of norepinephrine and epinephrine, e.g. β_1-adrenoceptors mediate the effects of these catecholamines on the heart, whereas β_2-adrenoceptors mediate arteriolar vasodilatation caused by the catecholamines.

The two divisions in general act by having opposite effects on target tissues. For example, the parasympathetic division when dominant stimulates GIT activity, while the sympathetic division inhibits, and this involves central and peripheral interactions between the two divisions. In the periphery, there is reciprocal inhibition of efferent impulse transmission (**C**). There is evidence that parasympathetic and sympathetic divisions send fibre branches to synapse pre-synaptically with those of the opposing division, so that activation of one actually inhibits neurotransmitter release from the nerve terminals of the other division. This form of innervation is termed pre-synaptic terminal innervation, and the reciprocal inhibitory system is termed heterotropic inhibition.

Some tissues, e.g. sweat glands and blood vessels, are innervated almost exclusively by the sympathetic division of the ANS, and in the vascular systems the effects of sympathetic stimulation vary with the vascular bed, e.g. sympathetic activity constricts cutaneous vascular beds, while dilating those in voluntary muscle. This makes sense, because during periods of 'fright or flight', when the organism is in danger, cutaneous vasoconstriction limits blood loss from the skin, while vasodilatation promotes blood flow and oxygen supply through the muscle.

Very many drugs have been developed to treat problems by blocking or enhancing the activity of one or other of the two divisions of the ANS, e.g. β-blockers slow the heart and thus help to reduce blood pressure.

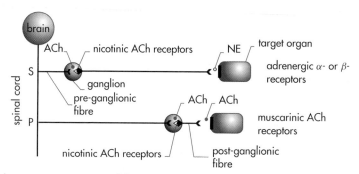

A. Schematic arrangement of the ANS (autonomic nervous system)

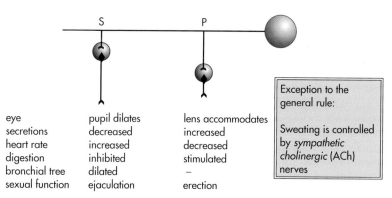

eye	pupil dilates	lens accommodates
secretions	decreased	increased
heart rate	increased	decreased
digestion	inhibited	stimulated
bronchial tree	dilated	–
sexual function	ejaculation	erection

Exception to the general rule:

Sweating is controlled by *sympathetic cholinergic (ACh) nerves*

B. Some examples of autonomic effects

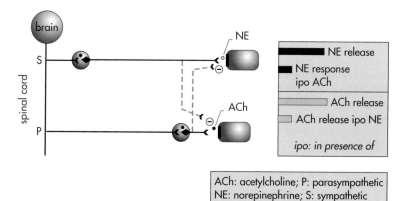

NE release
NE response ipo ACh

ACh release
ACh release ipo NE

ipo: in presence of

ACh: acetylcholine; P: parasympathetic
NE: norepinephrine; S: sympathetic

C. Reciprocal presynaptic regulation of ACh and NE release

18 The autonomic nervous system II: The sympathetic division

The sympathetic division is classically called the division of 'fight or flight'. It mobilises the body's defence mechanisms in emergency states, and its actions reflect this function. It stimulates the heart, increases blood supply to the muscles and decreases it to the skin. Digestive function is inhibited and the secretion of epinephrine (adrenaline) from the adrenal medulla is greatly increased. Airway resistance is reduced through bronchiolar dilatation. Generally, the sympathetic division opposes parasympathetic effects (see next spread). The effects of the sympathetic division on the cardiovascular and respiratory systems make it an important target for drugs that either oppose or enhance its actions.

Structurally, the efferent part of the sympathetic division consists of nerves with cell bodies that originate in the thoracolumbar region of the spinal cord. The cell bodies of these neurons lie in the lateral region of the cord and leave the cord in the ventral roots. Most of these nerves have **short pre-ganglionic fibres** that synapse in the bilateral sympathetic chain of ganglia with the cell bodies of the much **longer post-ganglionic nerve fibres** that run to the organs they innervate. (Note that in the diagram opposite only one chain is shown, for clarity.) Some preganglionic fibres synapse in the prevertebral coeliac, superior mesenteric and inferior mesenteric ganglia. Postganglionic fibres from the superior cervical ganglion innervate the eye and the salivary and lacrimal glands. The coeliac ganglion innervates the stomach, small intestine and associated organs. The superior and inferior mesenteric ganglia innervate the large intestine and genitourinary organs respectively. The arrangement is shown opposite. The **adrenal medulla**, which secretes epinephrine and norepinephrine, is a ganglion that has been modified to form an endocrine gland to which the pre-ganglionic fibres run.

Acetylcholine (ACh) is the major neurotransmitter released from pre-synaptic fibres in both sympathetic and parasympathetic ganglia, and it activates post-synaptic nicotinic receptors. The nicotinic ganglionic receptor in the sympathetic ganglion was the first target in the treatment of hypertension through the use of the nicotinic blocking drug hexamethonium; however, because it also blocked at parasympathetic ganglia it produced several severe side-effects including genitourinary blockade and is now of historical interest only. ACh is also the neurotransmitter released from postganglionic, post-synaptic nerve endings and binds to so-called **muscarinic** receptors, which are targets for drugs such as atropine, used to dry secretions, and hyoscine, used for travel sickness.

Norepinephrine is the neurotransmitter released from sympathetic post-ganglionic, postsynaptic nerve endings onto the target organ cell and it acts on **adrenergic** α- and β-receptors. These receptors are important targets for drugs used in the treatment of, for example, cardiovascular disorders and asthma. An exception to this general rule is that ACh is the sympathetic, post-ganglionic transmitter released at the sweat glands, where it acts on muscarinic receptors to promote sweating. This explains the toxic action of atropine in causing dry, reddened and warm skin by blocking ACh at the sweat glands.

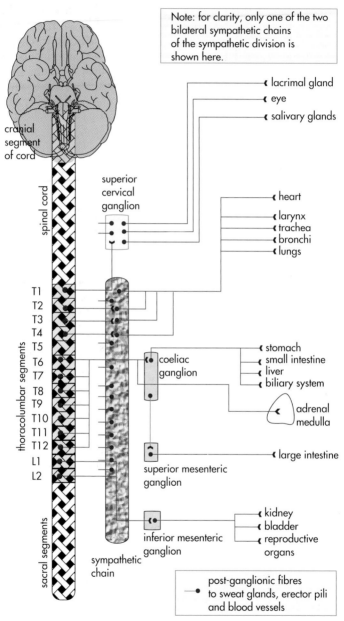

Note: for clarity, only one of the two bilateral sympathetic chains of the sympathetic division is shown here.

cranial segment of cord

spinal cord

superior cervical ganglion

lacrimal gland
eye
salivary glands

heart
larynx
trachea
bronchi
lungs

thoracolumbar segments

T1
T2
T3
T4
T5
T6
T7
T8
T9
T10
T11
T12
L1
L2

coeliac ganglion

stomach
small intestine
liver
biliary system

adrenal medulla

superior mesenteric ganglion

large intestine

inferior mesenteric ganglion

kidney
bladder
reproductive organs

sacral segments

sympathetic chain

post-ganglionic fibres to sweat glands, erector pili and blood vessels

Sympathetic division of the ANS

19 The autonomic nervous system III: The parasympathetic division

The parasympathetic division of the ANS (see opposite) is an important target for drugs that antagonise its actions. For example, muscarinic blocking drugs such as tropicamide dilate the pupil of the eye for examination purposes. Travel sickness tablets block the motility of the GIT and thus act as anti-emetics. Atropine may be used pre-operatively to inhibit secretions. Drugs such as carbachol, which stimulate muscarinic receptors, are used to contract the bladder in order to induce micturition post-operatively or after childbirth when there is no obstruction. Pilocarpine, another parasympathomimetic, is used as eye drops in acute angle-closure glaucoma, where it allows the drainage of aqueous humour through the duct of Schlemm and thus reduces intraocular pressure.

Structurally, the efferent part of the parasympathetic division consists of fibres that originate in the cranial and sacral regions of the central nervous system (CNS). In contrast to the sympathetic division, preganglionic fibres are long, and often the ganglia where they synapse lie in the tissue that they innervate. The **cranial** outflow originates in the midbrain and medulla of the brain. The third cranial nerve, which serves the eye, arises in the midbrain and the seventh (facial), ninth (glossopharangeal) and tenth (vagal) cranial nerves arise in the medulla. The vagus plays a vital role in the control of heart function. The **sacral** outflow originates in the second, third and fourth segments of the sacral region of the spinal cord and give rise to the pelvic nerves or nervi erigentes, which innervate the bladder, large intestine and reproductive organs.

As with the sympathetic division, ACh is the neurotransmitter released by preganglionic fibres in the ganglia, and it acts on nicotinic receptors on the postsynaptic, post-ganglionic fibre that runs to the organ. This similarity with the sympathetic nervous system accounts for the widespread and unacceptable side-effects associated with the targeting of drugs to the autonomic ganglia. Generally, postganglionic fibres are relatively short and may lie entirely on or within the organ that they innervate. These fibres also release ACh, which acts on **muscarinic** receptors on the target organ cell. Several subtypes of the muscarinic receptor have been identified on target tissues (see next spread) and these provide potential tools for the targeting of drugs to the parasympathetic division.

It is apparent from this and the preceding spread that the parasympathetic system, which controls autonomic systems associated with feeding and digestion, is essential to maintain life, while the sympathetic system is not. In addition, parasympathetic effects, through their more localised and limited systems of innervation, are highly localised to specific systems and organs, whereas the sympathetic division when activated affects virtually the whole body by preparing it for fight or flight. Its endocrine effect in causing the release of epinephrine from the adrenal medulla into the general circulation means that scarcely a tissue in the body is unaffected when the sympathetic division is activated.

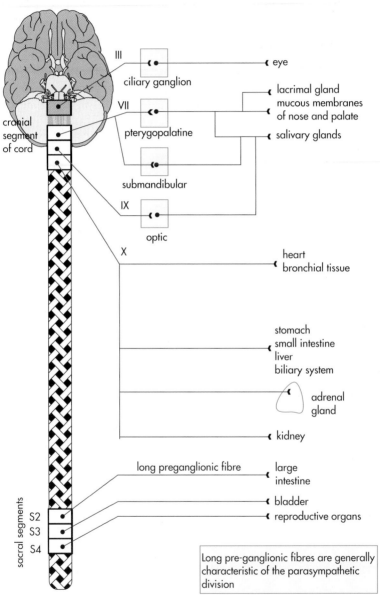

III
ciliary ganglion — eye

cranial segment of cord

VII
pterygopalatine
lacrimal gland
mucous membranes of nose and palate
salivary glands

submandibular

IX
optic

X
heart
bronchial tissue

stomach
small intestine
liver
biliary system

adrenal gland

kidney

long preganglionic fibre
large intestine

bladder
reproductive organs

sacral segments
S2
S3
S4

Long pre-ganglionic fibres are generally characteristic of the parasympathetic division

Parasympathetic division of the ANS

20 The autonomic nervous system IV: Receptors and drugs

Agonists activate receptors and **antagonists** block receptors so that agonists cannot produce their effects. This relationship between agonists and antagonists and the property of receptors to bind more than one drug provide the basis for much of drug action. Drugs can target ganglionic and postganglionic receptors, but, because receptors at both sympathetic and parasympathetic ganglia bind the same agonists, the effects of those drugs will be widespread with several side-effects. Although the body's own agonists, e.g. ACh and epinephrine, are formulated as drugs, their use is highly restricted because they are very unstable.

Sympathetic division: Drugs acting on sympathetic receptors are designed to target specific subtypes of α- or β-receptors (see opposite). For example, α_2-agonists such as clonidine inhibit sympathetic action by stimulating α_2-adrenoceptors on the presynaptic nerve terminal, which inhibits further norepinephrine release from the nerve terminal. This is, theoretically, a means of reducing blood pressure. A reduction of blood pressure can also be obtained by *blocking* α_1-adrenoceptors on the post-synaptic membrane with, for example, prazocin or indoramin. This manoeuvre causes a reflex tachycardia, which gives the patient palpitations.

Hypertension can be treated by blocking cardiac β_1-adrenoceptors. This reduces cardiac output. Propranolol was the first β-blocker but it also blocks lung β_2-adrenoceptors, which are the receptors that mediate dilatation of the bronchioles. Propranolol can therefore be dangerous in asthmatics, who have chronically narrow bronchioles, principally as a result of the action of endogenous constrictors, and any further constriction caused by β-blockers could be fatal. Selective β_1-blockers such as **atenolol** and **esmolol** have therefore been developed. β-Adrenoceptor agonists have been developed to treat asthma by dilating bronchioles. Isoprenaline was the first, but it proved dangerous because it also stimulates β_1-adrenoceptors on the heart and caused fatal arrhythmias. Selective β_2-agonists such as salbutamol are now used to treat asthma.

β_3-Adrenoceptors have been identified in adipose tissue, but their therapeutic potential awaits further elucidation.

Parasympathetic division: Very many drugs have been developed in order either to stimulate or to block the muscarinic ACh receptor on target organs, particularly in the GIT. Several different isoforms of the muscarinic receptor have been identified, and drugs are being developed to target these selectively. Systemic muscarinic agonists are of relatively little therapeutic use because they cause generalised stimulation of the parasympathetic division of the ANS and will slow the heart, cause increased peristaltic activity, thus causing cramps, and stimulate gastric and other secretions. Examples include pilocarpine, methacholine and carbachol. Pilocarpine is used topically in the eye to treat glaucoma (page 38).

Antimuscarinic drugs are more important therapeutically, and include the natural drugs atropine and hyoscine. Homatropine is a synthetic derivative of atropine. Other synthetic drugs include tropicamide and pirenzepine. Antimuscarinic drugs have been used preoperatively to reduce secretions and short-acting muscarinic blockers such as tropicamide are used to dilate the pupil for ophthalmic inspection of the eye. Atropine's actions on the eye are more long lasting and, because these drugs block accommodation, they will impair the patient's vision temporarily. Hyoscine is used to treat motion sickness by reducing peristalsis.

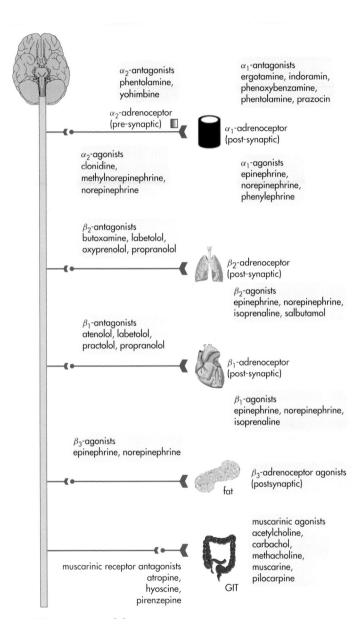

α₂-antagonists
phentolamine,
yohimbine

α_2-antagonists
phentolamine,
yohimbine

α_1-antagonists
ergotamine, indoramin,
phenoxybenzamine,
phentolamine, prazocin

α_2-adrenoceptor
(pre-synaptic)

α_1-adrenoceptor
(post-synaptic)

α_2-agonists
clonidine,
methylnorepinephrine,
norepinephrine

α_1-agonists
epinephrine,
norepinephrine,
phenylephrine

β_2-antagonists
butoxamine, labetolol,
oxyprenolol, propranolol

β_2-adrenoceptor
(post-synaptic)

β_2-agonists
epinephrine, norepinephrine,
isoprenaline, salbutamol

β_1-antagonists
atenolol, labetolol,
practolol, propranolol

β_1-adrenoceptor
(post-synaptic)

β_1-agonists
epinephrine, norepinephrine,
isoprenaline

β_3-agonists
epinephrine, norepinephrine

β_3-adrenoceptor agonists
(postsynaptic)

fat

muscarinic agonists
acetylcholine,
carbachol,
methacholine,
muscarine,
pilocarpine

muscarinic receptor antagonists
atropine,
hyoscine,
pirenzepine

GIT

ANS receptors and drugs

21 Cardiovascular system I: Stroke

This section starts with a patient history, to emphasise immediately the relevance of clinical pharmacology in cardiovascular medicine.

Case scenario: An 83-year-old lady was admitted to hospital after being found slumped in her chair at a local residential home. Her previous medical history was significant for atrial fibrillation, for which she took aspirin, and digoxin for angina. Warfarin had been deemed unsafe because of frequent falls. On examination in casualty, she had an expressive dysphasia and marked weakness in her right arm and right leg. Blood pressure was 180/80 and ECG showed atrial fibrillation with ventricular rate of 90 beats per minute. She was started on intravenous fluids and admitted to the ward. Overnight she developed a temperature of 37.8°C and was given rectal paracetamol. The next morning she was noted to be breathless and she was started on cefotaxime and metronidazole for aspiration pneumonia. She also had her swallowing assessed formally and a nasogastric tube was inserted. CT scan confirmed an ischaemic stroke of the left middle cerebral artery (**A**).

Points to include:

1. Control of blood pressure – continue usual medication but do not start any new ones.
2. Temperature assessment.
3. Swallowing assessment and nasogastric feed.
4. Thromboembolic deterrent (TED) stockings.
5. Regional guidelines for aspiration pneumonia.
6. Control of hyperglycaemia.
7. Aspirin is at 300 mg for 2 weeks and then 75 mg to continue.

Note that this is for ischaemic stroke only. There are two types of stroke: ischaemic and haemorrhagic. Obviously, for the latter, all antiplatelet drugs should be stopped and blood pressure control is important.

Stroke can affect many parts of the brain and some of the areas and consequences are shown in (**B**). An ischaemic stroke is caused by any occlusion that blocks blood flow to part of the brain and affects neurological function. Ischaemic stroke can occur as a result of an embolism caused by thrombus formation in the heart or by local development of an occlusion in the cerebral arteries. A haemorrhagic stroke results from the rupture of the blood vessel wall, allowing extravasation of blood into brain tissue. In this section the problems that cause stroke and other problems associated with blood coagulation are dealt with, as are the drugs that are used. The mechanisms of coagulation and the mechanism of action of anticoagulants and thrombolytic drugs are touched on. Drugs can be prescribed to dissolve existing clots or to lessen the risk of thrombus formation.

Clearly, cardiovascular disease has widespread implications for systems and organs of the body and the drugs used reflect this. The patient described above was prescribed anti-arrhythmic drugs, antiplatelet drugs, analgesics and antipyretics (aspirin and paracetamol), and antibacterials (cefotaxime and metronidazole). In addition, a pre-existing hyperglycaemia and hypertension needed to be managed. In this section the aetiology of cardiovascular disease, including myocardial infarction (MI), arrhythmias and hypertension, and treatments are described.

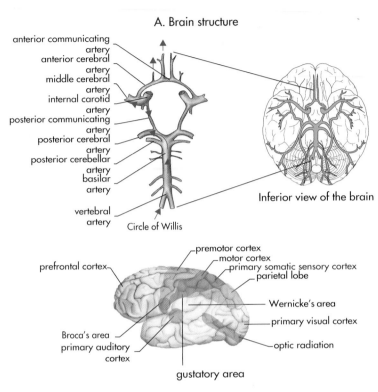

A. Brain structure

anterior communicating artery
anterior cerebral artery
middle cerebral artery
internal carotid artery
posterior communicating artery
posterior cerebral artery
posterior cerebellar artery
basilar artery
vertebral artery

Circle of Willis

Inferior view of the brain

prefrontal cortex
premotor cortex
motor cortex
primary somatic sensory cortex
parietal lobe
Wernicke's area
primary visual cortex
optic radiation
Broca's area
primary auditory cortex
gustatory area

B. Effects of stroke on cerebral areas	
Stroke-damaged region	**Signs**
Broca's area (speech)	Expressive dysphagia
Motor cortex (limb and facial areas – left side)	Right side paralysis of face, arm and leg
Optic radiation	Loss of right half of visual field if right optic radiation lost
Parietal cortex – left side	Right arm and leg coordination loss
Left sensory cortex (arm and facial areas)	Right side sensation loss in face and arm
Wernicke's area (language)	Receptive dysphasia

22 Cardiovascular system II: Essential heart function

The **heart** is a pump made mainly of muscle, which makes up the heart walls (**A**). Throughout life, the human heart contracts about 70 times per minute and pumps about 5 litres of blood each minute.

The function of the **cardiac cycle** is to ensure that blood is regularly pumped out of the heart and returned to it as an integrated part of normal physiological function. This is achieved through the cardiac cycle, which is a cyclical series of electrical, chemical and mechanical events. The first event of the cardiac cycle is the depolarisation of the atria, shown as the P wave of the ECG (**C**). This is followed by right and left atrial contraction. After the PR interval the ventricles are activated (QRS complex of the ECG) and the left ventricle begins to contract, followed soon after by the right ventricle. The consequent increase in ventricular pressure exceeds the atrial pressures and this closes first the mitral and then the tricuspid valves. Initially the ventricles contract with no volume change (isovolumetric contraction), until ventricular pressures exceed atrial pressures and the pulmonary and aortic valves open and blood is ejected from the ventricles. Then the ventricles start to relax and their pressures drop below aortic and pulmonary arterial pressures, and the aortic valve closes, followed soon after by the pulmonary valve. There is a short period of isovolumetric relaxation until ventricular pressures fall below atrial pressures and (vii) the tricuspid and mitral valves open.

The cardiac conduction system: The heart's pacemaker is the sinoatrial (SA) node, situated at the junction of the superior vena cava and the right atrium (**D**). The sequence of electrical events is: (i) depolarisation of **SA node tissue**; (ii) depolarisation of atrial myocardium; (iii) slow conduction of wave of depolarisation through the **atrioventricular** (**AV**) **node**, situated within the intra-atrial septum beneath the right atrial endocardium; (iv) conduction of the cardiac impulse along the bundle of His, which is a continuation of the AV node through the annulus fibrosus, insulating the atria from the ventricles; and (v) at the atrioventricular crest the bundle of His divides into right and left bundle branches, and the right bundle branch forms the Purkinje network, which carries the impulse throughout the right ventricular endocardium, whereas the left bundle branches (anterior and posterior) carry the impulse to the left ventricle.

Cardiac muscle resembles striated skeletal muscle; it is also striated and each cell contains sarcomeres with sliding filaments of myosin and actin (**E**). Cardiac muscle does, however, have unique properties designed to facilitate continuous pumping. The functional unit of striated muscle is the myofibril, and in the heart the myofibrils are branches, which interlock with branches of adjacent myofibrils through strong adherens junctions; this strengthens the heart so that fibres do not tear away from each other during contractions.

The **functional contractile units** of the **myocardial cell** (myocytes) are the myofibrils. Each myofibril is composed of a series of sarcomeres, which are made up of actin and myosin elements.

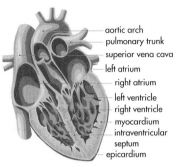

aortic arch
pulmonary trunk
superior vena cava
left atrium
right atrium
left ventricle
right ventricle
myocardium
intraventricular septum
epicardium

A. Heart anatomy

R

P   Q   S   T

P wave: atrial depolarisation
QRS complex: ventricular depolarisation
T wave: repolarisation of muscle

C. The ECG

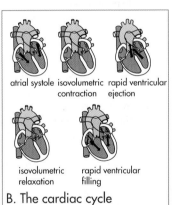

atrial systole   isovolumetric   rapid ventricular
                 contraction   ejection

isovolumetric   rapid ventricular
relaxation   filling

B. The cardiac cycle

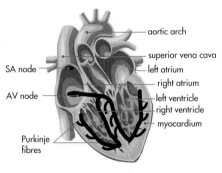

SA node

AV node

Purkinje fibres

aortic arch
superior vena cava
left atrium
right atrium
left ventricle
right ventricle
myocardium

D. Pacemakers and conducting tissue

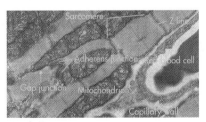

E. *Sarcomeres* – basic contractile units of striated muscle fibre

23 Coagulation I: Coagulation cascade

Coagulation of blood means the process of turning fluid blood into a solid clot. Coagulation is a part of **haemostasis**, which is an important defence mechanism to stop blood loss from damaged blood vessels. When a blood vessel is damaged, platelets adhere to macromolecules in subendothelial tissues and the platelets aggregate, forming a haemostatic plug. The platelets activate local coagulation factors that produce an insoluble protein called **fibrin**, which consolidates the platelet plug.

Coagulation can occur *in vivo* and *in vitro* (see opposite). The process consists of a cascade of enzyme reactions resulting finally in the conversion of soluble fibrinogen into an insoluble fibrous mass that traps blood cells to form the blood clot. The main components of the cascade are called 'factors', some of which are enzymes themselves; these are converted from inactive forms (zymogens) into active forms (proteases) by cleavage of peptide bonds in the zymogen. For example, factors IIa (thrombin), IXa, Xa, XIa and XIIa are all serine proteases ('a' indicates activated). The process is one of amplification, in that the activation of a relatively small amount of one factor catalyses a larger amount of the next in the cascade. A negatively charged phospholipid and Ca^{2+} are required for the action of three of the factors, namely those of factors VIIa and IXa on X, and of factors Xa on II. The peptides kallikrein and high-molecular-weight kininogens (HMWK) promote proteolysis of factor XII to XIIa.

Blood placed in a test tube coagulates within 4–8 minutes unless Ca^{2+} is inactivated by EDTA or citrate, and addition of excess Ca^{2+} will reactivate clotting. Plasma in the absence of platelets and presence of Ca^{2+} clots within 2–4 minutes. This is greatly speeded up to 60–85 seconds by the further addition of negatively charged phospholipids (PLs), and even more by addition of a particulate substance such as kaolin, to 21–32 seconds. The clotting produced by addition to plasma of a mixture of PLs, kaolin and Ca^{2+} is called the **activated partial thromboplastin time (APTT)** test. The most potent accelerator of plasma clotting in the presence of Ca^{2+} is **thromboplastin**, a saline brain extract that contains a lipoprotein called **tissue factor**. The clotting produced by addition to plasma of a mixture of Ca^{2+} and thromboplastin is called the **prothrombin time (PT)** test.

There are two pathways to coagulation, traditionally called the **intrinsic** and **extrinsic** pathways, based on results of the APTT and PT tests in patients with inherited bleeding disorders. Patients with a normal PT and a prolonged APTT are said to have a defect of the intrinsic pathway, because all the components except kaolin must normally be intrinsic to plasma. On the other hand, a normal APTT and a prolonged PT are said to imply a defect in the extrinsic pathway because tissue factor is extrinsic to plasma. If both the PT and the APTT are prolonged, this points to a defect in a common coagulation pathway. This is now somewhat dated, because both pathways are now known to share common members. Anticoagulant and antithrombotic drugs target the coagulation pathways.

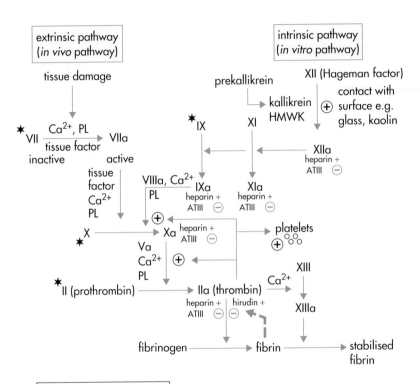

extrinsic pathway
(*in vivo* pathway)

tissue damage

★ VII $\xrightarrow[\text{tissue factor}]{Ca^{2+}, PL}$ VIIa
inactive   active

tissue
factor
Ca^{2+}
PL

★ X ──→ Xa $^{heparin\ +}_{ATIII}$ ⊖

Va
Ca^{2+} ⊕
PL

★ II (prothrombin) ──────→ IIa (thrombin) $\xrightarrow{Ca^{2+}}$ XIII
                         $^{heparin\ +}_{ATIII}$ ⊖ │ $^{hirudin\ +}$ ⊖
                                                    XIIIa

fibrinogen ──────→ fibrin ──────→ stabilised
                                   fibrin

intrinsic pathway
(*in vitro* pathway)

prekallikrein   XII (Hageman factor)

              kallikrein   contact with
              HMWK   ⊕ surface e.g.
        XI   glass, kaolin

★ IX   XIIa
                          $^{heparin\ +}$
                          ATIII ⊖

VIIIa, Ca^{2+} IXa   XIa
PL $^{heparin\ +}_{ATIII}$ ⊖ $^{heparin\ +}_{ATIII}$ ⊖
⊕

platelets
⊕ ∘∘∘

★ oral anticoagulants
  block synthesis of these factors
  HMWK: high-molecular-
  weight kininogen

Coagulation cascade

24 Coagulation II: Coagulation *in vivo*

Coagulation of blood *in vivo* is initiated by exposure of plasma to **tissue factor** and by the escape of **platelets** into the extravascular collagen-containing compartment. Tissue factor is a lipoprotein normally expressed (i) on the surface of cells such as macrophages and fibroblasts, which do not normally come into contact with plasma, and (ii) by endothelial cells of the blood vessel wall under the stimulation of some peptides involved in inflammation such as interleukin-1, tumour necrosis factor-α (TNF-α) or other endotoxins. Tissue factor greatly accelerates coagulation by binding to factor VIIa, which accelerates the formation of factor Xa at least 25000-fold. When bound to tissue factor, factor VIIa activates factor IX as well as factor X. Therefore tissue factor is an important part of the system that minimises blood loss from damaged blood vessels. The action of tissue factor is limited through the action of a plasma protein called **tissue factor pathway inhibitor** (**TFPI**), which is normally associated with plasma lipoproteins (see next spread).

Platelets (sometimes termed thrombocytes) are disc-shaped elements in the blood, about 1–2 µm in diameter. They possess receptors for a number of substances. One such receptor is called a glycoprotein (GP) Ia receptor. When a vessel wall is damaged, platelets are exposed to collagen and their GPIa receptors bind to it, which activates the platelets to degranulate and release thromboxane A_2, ADP and 5-HT, a potent vasoconstrictor. 5-HT constricts the vessel and ADP stimulates other platelets to produce pseudopodia, which make the platelets sticky and they aggregate, forming the platelet plug (**A**). The activated platelet surface promotes activation of factor X by a complex of factors IXa/VIIIa.

After formation of the plug, the platelet pseudopodia then retract, which causes the clot to shrink and become tough and elastic. This vasoconstriction and plug formation act to limit plasma loss. Platelet GPIb receptors bind to von Willebrand's factor (VWF), which occurs in plasma, platelets and the endothelial wall, and the plug begins to form (**B**). Congenital absence of VWF causes von Willebrand's disease. Platelet GPIIb/IIIa receptors bind to fibrinogen and other macromolecules. Binding of the platelets to the endothelial cell wall is limited by the release from the wall of the antiplatelet prostacyclin PGI_2.

Damaged endothelial tissue also activates the coagulation cascade (page 47) by causing release of thromboplastin which, via the extrinsic pathway, and together with factor VIIa, activates factor Xa, which in turn stimulates conversion of prothrombin to thrombin. Thrombin cleaves the fibrinogen molecule, producing sticky, insoluble strands of fibrin. These monomers polymerise in the presence of Ca^{2+} and factor XIII to produce the stable clot. This process takes seconds, compared with the activation of the intrinsic system, when factor XIIa is activated by exposed collagen. The thromboplastin/extrinsic pathway is slower, and takes minutes to complete.

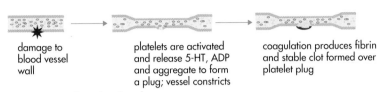

damage to
blood vessel
wall

platelets are activated
and release 5-HT, ADP
and aggregate to form
a plug; vessel constricts

coagulation produces fibrin
and stable clot formed over
platelet plug

A. Formation of a platelet plug

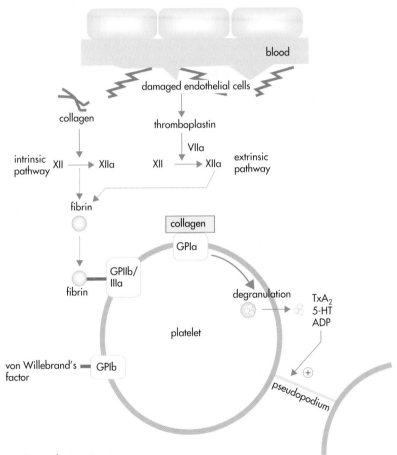

blood

damaged endothelial cells

collagen

thromboplastin

intrinsic
pathway
XII → XIIa

VIIa

XII → XIIa

extrinsic
pathway

fibrin

collagen

GPIa

GPIIb/
IIIa

fibrin

degranulation

TxA$_2$
5-HT
ADP

platelet

von Willebrand's
factor
GPIb

(+)

pseudopodium

B. Coagulation *in vivo*

25 Coagulation III: Haemostasis

Haemostasis is a term meaning the balance between coagulation and clot dissolution. The concept was introduced by Rudolph Virchow in the nineteenth century. He proposed a balance of stasis, vessel injury and hypercoagulability, which is still useful and is called Virchow's triad. Mechanisms exist, however, not only to form clots, but also (i) to prevent the cascade from freewheeling out of control, (ii) to localise them to sites of injury and (iii) to remove the clot.

The regulatory mechanisms of the coagulation cascade are mainly of a substrate feedback nature. Several of the activated proteases stimulate whereas others have a negative effect; this is summarised opposite. Localisation of clotting to the site of injury is achieved through two mechanisms: (i) selective activation of factor X by the factor IXa/VIIIa complex and activation of prothrombin by the factor Xa/Va complex only on the surfaces of activated platelets at the site of injury; and (ii) selective activation of factors X and IX by the VII/tissue factor complex on surfaces of smooth muscle cells situated immediately below the site of endothelial injury.

The action of tissue factor is limited through the action of a plasma protein **tissue factor pathway inhibitor** (**TFPI**). TFPI binds to factor Xa and blocks its action, which is to activate factor II (prothrombin; see opposite). The complex of factor Xa–TFPI binds to the VIIa–tissue factor complex and inhibits it, resulting in the shutdown of factor X and IX activation. The action of TFPI can be overcome if the original VIIa–tissue factor is generated to produce enough factor IXa to produce in turn enough Xa in the intrinsic pathway. The physiological and pathological significance of this is that the original VIIa–tissue factor complex may produce enough of factors IXa and X to initiate coagulation before being shut off, and factors VIIIa and IXa then generate sufficient Xa and thrombin to produce coagulation. An important feature of coagulation is the powerful positive and negative feedback actions of the factors on each other's activation, so that coagulation may occur rapidly enough to limit plasma loss, but be limited to the site of injury.

Antithrombin III (**AT-III**) is synthesised by endothelial and liver cells and binds to and inactivates thrombin and factors IXa, Xa, XIIa. Its action on thrombin is greatly enhanced by heparin. Other serine protease inhibitors include α_2-macroglobulin, heparin co-factor II and α-antitrypsin.

Thrombomodulin is a receptor on the endothelial cell that binds thrombin and changes its conformation so that it is no longer a protease. Instead, this altered form of thrombin activates a circulating protein, **protein C**, a vitamin K-dependent inhibitor of factors Va and VIIIa. Another circulating vitamin K-dependent plasma protein, **protein S**, enhances the activity of protein C. Thus thrombin can be converted from a promoter of coagulation into an anticoagulant. Thrombomodulin is part of the normal physiological system that removes any circulating thrombin and therefore prevents thrombus formation in undamaged blood vessels.

The **fibrinolytic system** degrades fibrin strands through a protein called plasmin. Plasminogen is the inactive form, synthesised in endothelial and liver cells and eosinophils, and is activated to plasmin by plasminogen activator.

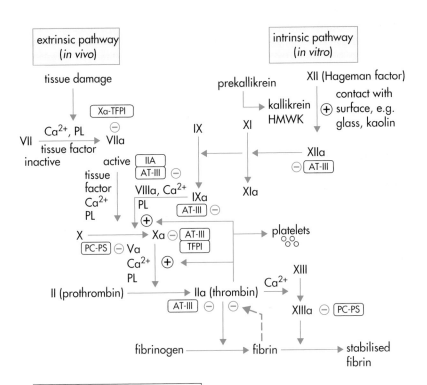

extrinsic pathway
(*in vivo*)

tissue damage

Xa-TFPI

$\ominus$

VII $\xrightarrow{\text{Ca}^{2+}, \text{PL}}$ VIIa
inactive $\quad$ tissue factor $\quad$ active

IIA
AT-III $\ominus$

tissue
factor
Ca^{2+}
PL

VIIIa, Ca^{2+}
PL
$\oplus$

IXa
AT-III $\ominus$

X $\xrightarrow{\quad}$ Xa $\ominus$
PC-PS $\ominus$ Va
Ca^{2+}
PL
$\oplus$

AT-III
TFPI

intrinsic pathway
(*in vitro*)

prekallikrein $\quad$ XII (Hageman factor)

kallikrein $\quad$ contact with
HMWK $\quad \oplus$ surface, e.g.
glass, kaolin

IX $\quad$ XI

XIIa
$\ominus$ AT-III

XIa

platelets

II (prothrombin) $\xrightarrow{\quad}$ IIa (thrombin) $\xrightarrow{\text{Ca}^{2+}}$ XIII
AT-III $\ominus \quad \ominus$ $\quad$ XIIIa $\ominus$ PC-PS

fibrinogen $\xrightarrow{\quad}$ fibrin $\xrightarrow{\quad}$ stabilised
fibrin

AT-III: antithrombin III
HMWK: high molecular weight kininogens
PC-PS: protein C-proteinS
TFPI: tissue factor pathway inhibitor

Haemostasis

26 Anticoagulants I: Heparin

Anticoagulants are used to inhibit thrombus formation. The main indications are: (i) unstable angina; (ii) pulmonary embolism; (iii) deep venous thrombosis in the leg; (iv) atrial fibrillation, mainly in elderly patients or those with mitral stenosis or impaired left ventricular function; (v) patients with mechanical prosthetic heart valves; (vi) pre-treatment of patients with acute coronary syndromes such as unstable angina who are to undergo angioplasty; and (vii) after a procedure in patients at high risk for in-stent thrombosis. The drug most often used is **heparin**, either unfractionated or as its low-molecular-weight fragments.

Mechanism of action of heparin: Heparin binds to antithrombin III and enhances antithrombin's reaction with the clotting factors, resulting in a prolongation of the clotting time.

Preparations of heparin used are unfractionated heparin and low-molecular-weight heparins. Unfractionated heparin can be split into fragments, not all of which are anticoagulant. The fragments that do have anticoagulant activity are called **low-molecular-weight heparins**, and include **dalteparin, enoxaparin, tinzaparin** and **certoparin**.

Advantages of low-molecular-weight heparins include: (i) no need for patient monitoring because of consistently controlled product preparation; (ii) that they do not cross the placenta and can be used in pregnancy; (iii) that they have a longer duration of action and can be given subcutaneously in single daily doses, which makes them more suitable for the treatment of, for example, deep venous thrombosis or pulmonary embolism; and (iv) that they are more suitable for use in preventing venous thrombosis in hip and knee replacement.

Administration: Unfractionated heparin infusion is given via a syringe pump. If a pump is not available the heparin can be added to 1 litre of saline or 5% dextrose and given as an infusion. Whichever method is used the infusion rate must be carefully controlled. The rate of infusion is monitored by measuring the kaolin cephalin time or APTT 6 hours after starting infusion and then at least once daily; these should be kept between two and three times the control value, depending on the indication.

Adverse effects of heparin include the following: (i) The most important adverse effect is **bleeding** because of overdose. This may often first appear as haematuria, but bleeding may occur from any site. The treatment is to stop the heparin. (ii) Prolonged use is associated with osteoporosis. (iii) Rarely, severe heparin-induced thrombocytopenia develops; platelet counts should be carried out if the patient receives heparin for more than 5 days.

Heparin antidote: Protamine sulphate is given intravenously, which may cause a fall in blood pressure and it has some anticoagulant effects. Patients with unstable angina are now routinely treated with low molecular weight hepatitis, with longer-lasting effects that are less easily reversed with protamine sulphate.

Clinical scenario: A 32-year-old woman went to her GP with chest pain, breathlessness and a cough. On examination, the GP noticed that her right calf was swollen. Also of concern was her 5-year history of oral contraceptive pill use. He sent her to casualty for assessment. There she became more breathless. O_2 saturations were 90% on air and arterial blood gases revealed a type I respiratory failure. ECG showed tachycardia and right bundle branch block. Chest X-ray and blood tests were normal. A deep vein thrombosis and subsequent pulmonary embolus were diagnosed on clinical grounds. The casualty doctor took blood for a thrombophilia screen and then started the patient on O_2, intravenous fluids and subcutaneous low-molecular-weight heparin. The diagnosis was confirmed using a ventilation perfusion scan and Doppler ultrasound. Following this the patient received warfarin for 6 months.

Risk factors for DVT:
Malignancy
Smoking
Immobilisation
History of DVT
Dehydration
Oral contraceptive pill
Factor V Leiden
Protein C deficiency
Protein S deficiency

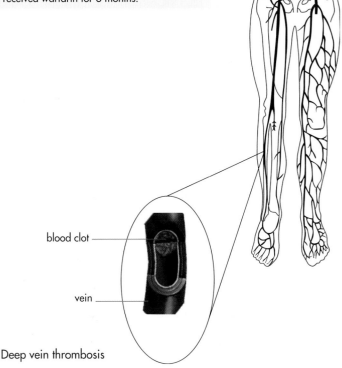

blood clot

vein

Deep vein thrombosis

27 Anticoagulants II: Warfarin

Warfarin is the most commonly used **oral anticoagulant** and is a synthetic derivative of bishydroxycoumarin, which is found in spoiled sweet clover. Warfarin is active orally and is therefore available to patients for long-term use. It is also used as a rat poison.

Mechanism of action: Warfarin is structurally similar to vitamin K and blocks the vitamin's reduction (**A**). Vitamin K is necessary for the post-translational γ-carboxylation of clotting factors II, VII, IX and X. Thus the onset of warfarin action is delayed until existing stores of these factors are depleted.

Administration and monitoring: Warfarin is given orally in tablet form, which is convenient for the patient, who can take warfarin at home. An initial loading dose is given, followed by lower maintenance doses. Because anticoagulant therapy has attendant dangers of haemorrhage the patient needs close and regular monitoring for blood coagulability. The prothrombin time is measured before initiating treatment, thereafter daily, and the dose is adjusted until the international normalised ratio (INR) is stabilised:

$$INR = \frac{\text{Patient's prothrombin time}}{\text{Normal prothrombin time}}$$

The dose is adjusted to keep the INR between 2.0 and 4.5 (depending on the clinical situation). This usually provides effective anticoagulation with a minimal risk of bleeding.

Precautions with warfarin: (i) Warfarin is metabolised in the liver, and liver disease or old age may result in dangerous levels of warfarin. (ii) Other drugs (see below), previous surgery and heart failure will increase patient sensitivity to warfarin. (iii) Patients must time dosage with strict accuracy.

Adverse effects and **contraindications:** Adverse effects include haemorrhage, jaundice, fever and skin rashes. Warfarin is teratogenic (see below). An INR above 5 indicates a haemorrhagic risk. Warfarin should be withdrawn immediately and, if required, an infusion of fresh frozen plasma will reverse warfarin's effects. Alternatively, or in addition, **vitamin K** can be administered, although this may take several days to take effect, even if given intravenously.

Warfarin and pregnancy: Warfarin crosses the placenta and is teratogenic in the first trimester. Heparin is used during this period and warfarin may be restored when the danger of teratogenicity has passed. Alternatively, heparin can be used throughout gestation. Maternal warfarin does not appear to gain access to mother's milk.

Drug interactions with warfarin: Many drugs either enhance or reduce the efficacy of a given dose and can even precipitate haemorrhage. The list of drugs that interact with warfarin is formidable, especially as warfarin circulates largely bound to plasma proteins, from which it is readily displaced by many other drugs (**B**), thus increasing the free and therefore physiologically active concentration of warfarin in blood. Drugs that alter the metabolism of warfarin will also affect its potency. Warfarin is metabolised by the cytochrome P450 liver enzyme systems in the liver, and drugs that induce the enzyme decrease the anticoagulant effects of warfarin. Those that inhibit the enzymes will increase warfarin's effects.

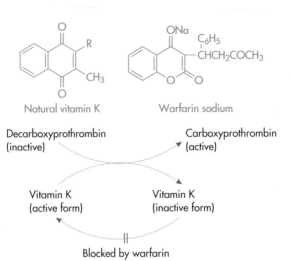

Natural vitamin K   Warfarin sodium

Decarboxyprothrombin   Carboxyprothrombin
(inactive)   (active)

Vitamin K   Vitamin K
(active form)   (inactive form)

Blocked by warfarin

A. Mechanism of action of warfarin

Examples of drugs that potentiate warfarin*	Examples of drugs that diminish warfarin action*
Aspirin	Antacids
Ciprofloxacin	Alcohol
Erythromycin	Barbiturates
Ibuprofen	Carbamazepine
Metronidazole	Griseofulvin
Omeprazole	Haloperidol
Simvastatin	Oral contraceptive pill
Sulfonamides	Rifampicin
	Vitamin K

*This list is not exhaustive

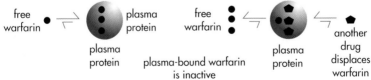

free   plasma   free   another
warfarin   protein   warfarin   drug
                                                                        displaces
            plasma   plasma   warfarin
            protein   plasma-bound warfarin   protein
                      is inactive

B. Warfarin drug interactions

28 Antiplatelet drugs

Platelet activation and aggregation are key events in normal haemostasis, but are also central to myocardial infarction (MI) and other atherothrombotic disorders, and drugs that block platelet activation are an integral part of treatment. Platelets promote blood vessel occlusion when activated by, for example, a ruptured atheromatous plaque (A). Several drugs are designed to block platelet activation and aggregation.

Key activators of platelets include (i) adhesion, e.g. to collagen, or (ii) contact with thrombin, fibrinogen, ADP or epinephrine. Ultimately thromboxane A_2 (TxA_2) is formed and activates the integrin GPIIb/IIIa receptor on the platelet. There are about 80 000 receptors per platelet and they cause platelet aggregation. Activated platelets release several inflammatory and other mediators, including: (i) platelet factor 4, a chemokine that mediates shear-resistant arrest of monocytes to endothelium; (ii) RANTES (MCP2), a chemokine that triggers shear-resistant monocyte arrest on inflamed or atherosclerotic endothelium; (iii) nitric oxide, which is anti-atherosclerotic; (iv) CD 154, a protein involved in endothelial cell function; and (v) thrombospondin, which interacts with a number of cell surface receptors involved in atherosclerosis (B).

Treatments: Low-dose (75 mg) aspirin blocks prostaglandin (and thus TxA_2) synthesis by irreversibly inhibiting the cyclo-oxygenase-1 (COX-1) enzyme. TxA_2 activates the GPIIb/IIIa-binding site on the platelet, which allows fibrinogen to bind, resulting in platelet aggregation. **Low-dose aspirin** is used for primary and secondary prevention of thrombotic cardiovascular or cerebrovascular disease. As soon as possible after an ischaemic event, a single dose of aspirin is given, preferably chewable or dispersed in water: 300 mg after an ischaemic (but not haemorrhagic) stroke; 300 mg after an MI. Maintenance thereafter is with 75–300 mg daily. Aspirin is also used following coronary bypass surgery, for primary prevention of vascular events when the estimated 10-year coronary heart disease risk is 10% or more, provided that blood pressure is controlled.

Clopidogrel and **ticlopidine** are used to prevent atherosclerotic events in patients with a history of symptomatic atherosclerotic disease. They are thienopyridines that are specific inhibitors of ADP-induced platelet aggregation at the platelet GPIIb/IIIa receptor. They block ADP binding to its platelet receptor, which would otherwise have caused activation of the GPIIb/IIIa receptor to bind fibrinogen followed by further platelet aggregation. Both are pro-drugs converted *in vivo* to active metabolites. Clopidogrel is safer than ticlopidine, which is associated with hepatic and renal impairment. Clopidogrel is associated, rarely, with thrombotic thrombocytopenic purpura (TTP), GIT bleeding and neutropenia.

GPIIb/IIIa antagonists prevent platelet aggregation by directly blocking the binding of fibrinogen to the receptor. **Abciximab** is a monoclonal antibody that binds to and dissociates slowly from the receptor. **Eptifibatide** is a peptide that binds to and dissociates rapidly from the receptor. Both drugs are administered by initial intravenous injection followed by intravenous infusion. Both are used only in hospital by specialists. **Tirofiban** is a non-peptide antagonist for oral use but its clinical efficacy by this route is not established.

Dipyridamole is a phosphodiesterase inhibitor that has an additive effect with aspirin in the secondary prevention of stroke.

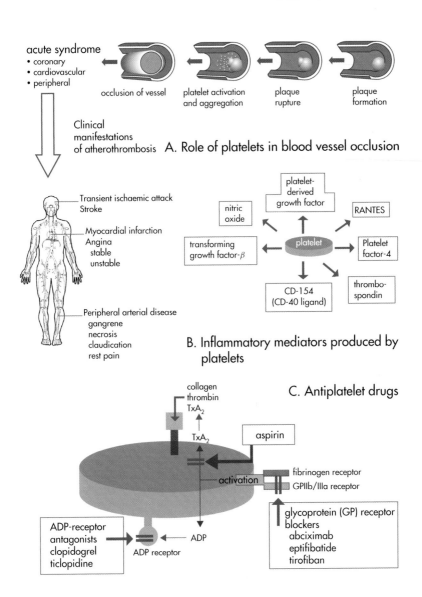

acute syndrome
- coronary
- cardiovascular
- peripheral

occlusion of vessel | platelet activation and aggregation | plaque rupture | plaque formation

Clinical manifestations of atherothrombosis

A. Role of platelets in blood vessel occlusion

Transient ischaemic attack
Stroke

Myocardial infarction
Angina
stable
unstable

Peripheral arterial disease
gangrene
necrosis
claudication
rest pain

platelet-derived growth factor

nitric oxide

RANTES

transforming growth factor-β

platelet

Platelet factor-4

CD-154 (CD-40 ligand)

thrombo-spondin

B. Inflammatory mediators produced by platelets

C. Antiplatelet drugs

collagen
thrombin
TxA_2

TxA_2

aspirin

activation

fibrinogen receptor
GPIIb/IIIa receptor

ADP-receptor antagonists
clopidogrel
ticlopidine

ADP

ADP receptor

glycoprotein (GP) receptor blockers
abciximab
eptifibatide
tirofiban

29 Thrombolytic and anti-fibrinolytic drugs

Physiological thrombolytic mechanisms exist (**A**) and these can be targeted by drugs to dissolve a thrombus. Essentially, when the coagulation system is activated, this triggers the fibrinolytic system through the production of several endothelial plasminogen activators, including tissue-type plasminogen activator (tPA), kallikrein, urokinase-type plasminogen activator (uPA) and neutrophil elastase. Plasmin digests the fibrin strands that form the framework of the clot, and releases fibrin degradation products. Conversely, anti-fibrinolytic agents (**B**) are used to inhibit the activation of plasminogen.

Thrombolytic agents: The most important are **alteplase, duteplase, reteplase, streptokinase** and **urokinase** (uPA). Alteplase and duteplase are both recombinant tPAs, the former being single chain and the latter double chain. Streptokinase is a non-enzymatic protein extracted from β-haemolytic streptococci. When infused intravenously it binds plasminogen and exposes serine residues, and plasmin is activated. The action is enhanced by aspirin. Streptokinase is an antigen and promotes production of antistreptoccal antibodies within about 4 days; thus it should not be re-used. Alteplase and duteplase are said to be 'clot selective' because they selectively target fibrin-bound plasminogen. They are not antigenic but have relatively short half-lives. Reteplase is similar in action to a tPA but has a longer half-life, and has been found useful for treating MI. Streptokinase, in contrast to a tPA, is not clot selective. Urokinase is prepared from human embryonic kidney cells. **Tenecteplase**, a more recent addition, is a modified derivative tPA with a longer half-life and can be given by bolus injection. Tenecteplase is claimed to bind fibrin specifically and with higher affinity.

Thrombolytic agents are used principally in MI, deep venous thrombosis and pulmonary embolism. Decisions for treatment are based on a balance between benefit and risk to the patient. In MI, treatment is indicated in patients with elevated ST segment or new left bundle-branch block. Streptokinase is used in life-threatening venous thrombosis and pulmonary embolism, and treatment needs to be prompt. The choice between streptokinase and tPA depends on several factors, including patient age, the risk of intracerebral bleeding, previous use of streptokinase and the size of the infarct.

Adverse effects, precautions and contraindications: Bleeding, nausea and vomiting are the most common adverse effects. Bleeding is usually confined to the injection site, but may occur elsewhere, e.g. at intracerebral sites. Bleeding can be treated with anti-fibrinolytic drugs (see opposite), and coagulation factors and thrombolytic treatment should be stopped. Reperfusion arrhythmias may occur when treating MI. Patients should not be thrombolysed if they have: (i) poorly controlled hypertension; (ii) GIT bleeding in the previous 3 months; (iii) pericarditis; (iv) pregnancy; (v) proliferative retinopathy; (vi) recent bowel resection or cardiovascular surgery; (vii) active haemorrhagic or bleeding disorders; and (viii) aortic dissection.

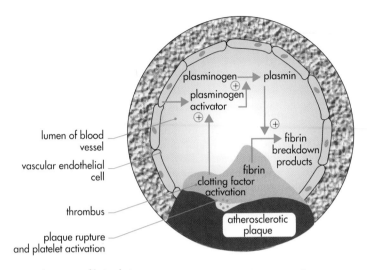

lumen of blood vessel

vascular endothelial cell

thrombus

plaque rupture and platelet activation

plasminogen → plasmin

plasminogen activator

fibrin breakdown products

clotting factor activation

fibrin

atherosclerotic plaque

A. Endogenous fibrinolytic system

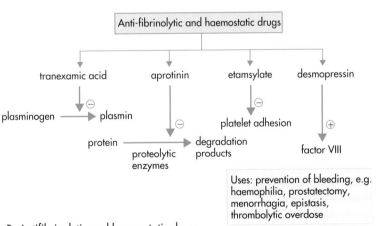

Anti-fibrinolytic and haemostatic drugs

tranexamic acid   aprotinin   etamsylate   desmopressin

plasminogen ⟶ plasmin

protein ⟶ proteolytic enzymes

degradation products

platelet adhesion

factor VIII

Uses: prevention of bleeding, e.g. haemophilia, prostatectomy, menorrhagia, epistasis, thrombolytic overdose

B. Antifibrinolytic and haemostatic drugs

30 Acute coronary syndromes I: Myocardial infarction

Myocardial infarction ('heart attack') is one of the most common and serious of all the medical emergencies. The classic presentation is crushing central chest pain with relatively rapid onset. **Triggers** include exercise, or preceding illness, but often the acute event is unheralded. **Associated symptoms** include breathlessness, pain in the left arm, neck and chin, and those associated with sympathetic drive, e.g. sweating and anxiety. In patients with diabetes or the elderly, symptoms may be less stereotypical and the patient may present with breathlessness caused by pulmonary oedema, or there may be even be no presenting symptoms – the 'silent myocardial infarction'. The outcome of MI depends on promptness of treatment. Public perception and understanding of heart attacks are very high and the response of the emergency services is usually prompt.

Diagnosis and treatment: As with all medical emergencies, initial history and examination are paramount, but vital information regarding further treatment comes from **ECG analysis**. Extensive studies have demonstrated that treatment with thrombolytic therapy is beneficial only in those patients with either ST-segment elevation or new left bundle-branch block. Assuming that there are no contraindications to thrombolysis, the **standard treatment** for the patient with an MI involves administration of **oxygen**, 300 mg of **dispersible aspirin**, thrombolysis and pain relief which is commonly **intravenous diamorphine** or **morphine**. With regard to the choice of thrombolytic agent, inferior MIs and those in the elderly are usually treated with **streptokinase**. The benefit of thrombolysis is directly proportional to the 'door-to-needle' time. Maximum benefit is gained in the first 3–6 hours after onset of symptoms. Twelve hours after onset of symptoms the benefit of thrombolysis is questionable. Some of the thrombolytic agents require concurrent treatment with **heparin**.

It may be necessary to provide inotropic support to the patient with an MI, and the agent of choice is **dobutamine** via a central line. Hypotension in an anterior MI is commonly due to myogenic shock. In an inferior MI, hypotension is often due to inadequate filling pressures and will respond to **fluid resuscitation**.

Common early complications of MI are arrhythmias. These are more common in inferior MIs due to the anatomy of the conducting system. Arrhythmias include ventricular ectopics, ventricular tachycardia, heart block and ventricular fibrillation. Ventricular fibrillation is always treated with **emergency electrical DC cardioversion** and may also necessitate **cardio-pulmonary resuscitation**. **Amiodarone** may be needed for symptomatic early arrhythmias, but often they settle as revascularisation occurs.

Following successful treatment for an MI, patients without specific contra-indications should receive treatment with regular **aspirin**, **β-blockers**, angiotensin-converting enzyme (**ACE**) **inhibitors** and a **statin**.

Percutaneous coronary intervention (PCI) is a procedure by which blood flow through a partially or completely obstructed arterial lumen is restored by means of **angioplasty** (inflation of a balloon) or insertion of a metal stent across the culprit lesion. Where the resources are available primary PCI is an alternative to thrombolysis. This procedure is usually accompanied by administration of **heparin, GPIIb/IIIa receptor antagonists** and **clopidogrel.**

Clinical scenario: The patient, a 50-year-old man with type 2 diabetes mellitus and hypertension, was admitted with a 6-hour history of central heavy chest pain, breathlessness, sweating and increasing nausea. An ECG showed ST-segment elevation in inferior leads with reciprocal ischaemia in anterior leads. He was treated with oxygen, 300 mg soluble aspirin and intravenous streptokinase. Intravenous diamorphine and metoclopramide were given for symptom relief.

Treatment: The three most important aspects of this patient's treatment are oxygen, the antiplatelet effect of aspirin and the thrombolytic effect of streptokinase. Diamorphine is a powerful analgesic and also causes a peripheral vasodilatation. Metoclopramide blocks central dopamine receptors and reduces nausea. These drugs can be given only to patients whose history is accompanied by ECG changes indicating an acute myocardial infarction. This is predominantly classic ST-segment elevation in contiguous leads, and less often the development of new left bundle-branch block or posterior myocardial infarction (dominant R waves in V1 and V2 with ST-segment depression). To achieve maximal benefit thrombolysis should be achieved within 6 hours of symptom onset. Its benefit diminishes from this point onwards and the treatment window closes at 12 hours. The thrombolytic agents currently in use are streptokinase, recombinant tissue plasminogen activator (rtPA), reteplase and tenecteplase. Streptokinase is the most commonly used agent at present.

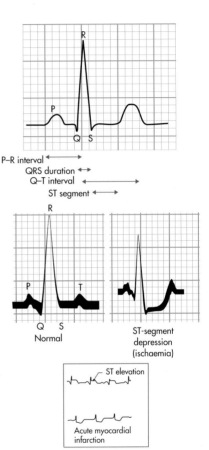

ST-segment depression (ischaemia)

Normal

ST elevation

Acute myocardial infarction

31 Acute coronary syndromes II: Unstable angina

The patient presents with chest pain that is more long lasting than that of stable angina, which often develops in an accelerating manner, is less responsive to medication and may occur when the patient is at rest.

Diagnosis is made using history, examination and ECG. Plasma troponin and creatine kinase (CK) or CK-MB provide corroboration. Other routine blood tests that should be carried out include total and low-density lipoprotein (LDL)-cholesterol, Hb, platelets and serum biochemistry. Twelve-lead ECG is done to determine if there is ST depression, which is an important determinant of mortality risk. Imaging studies, e.g. echocardiography for rapid assessment of left ventricular function, may be done.

Treatment: Unstable angina has a highly unpredictable and potentially dangerous course and, depending on the outcome of tests, may require aggressive management. Patients at moderate-to-high risk, e.g. with chest pain refractory to treatment, ST depression > 1 mm on the ECG and high troponin levels, may need cardiac catheterisation and possible angioplasty.

Drugs: Antiplatelet agents are given immediately. Early **aspirin** administration, alone or together with **clopidogrel**, reduces mortality by reducing the risk of fatal MI, strokes and vascular death. Aspirin is contraindicated in hypersensitive patients, hypoprothrombinaemia, asthma, patients younger than 16 years, vitamin K deficiency, peptic ulcer and liver damage, and should be used with caution if patients are taking anticoagulants. Urine alkalinity, corticosteroids and antacids will reduce aspirin efficacy, and aspirin will reduce the uricosuric efficacy of probenecid. Clopidogrel is contraindicated in hypersensitive patients, or in any case of active pathological bleeding. **Antithrombotic drugs** used include **heparin**. Low-molecular-weight heparin is given to almost all patients with unstable angina.

Statins are used to reduce plasma LDL-cholesterol. Statins, such as **atorvastatin**, which has a relatively long half-life, reduce the probability of MI and mortality, severe recurrent symptomatic ischaemia and resuscitated cardiac arrest. They are contraindicated in pregnancy, breastfeeding and patients with documented hypersensitivity.

Selective β_1-blocking drugs, e.g. metoprolol, are prescribed to reduce blood pressure and heart rate, thus reducing oxygen demand. Their use is known to reduce the incidence of MI and ischaemic symptoms. They should be avoided in patients with vasospastic angina or cocaine-induced coronary vasoconstriction

GPIIb/IIIa receptor antagonists, e.g. **tirofiban** and **eptifibatide,** may be infused, but must be used with caution in patients with hypertension and are contraindicated in patients with a history of bleeding disorders. Powerful platelet aggregation inhibitors, e.g. **abciximab,** are used in PCI.

Glyceryl trinitrate relieves pain by improving myocardial oxygen supply and decreases both preload and afterload. It can be given sublingually or intravenously. **Nicorandil** and **isosorbide mononitrate** are given once the patient has stabilised, and they reduce the frequency and severity of attacks.

Clinical scenario: The patient, a 47-year-old man, had been treated by his GP for cardiac chest pain. He had been started on aspirin and isosorbide mononitrate, but continued to experience pain and breathlessness on exertion. On the day of his admission, chest pain, nausea and vomiting lasted for 1 hour before settling. At presentation, although haemodynamically stable and pain free, an ECG showed ST-segment depression in lateral and septal leads. He was treated with 300 mg aspirin, full dose of a subcutaneous low-molecular-weight heparin and an oral β-blocker. Throughout the night he experienced fleeting chest pains which were unrelieved by sublingual nitrates, and by the morning he was receiving intravenous glyceryl trinitrate and was pain free. On the ward round in the morning he was commenced on atorvastatin based on presentation cholesterol measurements.

Clinical scenario: The patient, a 47-year-old man, had been treated by his GP for cardiac chest pain. He had been started on aspirin and isosorbide mononitrate, but continued to experience pain and breathlessness on exertion. On the day of his admission, he experienced sustained central chest pain with breathlessness and nausea. On examination he looked unwell, was hypoxic and had a tachycardia. ECG showed ST-segment depression in lateral and septal leads. Despite treatment with oxygen, diamorphine, metoclopramide, aspirin, low-molecular-weight heparin, intravenous glyceryl trinitrate and oral β-blocker, he remained in intermittent discomfort throughout the night. He was reviewed by a cardiology registrar in the morning, who noted a troponin T level of 0.13 μg/l and booked the patient for urgent percutaneous coronary angiography. Several hours later, the patient returned to the ward following insertion of an intracoronary stent. At this point he was receiving intravenous abciximab, a glycoprotein IIb/IIIa receptor antagonist, and was due to start 300 mg clopidogrel orally.

32 Transient ischaemic attack

A transient ischaemic attack (TIA) is a set of neurological symptoms that clears up completely within 24 hours. It is due to a temporary interruption of blood to a part of the brain by a tiny blood clot breaking off from an atheroma in a main blood vessel in the neck (see opposite). If the attack lasts longer than 24 hours but the neurological symptoms disappear within 7 days, it is sometimes called a reversible neurological deficit (RIND). It is a strong warning of a future, more serious stroke and patients must be treated urgently.

Risk factors: Gender (male > women) and advancing age are unavoidable risk factors. Treatable risk factors include hypertension, hypercholesterolaemia, smoking, lack of exercise, obesity, and a diet high in salt and fat. A full stroke is more likely within 3 months of a TIA in patients in whom the TIA lasted longer than 10 minutes, who were over 60 or have diabetes, or whose TIA symptoms included speech impairment and muscle weakness.

Symptoms of TIA include hemiparesis, hemisensory loss, dysphasia, amaurosis fugax (transient loss of vision), speech slurring (dysarthria) and reading problems (dyslexia). Visual problems include double vision (diplopia), vision loss in one eye (amaurosis fugax) and inability to see on one side of the body (hemianopia). Patients may experience sensation loss in part of the body or muscle weakness. **Diagnosis** relies on history, but also involves examination, including blood pressure measurement and ultrasound of the carotid arteries. Echocardiograms may be taken to check for the possibility of heart disease.

The main aim of **treatment** is to prevent a subsequent stroke. Carotid endarterectomy is indicated in patients in whom a greater than 70% stenosis is found.

Drugs: Antiplatelet drugs, e.g. **aspirin**, are prescribed and **warfarin** may be prescribed for patients in whom the clot resulted from a cardiac problem such as atrial fibrillation. **Dipyridamole** may be prescribed for patients who suffered TIA or stroke while on aspirin ('aspirin failure'). **Statins** may be prescribed to lower cholesterol levels and **antihypertensives** if needed. A recent study was done with TIA patients who took **perindopril**, a long-acting ACE inhibitor in combination with the antihypertensive indapamide. The results suggest that patients may need antihypertensive therapy in addition to antiplatelet drugs and statins.

Other preventive measures: Patients should consider the following alterations in lifestyle:

- Take regular exercise.
- Limit alcohol intake.
- Establish a high-fibre, low-salt diet.
- Limit intake of food with saturated fats.
- Stop smoking, as it promotes platelet aggregation and promotes occlusion of arteries.
- Find out the correct weight/height ratio and work towards attaining and maintaining it.
- If diabetic, achieve tight glycaemic control.

Note: Neurological evaluation of patients is recommended in view of the transient interruption of oxygen to a brain region.

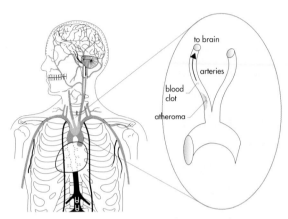

Site of blood clot formation in a transient ischaemic attack (TIA)

Case scenario: A 56-year-old man was seen in the rapid-access TIA clinic. He described waking up one morning and noticing a strange cold sensation creeping up his right arm. This was then followed by an almost complete loss of function in the affected arm. Symptoms lasted approximately 8 hours and his speech, smell, taste and vision were not affected. His previous medical history was significant for diet-controlled diabetes mellitus. On examination he was hypertensive, with a blood pressure of 170/90. There was a carotid bruit on the left with normal heart sounds. ECG showed left ventricular hypertrophy but was in sinus rhythm. He was commenced on aspirin and bendrofluazide. Carotid Doppler ultrasounds later confirmed 80% stenosis of the internal carotid artery and he was referred to a vascular surgeon.

33 Dysrhythmias I: Causes of dysrhythmias

Dysrhythmias are interruptions of normal cardiac rhythm, caused by disturbances of normal cardiac impulse formation, conduction or both (**A**). The patient may experience palpitations, dizziness, light-headedness or nausea, and may faint. The symptoms, understandably, may produce fear as well. **Bradycardia** is a slowing of the heart, and **tachycardia** is a speeding up of heart rate.

Dysrhythmias are generally classified according to their site of origin, i.e. atrial, nodal or ventricular. Causative factors include: (i) plasma pH disturbances; (ii) cardiac ischaemia; (iii) drug toxicity; (iv) electrolyte imbalances; (v) excess sympathetic activity, including raised plasma epinephrine; and (vi) scarring and stretching of cardiac muscle.

Disturbances of impulse formation arise through alterations in the duration of (a) the action potential and, more importantly, (b) the diastolic intervals (**B**). Pacemaker rate will be increased by a shortening of (a) or (b) or both.

Note: The interval between pacemaker depolarisations = duration of the diastolic interval + duration of the action potential

The diastolic intervals are determined by: (i) the threshold potential; (ii) the slope of phase 4 depolarisation; and (iii) the maximum diastolic potential. Pacemaker activity is slowed, e.g. by β-blockers such as propranolol or increased vagal discharges, by making the maximum diastolic potential more negative. This in turn reduces the slope of phase 4 depolarisation. Pacemaker activity can be speeded up by tissue injury, fibre stretch, β-adrenoceptor activation, hypokalaemia or acidosis.

Disturbances of impulse conduction arise from a block, either anatomical or physiological, to the conducting system or the tissue through which the impulse passes. This may be a simple bundle-branch block (by far the most common), an atrioventricular nodal block or conduction abnormality (**C**). There are three 'bundles': right, left anterior and left posterior. Right bundle branch may be a normal finding. Bifascicular block, involving the right and one of the left branches, warrants investigation and can lead to trifascicular, or complete, heart block.

Re-entry circuits may be highly localised to a small area of atrial or ventricular tissue, or may have multiple re-entry sites, e.g. the Wolff–Parkinson–White (WPW) syndrome, where there are re-entry circuits at the AV node, in atrial and ventricular tissue, and at so-called 'by-pass tracts'. Large parts of the atrial and/or ventricular walls may have re-entry circuits.

Several different types of dysrhythmias are classified and require specific drug treatments, which will be covered in other spreads. These are, very broadly speaking, classified as either supraventricular or ventricular.

34 Dysrhythmias II: Vaughan Williams classification of anti-dysrhythmic drugs

Dysrhythmic drugs correct disturbances of cardiac rhythm. The aim is to correct abnormal pacemaker activity and/or abnormal propagation of impulses through the heart. **The four main mechanisms:** (i) They block sympathetic cardiac activity; (ii) they block Na^+ channels; (iii) they prolong the effective refractory period; (iv) they block Ca^{2+} channels.

Note: Emergency treatment of dangerous dysrhythmias is usually mechanical, using electrical cardioversion or pacing.

Dysrhythmic drugs are classified into four main classes in terms of their effects on different phases of the cardiac action potential. **Class I** drugs, e.g. lidocaine (lignocaine) and flecainamide, block Na^+ channels, and are subdivided into Ia, Ib and Ic and all depend on the principle of use-dependent blockade of Na^+ channels. **Class II** are the β-blocking drugs, e.g. **atenolol**. **Class III** drugs, notably **amiodarone** and **sotalol**, significantly prolong the action potential (pro-longed QT interval), which is associated with a prolongation of the refractory period. The exact mechanism is not known but may involve the blockade of K^+ channels. **Class IV** drugs, for example **verapamil**, selectively target voltage-sensitive Ca^{2+} channels. They slow conduction in the SA and AV nodes. This slows the heart and corrects supraventricular tachycardias through a partial AV block.

Uses of antidysrhthmic drugs: **Class Ia: Disopyramide** is now very occasionally used for recurrent paroxysmal atrial fibrillation with vagal over-activity because it has atropine-like actions. **Ib: Lidocaine** is a second-line agent used intravenously after amiodarone in the treatment of ventricular tachycardia. It has CNS side-effects, including convulsions, drowsiness and disorientation. **Ic: Flecainide** is an effective agent used orally and intravenously in the treatment of acute atrial fibrillation to achieve chemical cardioversion to sinus rhythm. It should not be used in ventricular fibrillation that is due to ischaemic or structural heart disease. It has been used to treat ectopic ventricular beats but is associated with increased incidence of fatal ventricular fibrillation after MI. Flecainide has a role to play in younger patients who do not have established ischaemic heart disease. **Class II:** β-blockers, e.g. propranolol, atenolol and timolol, reduce mortality after MI and they help to reduce recurrent paroxysmal atrial fibrillation when caused by increased sympathetic activity. **Class III: Amiodarone** is, after digoxin, the most commonly used medication in atrial fibrillation and is used to restore sinus rhythm. It may be used either orally or intravenously. When given through a peripheral intravenous line it causes thrombophlebitis and therefore has to be given either through a long line or a central line. Amiodarone reduces (i) tachycardia associated with the Wolff–Parkinson–White syndrome (see opposite); (ii) atrial fibrillation; (iii) chronic malignant ventricular tachycardia associated after MI. It has several adverse effects, including hypo- or hyperthyroidism (it contains iodine), skin disorders, e.g. photosensitivity, irreversible pulmonary fibrosis and GIT and neurological disturbances. **Sotalol,** a non-selective β-blocker, has similar efficacy to amiodarone for treatment of ventricular dysrhythmias and has fewer adverse effects, but is contraindicated in asthma. **Class IV:** Verapamil and diltiazem are the calcium channel blockers with negative chronotropic effects. Verapamil can be given acutely to slow or cardiovert supraventricular tachycardia. It should not be given to patients who are already taking (3-blockers due to the risk of complete heart block. Ca^{2+} antagonists are dangerous and ineffective in ventricular dysrhythmias.

Case scenario: A 30 year-old man was admitted to hospital with palpitations, which had started in the evening of the previous day. He had spent that day at the races with his friends and had consumed 12 pints of lager. His normal alcohol intake was between 40 and 60 units of alcohol per week. On examination his pulse was 80 beats per minute, equal at the apex and the wrist, but irregular in nature. ECG confirmed atrial fibrillation with a controlled ventricular rate. He was admitted to the coronary care unit where he cardioverted to sinus rhythm on an infusion of flecainide. He was discharged the following day with caution regarding alcohol and an appointment for a 24-hour tape.

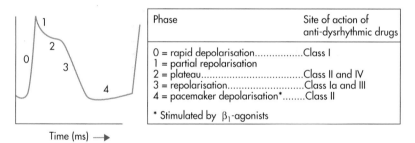

Phase	Site of action of anti-dysrhythmic drugs
0 = rapid depolarisation	Class I
1 = partial repolarisation	
2 = plateau	Class II and IV
3 = repolarisation	Class Ia and III
4 = pacemaker depolarisation*	Class II
* Stimulated by β_1-agonists	

Time (ms) ➔

Dysrhythmic drugs and the Purkinje fibre action potential

35 Dysrhythmias III: Other anti-dysrhythmic drugs

Important drugs that do not fall within the Vaughan Williams' classification include **adenosine** and **digoxin**.

Adenosine is an endogenous nucleoside involved in, for example, cardio-vascular, respiratory and platelet function. Through its A_1-receptor it slows the rate of rise of the pacemaker potential in the AV node via a mechanism linked to the muscarinic M_2-receptor, which hyperpolarises cardiac muscle.

Therapeutic use: Adenosine is used intravenously to terminate supra-ventricular tachycardia after manoeuvres such as the Valsalva have failed and is currently the treatment of choice for this. Its action is short-lived (20–30 s for a bolus dose) through its rapid metabolism by enzymes of the vascular luminal endothelium and its uptake by red cells. Even that short period of action may restore normal rhythm after the drug is inactivated. This makes it safer than verapamil. **Adverse effects** include dizziness, nausea, chest pain and shortness of breath, but these resolve rapidly due to inactivation of the drug. **Drug interactions** include blockade of adenosine's effects by theophylline, which like other xanthines blocks the adenosine receptor. Dipyridamole, on the other hand, enhances adenosine's actions and side-effects by blocking its uptake into red blood cells.

Digoxin is a cardiac glycoside originally extracted from the foxglove (*Digitalis purpura*) and is used to slow ventricular rate in AF (see opposite). It acts in two ways. The first is by blocking the Na^+/ATPase pump, which increases intracellular Na^+. Consequently, intracellular Ca^{2+} is increased, resulting in an increased force of contraction. This action has been used to treat congestive heart failure. The second way is by central stimulation of vagal activity, thus slowing the heart. Digoxin is administered orally or intravenously in emergencies. **Adverse effects** include nausea, vomiting, confusion and arrhythmias. Digoxin has a low therapeutic index, making it a dangerous drug in overdose, and plasma monitoring is advisable with repeated use. **Drug interactions:** digoxin toxicity is precipitated by hypokalaemia and its action is potentiated by drugs associated with K^+ loss, e.g. furosemide (frusemide). This is because there is reduced extracellular K^+ to compete with digoxin for binding sites on the Na^+/ATPase pump. Amiodarone and verapamil potentiate digoxin by decreasing its excretion and binding to tissues.

Principles underlying the clinical use of anti-arrhythmic agents: (i) All anti-arrhythmic agents and other drugs, e.g. some antipsychotics, erythromycin in high doses, terfenadine and tricyclic antidepressants, can precipitate arrhythmias. (ii) Electrolyte disturbances, e.g. low plasma K^+ or Mg^{2+}, can precipitate arrhythmias. (iii) Arrhythmias may occur in patients with, for example, hyperthyroidism, and treatment with anti-arrhythmic drugs may be inappropriate, ineffective and even precipitate serious arrhythmias. (iv) Verapamil should not be prescribed unless the arrhythmia is definitely of supraventricular origin. A mistaken diagnosis and verapamil treatment could result in profound hypotension and cardiac arrest.

Other therapies to treat arrhythmias include DC electrical cardioversion, the delivery of a brief electrical shock to the heart to convert either supraventricular or ventricular tachycardia back to a normal rhythm. A synchronised electrical shock is delivered through the chest wall to the heart. This disrupts the abnormal electrical circuit(s) in the heart and restores a normal heart beat. It is the most appropriate intervention when the patient is in extremis.

Atrial fibrillation: The treatment of atrial fibrillation is concerned with controlling ventricular rate, achieving cardioversion and restoring sinus rhythm, and prevention of thromboembolism. Atrial fibrillation can cause acute cardiovascular compromise when associated with a rapid ventricular response. If the patient's blood pressure is within normal limits rate control is usually achieved with digoxin, either intravenously or orally. A loading dose of either 500 mcg or 1 mg is followed by a smaller daily dose. If the patient's blood pressure is compromised then emergency electrical cardioversion is indicated. Amiodarone and flecainide can be used to restore sinus rhythm. If, however, atrial fibrillation has been present for a long time then restoration of sinus rhythm is unlikely to be maintained and the emphasis of treatment lies with rate control. Patients with atrial fibrillation who are over the age of 75 or have structural heart disease benefit from anticoagulation with warfarin. In other patients, however, the risk of haemorrhage from warfarin treatment outweighs the risk of embolism from atrial fibrillation and aspirin should be prescribed instead.

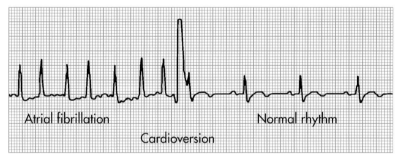

Electrical cardioversion ECG

36 Hypertension I: Guidelines for treatment

Hypertension is a common cardiovascular problem that, if left untreated, can result in renal failure, heart failure, stroke and coronary heart disease. Hypertension may be secondary to endocrine disorders, e.g. Cushing's disease and Conn's syndrome, and disorders such as phaeochromocytoma and renal causes (renal artery stenosis). Most cases of hypertension, however, are of unknown aetiology and are historically called essential hypertension. Essential hypertension is **treated** through lifestyle changes and diet, e.g. encouraging the patient to eat more fruit and vegetables, and restrict salt and alcohol intake, and, when necessary, through the use of appropriate drugs.

Guidelines for therapy: Extensive clinical history has established that hypertension is often undiagnosed and when discovered is generally poorly controlled, despite the availability of disparate therapeutic strategies. A major reason for this appears to be the persistent practice of monotherapy, i.e. use of only one drug. Guidelines for the management of hypertension have been published by the British Hypertension Society, based on the principle of dual or triple therapy and on the age and racial origin of the patient. The strategy is called AB/CD (A = angiotensin-converting enzyme [ACE] or angiotensin receptor inhibitor; B = β-blocker; C = Ca^{2+} channel blocker; D = diuretic), and is based on the difference between renin-dependent and renin-independent hypertension. Young white patients (< 55 years) typically have renin-dependent hypertension that usually responds to ACE inhibitors, angiotensin receptor blockers and β-blockers, whereas older white patients and black patients have predominantly renin-independent hypertension and respond to Ca^{2+} channel antagonists and diuretics. Because the latter drugs activate the renin–angiotensin system these patients can, if necessary, be given adjunct renin-suppressive activity. The guidelines also emphasise the need to adopt the approach of 'the lower the pressure the better'.

Treatment strategies: Recent important studies indicated that β-blockers, although potent antihypertensives, compare unfavourably with amlodipine and ACE inhibitors as protectants against stroke or heart failure and may increase the risk of diabetes development.

Aims of treatment: There is no definitive optimal target for blood pressure, although the European Society for Hypertension recommends a blood pressure target of 140/90 mmHg as an 'audit standard', but supports a policy of 'the lower the better' for diabetic patients and those at high risk for cardiovascular disease.

Lifestyle changes: There is evidence that lifestyle measures can lower blood pressure. These include limiting alcohol consumption, regular aerobic physical exercise, reduction in fat intake and plenty of fresh fruit and vegetables. There should be a reduction in salt intake to less than 6 g/day, alcohol consumption to less than 25 units per week for men and 14 units for women, as well as maintenance of a normal adult body mass index of 20–25 kg/m^2.

Blood pressure category	Systolic blood pressure (mmHg)	Diasystolic blood pressure (mmHg)
Optimal	> 120	> 80
Normal	< 130	< 85
High normal	130–39	85–89
Hypertension grade 1 (mild)	140–159	90–99
Hypertension grade 2 (moderate)	160–179	100–109
Hypertension grade 3 (severe)	≥ 180	≥ 110
Isolated systolic hypertension		
Grade 1	140–159	< 90
Grade 2	≥ 160	< 90

Hypertension classification

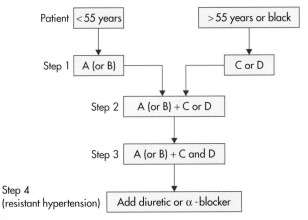

AB/CD strategy

Case scenario: On a routine 'well woman' general practice initiative clinic, a patient was noted to have hypertension with a blood pressure of 175/112. Bendrofluazide was commenced at a dose of 2.5 mg daily and a repeat appointment was made for 3 months. At her next appointment, the patient's blood pressure was at similar levels and atenolol at 50 mg daily was added. At this point, routine investigations – electrolytes, urea and creatinine levels, an ECG and a renal tract ultrasound – were ordered. Three months later, although her blood pressure was now 154/92, she complained of sleep disturbance. The atenolol was reduced to 25 mg daily and 5 mg amlodipine daily was added to her regimen.

Case scenario

37 Hypertension II: Anti-hypertensive drugs

Hypertension is treated with drugs that reduce cardiac output or lower the peripheral resistance. Cardiac output can be lowered by drugs that (i) directly block sympathetic action on the heart, i.e. the β-blockers such as **propranolol** and **atenolol**, or, less commonly, (ii) reduce sympathetic drive, e.g. **clonidine** and **methyldopa**. The peripheral resistance can be lowered by (i) directly dilating arterioles with vasodilators such as Ca^{2+} channel blockers, e.g. **amlodipine**, or α_1-receptor blockers, e.g. **prazocin**; (ii) using ACE inhibitors, e.g. **ramipril** to block the conversion of angiotensin I to angiotensin II, or angiotensin II receptor blockers such as **losartan** to dilate arterioles by blocking angiotensin II. The peripheral resistance can also be lowered (iii) by reducing the blood volume with diuretics such as the **thiazides** or **furosemide**.

Use of antihypertensive drugs: If there are no special considerations, then the use of the AB/CD algorithm should be used. For every class of drug there will be indications, precautions and contraindications depending on factors such as the patient's age, organ status (e.g. the kidney or heart), the severity of the hypertensive state and any other medical problems. Patients may have not just hypertension but other disorders, e.g. of the cardiovascular and renal systems, or they may have diabetes, which also produces cardiovascular, nervous and renal pathological states.

ACE inhibitors are indicated in hypertensive patients or post-MI, with heart failure, left ventricular dysfunction or secondary stroke prevention. Caution and monitoring are necessary in patients with renal disease and they are contraindicated in pregnancy and bilateral renal artery stenosis. **Adverse effects** include a dry cough attributed possibly to inhibition of bradykinin breakdown, hyperkalaemia due to inhibition of aldosterone production and, less commonly, hypersensitivity manifested as angioneurotic oedema.

Angiotensin II receptor blockers are used to treat heart failure after MI in patients intolerant to ACE inhibitors and in type II diabetic nephropathy. They do not block bradykinin breakdown. They should be used with caution in renal artery stenosis and are contraindicated in pregnancy, breastfeeding and renovascular disease. **Adverse effects** are few and include occasional symptomatic hypotension and angio-oedema.

β-Blockers are indicated in angina and MI and in stable, chronic heart failure, although they may worsen acute heart failure. They should be used with caution in heart failure, diabetes (except with coronary heart disease) and peripheral vascular disease. They are contraindicated in asthma (see also page 72).

Calcium channel blockers are indicated in angina, elderly patients and isolated systolic hypertension. **Amlopidine** dilates coronary and other arteries and relaxes vascular smooth muscle. Short-acting nifedipine preparations are not recommended for long-term management of hypertension; this usage is associated with reflex tachycardia resulting from the large changes in blood pressure. **Adverse effects** of calcium channel-blocking drugs include ankle swelling, headaches and flushing, which are associated with vasodilatation.

Diuretics are indicated in elderly patients, patients with heart failure and isolated systolic hypertension, and for secondary stroke prevention. **Thiazides**, e.g. bendrofluazide and **indapamide**, are often prescribed for essential hypertension. They cause K^+ loss and are contraindicated in, for example, Addison's disease.

74

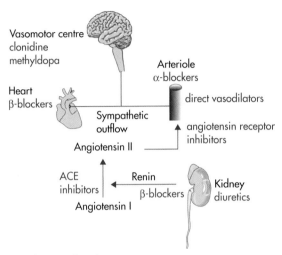

Vasomotor centre
clonidine
methyldopa

Arteriole
α-blockers

Heart
β-blockers

direct vasodilators

Sympathetic
outflow

angiotensin receptor
inhibitors

Angiotensin II

ACE
inhibitors

Renin
β-blockers

Kidney
diuretics

Angiotensin I

Sites of action of antihypertensives

Clinical scenario: Hypertension is usually symptomless in the early stages and routine medical examination often reveals it. Abnormally high diastolic readings made on three separate occasions confirm hypertension. Hypertension may be present in some other problem, e.g. renal or hormonal, when it is referred to as secondary hypertension. Essential hypertension, which is very common in Western societies, is abnormally raised pressure without any identifiable cause. It may be due, at least in part, to a disturbance of the central regulatory control systems that control blood pressure. It is often associated with arterial hardening and narrowing, which put extra workload on the heart. Risk factors include high salt intake, obesity, excessive, chronic stress and possibly a sedentary lifestyle. If left untreated, hypertension leads to kidney problems, retinal damage, and eventually heart failure and stroke.

38 Congestive heart failure

Congestive heart failure (CHF) is the result of cardiac disease which causes impairment of ventricular filling or of blood ejection. This results in breathlessness, fatigue and fluid retention which can cause pulmonary and peripheral oedema. A common cause of heart failure is left ventricular dysfunction, and other causes include most disorders of the endocardium, myocardium, pericardium or the valves. Left ventricular dysfunction is caused by coronary artery disease in about two-thirds of patients. Causes of a non-ischaemic cardiomyopathy include hypertension, valvular disease, thyroid disorders, alcohol and myocarditis.

CHF is progressive with involvement of non-cardiac factors, e.g. changes in neurohormonal and autonomic activity and alteration of peripheral vascular function. The left ventricle undergoes structural changes, initially dilatation and hypertrophy, eventually becoming spherical. This remodelling is fuelled by increases in norepinephrine, aldosterone, endothelin, antidiuretic hormone (ADH) and angiotensin II. These cause sodium retention and peripheral vasoconstriction, as well as directly acting on cardiac cells.

Treatment is based on accurately assessing changes in exercise tolerance and volume status, and identifying and treating predisposing factors and structural defects. Pharmacological intervention addresses avoidance and initiation of medication.

Drugs: Three routine classes of medication are used, namely diuretics, ACE inhibitors and β-blockers.

Diuretics promote urine flow by increasing Na$^+$ excretion. In heart failure they increase urinary Na$^+$, reduce fluid overload, jugular venous pressure, pulmonary congestion, peripheral oedema and body weight. The most commonly used diuretics in heart failure are **furosemide** and **bumetanide.** These block **Na$^+$** reabsorption in the ascending limb of the loop of Henle. Other diuretics include **metolazone, spironolactone** and the **thiazides.**

Under-use of diuretics reduces the cardiac response to ACE inhibitors and increases risks associated with β-blocker use. **Over-use** of diuretics causes hypokalaemia and hypovolaemia which accentuates the hypotension caused by ACE inhibitors.

Angiotensin-converting enzyme reduces the heart's workload through peripheral vasodilatation and also directly improves left ventricular function. ACE inhibitors reduce mortality and hospitalisation in patients with heart failure as well as improving symptoms and clinical status.

β-Blockers used include carvedilol and timolol.

Drugs to avoid in heart failure include: (i) **antiarrhythmic agents** which can cause proarrhythmic and cardiodepressant effects. Only **amiodarone** has been shown not to reduce survival, although it may cause peripheral oedema which may complicate clinical assessment. The remainder exacerbate heart failure and are associated with increased risk of cardiovascular morbidity. (ii) **NSAIDs** and COX-2 inhibitors cause sodium (and therefore water) retention and a peripheral vasoconstriction. The resulting electrolyte disturbances increase the toxicity of ACE inhibitors and other diuretics. **Rofecoxib** and **celecoxib** are highly selective COX-2 inhibitors and have been shown in trials to be associated with both fatal and non-fatal MI; not all NSAIDs, however, have this adverse effect. (iii) **Calcium channel blockers**, verapamil and diltiazem, should not be used in patients with CHF.

Case scenario: The patient, a 67-year-old man, was referred to the local chest clinic for investigation of breathlessness. Over the 3 months preceding consultation he had noticed that, after walking for two blocks down the street, he would have to stop because of breathlessness. He was also breathless throughout the night and would wake periodically with a cough. There had been some swelling of his ankles and feet. On examination he was hypertensive with a blood pressure of 170/90. There was pitting oedema of both ankles and his jugular venous pressure was raised. His pulse was 110 and regular. Heart sounds revealed a gallop rhythm. ECG showed a sinus tachycardia with left axis deviation and an interventricular conduction defect. Chest X-ray showed pulmonary congestion and a small right pleural effusion.

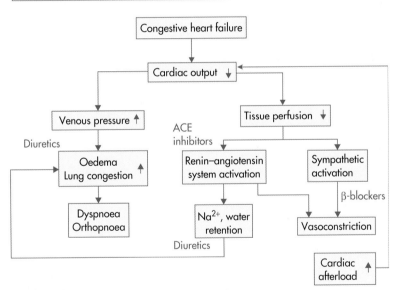

Consequences of congestive heart failure and treatments

39 Infective endocarditis

Infective endocarditis is infection of the mural surface of the endocardium or the cardiac valves. Adherent organisms and thrombotic debris form what is termed a 'vegetation'. Infecting organisms are often bacterial, rarely fungi, rickettsial or chlamydial, but never viral (as far as is known). Oral flora are an important source of bacteraemia. Some bacteria, e.g. *Streptococcus viridans*, attach themselves to fibrin and endothelial surfaces. Valves on the left side of the heart are more commonly affected due to the higher pressure gradient. An exception to this rule occurs in endocarditis associated with intravenous drug abuse and intravenous long lines.

The infected vegetation releases bacteria into the circulation, usually resulting in fever. A heart murmur may be heard. Immune complexes may be deposited in the kidneys and reticuloendothelial system, causing haematuria and splenomegaly. Occasionally a fragment of the vegetation may enter the circulation, causing systemic emboli, which may present as a cerebrovascular accident or limb ischaemia.

Signs of infective endocarditis include weight loss, anorexia, raised erythrocyte sedimentation rate (ESR) and C-reactive protein (CRP), murmurs at auscultation, retinopathy (Roth spots), hepatosplenomegaly, splinter haemorrhages in the hands or feet, and painful Osler's nodes. Later symptoms include renal infarcts, stroke and arterial occlusion, and in extremis valve rupture and acute heart failure.

Prophylactic treatment is initiated in higher-risk patients, e.g. with prosthetic heart valves, cyanotic congenital heart disease or coarction, whereas patients at intermediate risk include those with mitral valve prolapse with regurgitation or tricuspid and pulmonary heart disease. Patients at risk who are undergoing dental, obstetric, GIT, genitourinary or upper respiratory tract procedures are prescribed oral amoxicillin. Penicillin-allergic patients, or those prescribed more than a single dose of penicillin in the previous month, are prescribed either gentamicin or vancomycin.

Treatment of infective endocarditis: Patients with streptococci, e.g. *S. viridans*, are prescribed benzylpenicillin plus low-dose gentamicin. Treatment for 4 weeks is recommended. Penicillin-resistant patients can be prescribed vancomycin for 4 weeks plus low-dose gentamicin for the first 2 weeks (although all these decisions should involve consultations with a microbiologist). Endocarditis caused by enterococci, e.g. *Enterococcus faecalis*, is treated as above, except that amoxicillin is used instead of benzylpenicillin. Patients should be treated for 4 weeks and, if resistant to gentamicin, streptomycin can be used instead and treatment should be for at least 6 weeks. Endocarditis caused by staphylococci, e.g. *Staphylococcus aureus* or *S. epidermidis*, is treated with flucloxacillin plus gentamicin or fusidic acid. Vancomycin can be used instead of flucloxacillin if patients are allergic to penicillin or if their staphylococcal infection is resistant to methyl-penicillin.

Alternatives to antibiotics: Some patients not responding to antibiotic treatment require valve replacement. It is preferable to attempt to bring the infection under control first because operating on an infected valve is associated with a high mortality.

Case scenario: A 40-year-old woman was seen in the rheumatology clinic with a 3-week history of a painful swelling in her foot, generalised lethargy and night sweats. In addition she was stiff in the morning for at least 1 hour and had polyarthralgia through the day. On examination there was a painful tendinitis on the dorsum of her left foot. However, on examination of her heart, she had a pansystolic murmur that was heard loudest at the apex. The doctor arranged a transthoracic echocardiogram, which suggested a vegetation on her mitral valve, and she was admitted to the cardiology ward. Serial blood cultures were taken and later grew *Streptococcus pneumoniae*. Initial treatment was with intravenous benzylpenicillin and gentamicin. Later treatment was guided by the microbiology department. Subsequently it transpired that some months previously she had undergone extensive dental restorative treatment.

Predisposing factors

- Cardiac surgery
- Congenital heart disease
- Degenerative heart disease
- Intravenous drug abuse
- Mural thrombosis
- Prosthetic valves
- Rheumatic heart disease
- Septal defects (mainly ventricular)

Infective organisms	Case (%)
Streptococcus spp.	about 65
Staphyloccocus spp.	about 20
Other organisms	about 15

Treatment aims

- Permanent sterilisation of the vegetation
- Initiation of appropriate treatment a.s.a.p. without compromising diagnosis
- Prolonged treatment with high doses of antibiotic

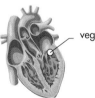

vegetation

40 Disorders of lipid metabolism I: Lipid metabolism

Myocardial infarction risk rises sharply with relatively small increases in total cholesterol. Plasma-insoluble triglycerides and cholesterol circulate bound to lipoproteins consisting of proteins, phospholipids and lipids. Lipoproteins bind to receptors on cells and are also enzyme co-factors. Two pathways for transport of lipids are known: (i) **exogenous pathway**, for transport of ingested lipids and cholesterol from the gut as chylomicrons to the capillaries in muscle and adipose tissue; and (ii) **endogenous pathway**, for transport of newly synthesised triglycerides and cholesterol from the liver as VLDL to muscle and adipose tissue.

Types of lipoproteins: Four main types exist: high-density lipoproteins (HDLs), low-density lipoproteins (LDLs), very-low-density lipoproteins (VLDLs) and chylomicrons. **Chylomicrons** carry dietary lipids from the GIT to the liver in the portal circulation, in which lipoprotein lipase releases free fatty acids from the chylomicrons. **VLDLs** carry some of the triglycerides and cholesterol from the liver to the other tissues. Lipoprotein lipase also hydrolyses the triglyceride core of the VLDLs to release free fatty acids, leaving remnants of VLDL, called intermediate-density lipoprotein.

LDL is formed from intermediate-density lipoprotein by hepatic lipase; its synthesis is regulated by the cellular requirements for cholesterol through a negative feedback effect on the LDL receptor. When intracellular cholesterol supplies are adequate, the cell switches off synthesis of its LDL receptor, thus reducing cellular uptake of LDL-cholesterol. Conversely, when intracellular cholesterol levels fall, LDL-receptor expression is switched back on. Lipoprotein (a) (Lp(a)) is a form of LDL that inhibits fibrinolysis and enhances atherosclerotic plaque formation. Lp(a) is an independent risk determinant for ischaemic heart disease. **HDL** is synthesised in the liver and GIT. HDL takes up cholesterol from the intracellular compartment and transports it from the tissues to the liver.

> **Note:** HDL is protective against coronary heart disease, whereas raised LDL is associated with increased risk. A total cholesterol:HDL ratio > 4.5 flags increased risk.

Hyperlipidaemia is an abnormally high concentration of plasma fats. Several different types exist, broadly classified as primary and secondary. **Primary hyperlipidaemias** are grouped according to the lipid profile as: (i) **primary hypercholesterolaemia** (without hypertriglyceridaemia); (ii) **primary hypertriglyceridaemia** (without hypercholesterolaemia); and (iii) primary mixed (or combined) hyperlipidaemia. **Secondary hyperlipidaemias** are caused by, for example, alcoholism, cholestasis, chronic renal failure, diabetes mellitus, high doses of estrogens, hypothyroidism, liver disease, obesity and smoking.

Primary hypercholesterolaemia may be (i) familial, a monogenic problem caused by malfunction of the LDL receptor – several different mutations exist, most of which are heterozygous. (ii) **Polygenic hypercholesterolaemia**: the exact nature of the mutations is at the time of writing unknown. Patients are at risk of premature atherosclerosis. **Primary hypertriglyceridaemia** usually presents in childhood with hepatosplenomegaly, pancreatitis, retinal vein thrombosis, eruptive xanthomata and lipaemia retinalis. Hypertriglyceridaemia may be polygenic with elevated VLDL, occasionally familial, or rare apoprotein CII or lipoprotein lipase deficiency. Failure to metabolise chylomicrons results in hypertriglyceridaemia.

Exogenous pathway

Endogenous pathway

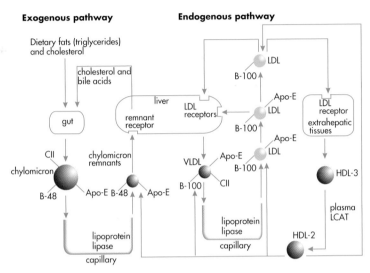

1. Apoprotein CII on chylomicron surface activates lipoprotein lipase in muscle and adipose tissue capillaries → HOH of TG
   uptake into tissues ← FFA ←

2. Apo-E and B-48 on chylomicron remnant interact with remnant receptor on hepatocyte to deliver cholesterol to the liver

3. The liver releases cholesterol and bile acids
   Gut ←

FFA: free fatty acids
HOH: hydrolysis
TG: triglyceride

1. In the liver (apoproteins B-100, CII and E + TG + cholesterol esters) → VLDL → circulation

2. CII on VLDL activates circulating lipoprotein lipase
   liberates TG + cholesterol-enriched LDL ←

3. Apo B-100 on LDL interacts with LDL receptors on tissues
   uptake of LDL cholesterol into tissues ←
   cholesterol into tissues for membrane and hormone synthesis (e.g. steroid hormones)

4. Liver LDL receptor takes up LDL-cholesterol and eliminates it in the bile.

REGULATION OF LIVER LDL RECEPTOR REGULATES PLASMA LDL LEVELS.

5. HDL synthesised by the gut and liver is converted to VLDLand LDL, which are taken up by the liver and so HDL removes excess LDL from the circulation

41 Disorders of lipid metabolism II: Lipid-lowering drugs

Lipid-lowering drugs are part of a wider strategy involving consideration of other risk factors, e.g. diet, weight, alcohol, smoking, hypertension and diabetes.

Statins, e.g. **atorvastatin, fluvastatin, pravastatin, rosuvastatin** and **simvastatin**, inhibit hydroxymethylglutaryl-coenzyme A (HMG-CoA) reductase, the rate-limiting step in cholesterol synthesis. They are usually the drugs of choice for patients most at risk of coronary heart disease, provided that there are no contraindications. **Adverse reactions** include rashes, headaches, GIT upsets, muscle pain and upper respiratory tract infections. More severe reactions include myopathy, presenting as severe myalgia, myoglobinuria, rhabdomyolysis, renal failure and, rarely, death. Increased risk of myopathy occurs with increased dose, hepatic disease and drug reactions, especially with other classes of lipid-lowering agents, e.g. fibrates. Statins should never be prescribed with the fibrate gemfibrozil. **Contraindications** include pregnancy, breastfeeding and active liver disease.

Fibrates include **bezafibrate, ciprofibrate, fenofibrate** and **gemfibrozil**. They reduce triglyceride levels by increasing plasma clearance. They lower LDL and raise HDL levels and are indicated for hyperlipidaemias of types IIa, IIb, III and IV. They may be used with a statin to control combined hypertriglyceridaemia and hypercholesterolaemia (but bear in mind the risk of myopathies). **Adverse reactions** include increased biliary saturation with cholesterol, which can cause cholelithiasis (especially if used together with ezetimibe), myositis and hepatitis. Other **drug interactions** include potentiation of oral hypoglycaemic drugs and warfarin. Fibrates are **contraindicated** in pregnancy, breastfeeding, hepatic disease, primary biliary cirrhosis, hypoalbuminaemia, nephrotic syndrome and gall bladder disease.

Anion exchange resins colestyramine and **colestipol hydrochloride** bind to gut bile acids and block their reabsorption. In response, the liver increases cholesterol breakdown to bile acids, which in turn stimulate hepatic LDL receptors, thus increasing breakdown of LDL. The negative effect is an aggravation of hypertriglyceridaemia. They are used to treat hyperlipidaemias, especially type IIa, and in patients who do not respond to dietary management. **Adverse effects** reflect local action in the gut and include constipation, diarrhoea, heartburn and increased triglyceride levels in patients with hypertriglyceridaemia. **Drug interactions** are frequent due to interference with drug absorption and absorption of fat-soluble vitamins.

Cholesterol absorption inhibitors, e.g. **ezetimibe**, block cholesterol uptake from the small intestine. It is prescribed orally as an adjunct to dietary management, and with or as an alternative to statins when these are contraindicated for primary hypercholesterolaemia. **Adverse reactions** are similar to those with statins, e.g. upper respiratory tract infections, although there are no reports of increased risk of myopathies when used with statins. Important **drug interactions** include risk of cholelithiasis with fibrates and decreased absorption when used with colestyramine.

Nicotinic acid and its derivatives reduce lipolysis in adipose tissue, thereby reducing plasma triglycerides. Its **main use** is with a statin for treatment of hypercholesteraemia with or without triglyceridaemia. Its use is limited by several **adverse effects**, especially vasodilatation and GIT upsets, prevented by reducing the dose or giving aspirin just beforehand. **Contraindications** include pregnancy, breastfeeding and peptic ulcer.

Omega-3 triglycerides (fish oil) can lower plasma triglycerides although they may aggravate hypercholesterolaemia.

Management of hyperlipidaemia

- Primary aim of treatment is reduction of serum cholesterol to > 6.5 mmol/l
- Serum triglyceride levels < 2mmol/l = normal
- Serum triglyceride levels within 2–6 mmol/l in patients require no intervention unless patient has hypercholesterolaemia; then reduce levels to < 2 mmol/l
- Initial treatment includes dietary control and usually requires additional therapy:
  - Familial hypercholesterolaemia usually needs drug intervention
  - Co-existing cardiovascular risk factors must be addressed:
    - Obesity
    - Smoking
    - Hypertension
  - Dietary control involves
    - Limiting intake of fatty foods, e.g.
      - poultry
      - red meat
      - fried food
      - dairy products
      - offal
    - Increased grilling rather than frying
    - Increased consumption of high-fibre foods, e.g. legumes and pulses, which reduce plasma cholesterol
    - Substitution with low-fat cheese, skimmed milk
    - Increased use of polyunsaturated fats in (e.g.) soya oil and corn oil
  - Reducing or limiting smoking and alcohol intake
  - Lipid-lowering drugs:
    - Fibrates
    - Statins
    - Bile acid-binding resins
    - Nicotinic acid
    - Fish oils

42 Non-steroidal anti-inflammatory drugs (NSAIDs): Mechanisms

Non-steroidal anti-inflammatory drugs (NSAIDs) reduce pain and inflammation by blocking the cyclo-oxygenase (COX) enzyme system, which converts arachidonic acid to prostaglandins (see opposite). The prostaglandins and other related substances are termed the eicosanoids. The system has two structurally distinct enzymes, COX-1 and COX-2. COX-1 generates prostaglandins that mediate gastric cytoprotection, platelet aggregation and renal perfusion, and is constitutively expressed, i.e. it is always expressed, whereas COX-2, which is inducible by, for example, cytokines, endotoxins and growth factors, produces prostaglandins that mediate the inflammatory process. This enzyme duality has stimulated a search for specific blockers of COX-2.

Aspirin (acetylsalicylic acid) blocks both COX-1 and COX-2 irreversibly by binding to a serine residue near the active site of the COX enzymes, thereby reducing synthesis of prostaglandins and thromboxane. Thus it reduces fever, inflammation and pain, and also platelet-mediated blood clotting. It is taken orally and is absorbed in both the stomach and the small intestine. Being a weak acid it is largely unionised in the stomach and thus crosses rapidly into the portal blood system, but it is also well absorbed from the large surface area of the small gut despite the more basic pH. Much of an oral dose is destroyed in the liver and that which escapes as salicylate into the general circulation is largely bound to plasma proteins, which may cause drug interactions through drug displacement from plasma proteins. Aspirin and salicylate may be excreted in the urine or conjugated in the liver and excreted in the bile.

Actions of aspirin: Aspirin is antipyretic, anti-inflammatory, analgesic and antithrombotic in action. It lowers fever temperature by targeting prostaglandin synthesis in the temperature control area of the hypothalamus in the brain. Aspirin does not appreciably affect normal body temperature. The anti-inflammatory and analgesic actions, on the other hand, are effected at peripheral sites of tissue damage, e.g. in arthritic joints where inflammatory prostaglandins are synthesised. Aspirin also lowers platelet aggregation by inhibiting thromboxane synthesis. Aspirin blocks COX-2 in cancer cells, which express high levels of the enzyme, and there is evidence that aspirin may lower the risk of colorectal cancer.

Aspirin's **adverse affects** reflect its mode of action. It inhibits production of gastric mucus, damages the gastric mucosa and causes bleeding, which can be serious in patients with liver disease or on anticoagulants, with haemophilia or alcohol problems. Additionally, the antiplatelet action of aspirin compounds the bleeding risk. Aspirin should not be given to children under 12 years of age as it can (rarely) precipitate Reye's syndrome, a potentially fatal problem involving coma and liver damage. The UK's Committee on Safety of Medicines (CSM) has recommended that aspirin should not be given to feverish children aged 12–15. Aspirin can cause **allergies** through its action as a hapten. It may acetylate a plasma protein to which it is bound, thereby creating a protein recognised as foreign by the immune system.

Drug interactions with aspirin are due mainly to its ability to displace drugs such as warfarin, thereby increasing the free, pharmacologically active plasma level of warfarin. Aspirin may reduce the action of high-ceiling diuretics by inhibiting prostaglandin synthesis. The toxicology of aspirin is covered more fully on page 86.

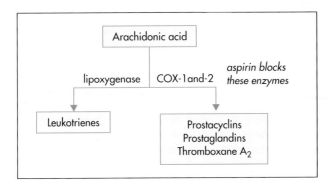

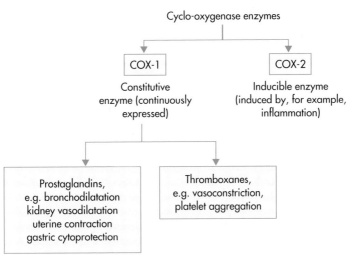

Eicosanoid synthesis

43 Therapeutic use of aspirin

Aspirin is the prototype analgesic, antipyretic and anti-inflammatory drug. It is indicated for dysmenorrhoea, headache, pyrexia and transient musculoskeletal pain. Non-proprietary oral preparations of aspirin are usually prepared as 300-mg tablets. This dose may also be taken in suppository form. The *British Pharmacopoeia* directs that 300 mg aspirin tablets should be dispensed if no strength is stipulated. If so-called soluble aspirin is prescribed, then dispersible aspirin should be dispensed. Aspirin for analgesic purposes is also combined with caffeine, and with codeine phosphate as co-codaprin, containing codeine phosphate 8 mg and aspirin 400 mg.

Cardiovascular actions: Aspirin is now prescribed for its cardiovascular protective effects. Aspirin therapy is generally accepted to be of proven value in the treatment of acute MI. It is also now in long-term use in patients who exhibit prior manifestations of cardiovascular disease. It is believed that the use of aspirin contributes to reductions in cardiovascular disease and mortality. Other patients at risk include those with unstable or stable angina, or patients who have had coronary angioplasty or artery bypass grafting. Other candidates for aspirin include those at risk of systemic embolism with other high-risk conditions such as carotid artery disease and diabetes. Aspirin is used as: (i) an antiplatelet drug (see also page 56); (ii) in the management of MI; and (iii) in angina. As an antiplatelet drug, it is used for the secondary prevention of thrombotic diseases. Unless otherwise indicated, aspirin is prescribed immediately after the occurrence of an ischaemic event. A low dose of aspirin is usually given after coronary bypass surgery. In the management of MI aspirin may be prescribed before the patient is admitted to hospital and the admitting staff should be informed of this. Aspirin may be prescribed in lower doses (75–150 mg) in stable angina in addition to other drugs such as glyceryl trinitrate and β-blockers. It is now accepted that asymptomatic patients who are at increased risk of a coronary heart disease event may reduce the risk by taking low-dose aspirin. Nevertheless, the prescriber needs to weigh the potential benefit against hazards of, for example, bleeding.

Aspirin toxicity may range from mild to very severe. Patients who have taken a mild overdose may complain of dizziness, GIT upsets, headache, tinnitus and blurred vision. There may be hyperventilation, which reduces the P_{CO_2} and causes a respiratory alkalosis. More severe poisoning results in a metabolic acidosis with accumulation of salicylate and an increased body temperature, attributed to the uncoupling of oxidative phosphorylation. In the advanced stages of extreme aspirin toxicity, the patient experiences febrile seizures with temperatures in excess of 103°C and severe metabolic and respiratory acidosis. There is GIT bleeding, diarrhoea and vomiting, followed by coma and death.

The treatment of aspirin toxicity consists of: (i) promoting salicylate excretion by administration of bicarbonate to alkalinise the urine – this allows ionisation of salicylate in the urine, and less is reabsorbed; (ii) temperature reduction by applying cooling; (iii) intravenous maintenance of plasma K^+ and bicarbonate and of urinary osmotic pressure with diuretics and fluid; and (iv) constant monitoring of the patient's vital signs.

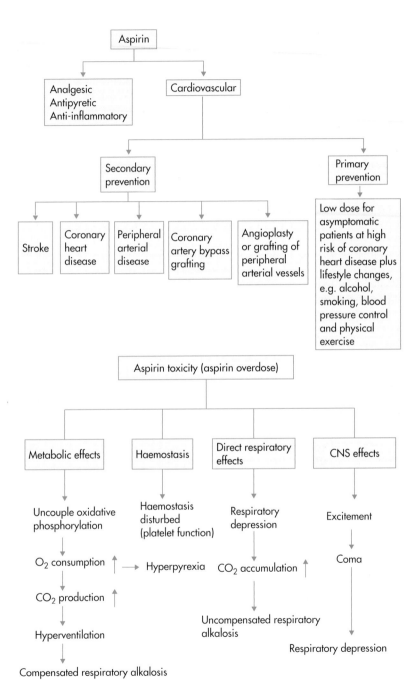

Therapeutic use of aspirin

44 Other non-steroidal anti-inflammatory drugs (NSAIDs)

Aspirin was the first NSAID and there are now many others in use. NSAIDs inhibit the COX enzymes, thus producing analgesic and anti-inflammatory effects. Being non-specific, they inhibit both COX-1 and COX-2 and produce several side-effects, especially GIT upsets, because prostaglandins protect the gastric mucosa, and NSAIDs also interfere with normal renal blood flow. For short-term pain relief, especially in elderly patients, it may be preferable to prescribe paracetamol, but, for more prolonged use, the NSAIDs are more suitable for analgesic and anti-inflammatory action, particularly in inflammatory arthritides such as rheumatoid arthritis.

NSAIDs include **propionic acid derivatives**, e.g. ibuprofen, fenbufen, fenoprofen, naproxen, ketoprofen and teoprofenic acid. They vary both quantitatively and qualitatively in side-effects. For example, fenbufen is reported to cause less GIT upset than other NSAIDs, but may cause skin rashes. A number of other drugs with therapeutic properties similar to those of propionic acid derivatives are used, including azapropazone, diflunisal, a derivative of aspirin, indometacin, lornoxicam and piroxicam. The reader is referred to the BNF for a more comprehensive list. The choice of NSAID is dictated by the response of the patient in terms of pain relief and occurrence of side-effects, and is currently largely a matter of trial and error.

The **side-effects** of NSAIDs are mainly GIT discomfort, e.g. nausea, and occasional ulceration and bleeding. Therefore patients who need an NSAID and who are at risk of ulceration, either gastric or duodenal, may need a selective NSAID (see next spread) as well as GIT protection. The CSM has published guidelines on the use of NSAIDs with respect to the relative risk of GIT side-effects. Azapropazone is considered high risk, while intermediate-risk NSAIDs include diclofenac, indometacin, ketoprofen, naproxen and piroxicam. Ibuprofen and selective COX-2 inhibitors (see next spread) have been classed as low risk, but at the time of writing COX-2 inhibitors are increasingly associated with cardiovascular accidents. Other common side-effects that may occur include hypertension, fluid retention and skin rashes. Central effects include vertigo, depression, anxiety, hearing disturbances and drowsiness. Relatively rare side-effects include hepatic damage and renal failure due to pre-existing kidney disease or through interstitial fibrosis and papillary necrosis. Patients may experience ocular changes, pancreatitis, toxic epidermal necrolysis, alveolysis or pulmonary eosinophilia. NSAIDs should always be used with caution in the elderly. The prolonged use of NSAIDs can cause infertility in women but this effect is reversed on stopping the treatment. Phenylbutazone, one of the earlier NSAIDs, causes dangerous blood dyscrasias and is now used only for ankylosing spondylitis and when all other drugs have failed to treat the pain and inflammation.

Contraindications include pregnancy, breastfeeding and patients with a history of hypersensitivity to aspirin or who have defects of coagulation.

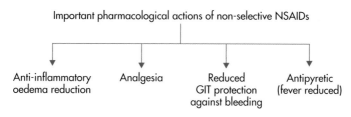

Aspirin   Ibuprofen

Important pharmacological actions of non-selective NSAIDs

| Anti-inflammatory oedema reduction | Analgesia | Reduced GIT protection against bleeding | Antipyretic (fever reduced) |

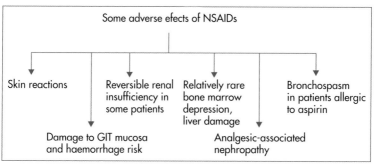

Some adverse efects of NSAIDs

Skin reactions | Reversible renal insufficiency in some patients | Relatively rare bone marrow depression, liver damage | Bronchospasm in patients allergic to aspirin

Damage to GIT mucosa and haemorrhage risk | Analgesic-associated nephropathy

45 Paracetamol

Paracetamol (called acetaminophen in the USA) is an orally active analgesic and antipyretic drug with very weak anti-inflammatory activity. Chemically it is an aminophenol derivative (see opposite). It is now used instead of aspirin in young teenagers and children. Its mechanism of action is unknown. It is a very weak inhibitor of the COX enzymes and its poor anti-inflammatory action militates against an action via the COX-1 and -2 enzyme systems. It is usually prescribed for pyrexia and for mild-to-moderate pain.

Clinical use: For adults, paracetamol is usually prescribed as 500 mg tablets, one or two to be taken every 4–6 hours up to a maximum of 4 g daily. For children, paracetamol is usually prescribed as an oral solution of 120 mg/5 ml and should be used only with the doctor's advice in children under 2 months of age. Paracetamol is also available in suppository form.

Paracetamol toxicity: Side-effects with paracetamol are rare, although skin rashes and blood disorders may occur. More importantly, paracetamol is potentially hepatotoxic in doses not far above therapeutic doses. Two to three times the maximum therapeutic dose causes a serious and potentially fatal hepatotoxicity, and renal damage may also occur. This happens because paracetamol is normally conjugated in therapeutic doses to form a more soluble sulphate and glucuronide. At higher doses, paracetamol is metabolised by mixed function cytochrome P450 oxidases to a toxic metabolite, N-acetyl-p-benzoquinone, which at lower doses is rendered harmless by a reaction with glutathione, and the metabolite is finally excreted as mercapturic acid (see opposite). If the available glutathione stores are exhausted, e.g. at high doses of paracetamol, or through alcohol or salicylate, then this toxic metabolite accumulates in the hepatocyte and reacts with nucleophilic constituents in the cell, resulting in liver and kidney cell necrosis.

Symptoms and treatment of paracetamol poisoning: The initial symptoms are nausea and vomiting. The symptoms of hepatotoxicity are manifested 24–48 hours later. As soon as possible after the overdose oral activated charcoal should be administered. Treatment with oral methionine or intravenous N-acetylcysteine, both of which increase glutathione levels as metabolic precursors, should be initiated as soon as paracetamol poisoning is identified. If given soon after the overdose is taken, liver damage can be prevented. These antidotes may be of little or no use if they are administered more than 12 hours after the overdose, and may cause adverse effects, e.g. nausea and vomiting. Glutathione is part of the REDOX cycle, which maintains the balance between oxidation and reduction in the cell. The glutathione REDOX cycle is protective against cell damage because it minimises oxidative stress. Overactive oxidation reactions in the cell promote the accumulation of toxic metabolites, such as that generated by the metabolism of paracetamol.

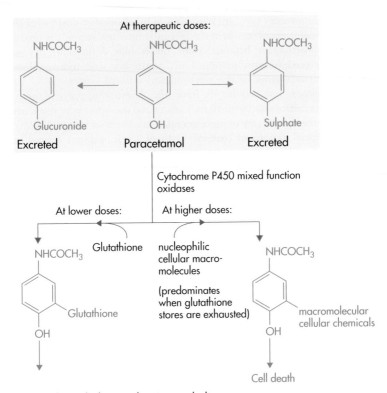

At therapeutic doses:

NHCOCH₃ — Glucuronide — Excreted

NHCOCH₃ / OH — Paracetamol

NHCOCH₃ — Sulphate — Excreted

Cytochrome P450 mixed function oxidases

At lower doses:

At higher doses:

Glutathione

nucleophilic cellular macro-molecules

(predominates when glutathione stores are exhausted)

NHCOCH₃ — Glutathione — OH

NHCOCH₃ — macromolecular cellular chemicals — OH

Cell death

Paracetamol metabolism and toxic metabolites

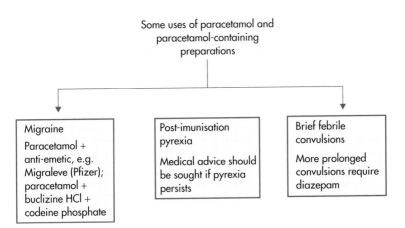

Some uses of paracetamol and paracetamol-containing preparations

Migraine	Post-imunisation pyrexia	Brief febrile convulsions
Paracetamol + anti-emetic, e.g. Migraleve (Pfizer); paracetamol + buclizine HCl + codeine phosphate	Medical advice should be sought if pyrexia persists	More prolonged convulsions require diazepam

46 Steroidal anti-inflammatory drugs I: Cortisol

When first introduced in the 1950s, anti-inflammatory steroids were hailed as a major breakthrough – until the serious adverse effects of their long-term use became apparent. They are now used in much smaller doses over shorter periods of time if possible. The main anti-inflammatory steroids in clinical use include **beclomethasone, betamethasone, budesonide, deflazacort, dexamethasone, methylprednisolone, prednisolone, prednisone** and **triamcinolone**. All are synthetic analogues of the physiological adrenal corticosteroid **cortisol** (hydrocortisone) and, while all have the immunosuppressive and anti-inflammatory actions of cortisol, they also have the other actions of cortisol, resulting in the side-effects of these agents.

Physiological actions of cortisol: Cortisol is released in a diurnal pattern from the adrenal cortex. It is part of the body's response to stress. In the body's resting state it also has a so-called 'permissive' role in allowing other hormones to exert their actions. It acts on virtually all tissues of the body. In the liver, cortisol mobilises glucose. In fat it causes lipolysis. In the longer term it mobilises energy from muscle through proteolysis and so is atrophic to muscle. It inhibits growth through an action on connective tissue and causes atrophy of lymphoid tissue. It is anti-inflammatory and immunosuppressive, two actions exploited therapeutically. Cortisol regulates its own release by inhibiting the release from the anterior pituitary gland of **adrenocorticotrophic hormone (ACTH)**, and of the hypothalamic peptide corticotrophin-releasing hormone (CRH; page 93). ACTH causes the release of the adrenal steroids and its release in turn is promoted by the hypothalamic peptide CRH, and also by the action of vasopressin in the hypothalamus (see opposite). These suppressive actions of the synthetic analogues of cortisol on CRH and ACTH need to be taken into account when stopping treatment (page 96). A deficiency of adrenal corticosteroid production causes Addison's disease (page 180). The adrenal cortex also secretes the mineralocorticoid aldosterone (page 174) and the adrenal androgens (page 180). If allowed, cortisol would have an aldosterone-like action in the kidney tubule (it is potentially equipotent in this respect with aldosterone), but it is inactivated in the tubule by an enzyme, 11β-hydroxysteroid dehydrogenase, through conversion to the inactive steroid cortisone.

Mechanism of action of cortisol: Cortisol, in common with many other steroid hormones, passes freely into the cytoplasm, where it combines with a protein receptor and the complex is translocated to the nucleus, where it binds to specific response elements, resulting in RNA and protein synthesis. The steroid–receptor complex binds to specific response elements on the DNA and *de novo* protein synthesis is initiated. The fact that protein synthesis needs to be initiated explains the lag phase between initial corticosteroid administration and the onset of a detectable therapeutic effect. There is evidence that some of the rapid actions of cortisol, e.g. on the release of CRH in the brain and of ACTH in the anterior pituitary gland, are through cell membrane receptors for cortisol. Through its cellular actions, cortisol inhibits the production of a wide range of macrophages and other white cells, as well as the cytokines involved in inflammation.

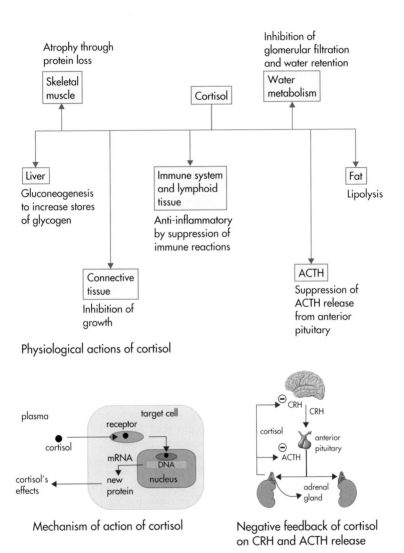

Atrophy through
protein loss

Skeletal
muscle

Cortisol

Water
metabolism

Inhibition of
glomerular filtration
and water retention

Liver

Gluconeogenesis
to increase stores
of glycogen

Immune system
and lymphoid
tissue

Anti-inflammatory
by suppression of
immune reactions

Fat

Lipolysis

Connective
tissue

Inhibition of
growth

ACTH

Suppression of
ACTH release
from anterior
pituitary

Physiological actions of cortisol

Mechanism of action of cortisol

Negative feedback of cortisol
on CRH and ACTH release

47 Steroidal anti-inflammatory drugs II: Therapeutic use

Anti-inflammatory glucocorticoids act not only by inhibiting inflammation, but also by immunosuppression. They block not only the initial inflammatory response but also the later stages, i.e. cellular proliferation of chronic inflammation and wound healing. Glucocorticoids act by inhibiting genes resulting in the production of COX-2. They inhibit transcription of genes that code for cell adhesion molecules and several of the cytokines, e.g. for interleukin (IL) IL-2 and its receptor, and for IL-3, -4, -5, -6 and -8 and for TNF-α. They inhibit extravasation of neutrophils to the tissues. They delay healing by inhibiting the synthesis of the glycosaminoglycans and of collagen. They also have several serious adverse effects resulting from prolonged use.

Therapeutic uses: Glucocorticoids are used: (i) for replacement therapy in diseases of adrenocortical insufficiency such as hypopituitarism and Addison's disease; (ii) for tests of ardenocortical function; (iii) for acute allergic reactions and status asthmaticus; and (iv) for anti-inflammatory use in, for example, Crohn's disease, rheumatic fever, rheumatoid arthritis, systemic lupus erythematosus (SLE), ulcerative colitis and chronic active hepatitis. They may be administered orally, parenterally or topically.

Tests of adrenocortical function: Cortisol regulates its own production and release from the adrenal cortex by inhibiting release of the hypothalamic factor CRH and of the anterior pituitary hormone ACTH from the anterior pituitary. Thus injection of a corticosteroid such as **dexamethasone** or **prednisolone** should decrease circulating levels of ACTH if the negative feedback mechanism is operating properly. There may be an ACTH-producing tumour in the body, in which case dexamethasone would have no effect on ACTH release.

Adrenocortical insufficiency: The aim is to restore levels of both glucocorticoid and mineralocorticoid activity and this is generally achieved with parenteral cortisol (hydrocortisone), which in therapeutic doses has adequate Na$^+$-retaining activity.

Anti-inflammatory uses: Anti-inflammatory glucocorticoids are now reserved for conditions unresponsive to other approaches and, if used over longer periods, e.g. rheumatoid arthritis (RA), are given in much smaller doses (e.g. 7.5 mg prednisolone daily). Even with these smaller doses, it is not recommended to continue therapy for more than 2–4 years due to longer-term adverse effects (see next spread). The modern approach to RA is to tackle the disease at an early stage with disease-modifying anti-rheumatic drugs (DMARDs). Other conditions treated with glucocorticoids include giant cell (temporal) arteritis, polyarteritis nodosa, polymyositis and SLE.

Acute inflammatory conditions and emergencies, e.g. painful joints and acute asthma attacks, are treated with high doses of a glucocorticoid, which is then discontinued as soon as possible. Local injections of glucocorticoids are given intra-arterially to treat inflamed joints, reduce joint damage and increase mobility. Steroids used for this purpose include **hydrocortisone acetate** and **triamcinolone hexacetonide.**

Note: Glucocorticoids should not be used long term to treat ankylosing spondylitis, but only as an emergency treatment for very active and unresponsive disease.

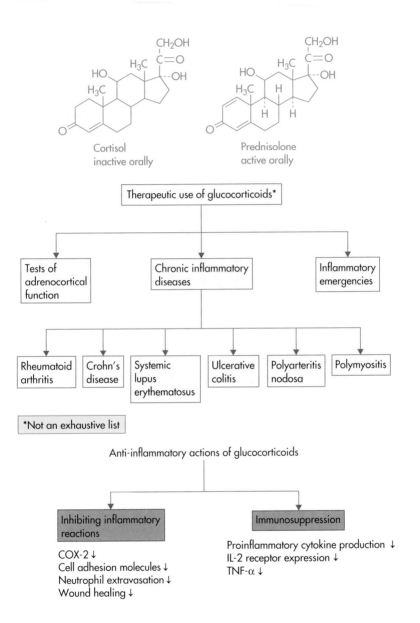

Cortisol
inactive orally

Prednisolone
active orally

Therapeutic use of glucocorticoids*

Tests of adrenocortical function

Chronic inflammatory diseases

Inflammatory emergencies

Rheumatoid arthritis

Crohn's disease

Systemic lupus erythematosus

Ulcerative colitis

Polyarteritis nodosa

Polymyositis

*Not an exhaustive list

Anti-inflammatory actions of glucocorticoids

Inhibiting inflammatory reactions

Immunosuppression

COX-2 ↓
Cell adhesion molecules ↓
Neutrophil extravasation ↓
Wound healing ↓

Proinflammatory cytokine production ↓
IL-2 receptor expression ↓
TNF-α ↓

Steroidal anti-inflammatory drugs II   **95**

48 Steroidal anti-inflammatory drugs III: Unwanted effects

Unwanted effects of glucocorticoids become apparent after prolonged use of large doses and result from three main pharmacological actions, namely: (i) metabolic effects; (ii) suppression of the hypothalamus–anterior pituitary–adrenal axis, resulting in cessation of production of corticosteroids; and (iii) suppression of the immune system and healing processes. Glucocorticoids also affect CNS function and can cause mood changes.

Metabolic effects include **osteoporosis** through interference with collagen synthesis, inhibition of osteoblast function, enhancement of collagen breakdown, and disturbances of calcium and phosphate metabolism, partly by blocking the action of vitamin D on calcium absorption. Inhibition of calcium absorption from the GIT stimulates parathyroid hormone secretion, which in turn promotes calcium resorption from bone. The net result is osteoporosis and danger of fractures. Glucocorticoids are diabetogenic and can precipitate full-blown diabetes. This, together with increased appetite, causes obesity. Glucocorticoids have variable aldosterone-like properties and this promotes salt and water retention, resulting in oedema and cardiovascular disease, particularly hypertension. Furthermore, high doses of glucocorticoids produce the same metabolic disturbances caused by hyperactivity of the adrenal cortex, namely Cushing's syndrome.

Suppression of the hypothalamus–anterior pituitary–adrenal axis: Glucocorticoids mimic the physiological regulatory action of cortisol in suppressing CRH and ACTH production, resulting in virtually complete suppression of adrenal steroids, including cortisol. This is potentially dangerous for the patient, particularly if steroid therapy is abruptly stopped, since it leaves the patient defenceless against stress and trauma, which are normally countered through the response of the hypothalamus–anterior pituitary–adrenal system. It takes time (up to 2 months) for the system to restore normal cortisol production after long-term suppression by glucocorticoids, and patients should be weaned gradually off glucocorticoids with tapering doses to allow the gradual restoration of cortisol secretion.

Suppression of the immune system and of healing processes: Glucocorticoids have wide-ranging suppressive effects on the immune system and on healing. They affect white cell concentrations, activity and distribution. Plasma concentrations of lymphocytes (B and T cells), basophils, eosinophils and monocytes fall through a migration from the vascular bed to lymphoid tissue, and plasma neutrophils rise due to an increased movement from bone marrow to blood and a reduced migration away from blood to sites of infection. Glucocorticoids actually reduce the functional capacity of tissue macrophages and leukocytes. The drugs reduce the ability of these cells to respond to mitogens and antigens. Macrophages can no longer efficiently produce a wide variety of factors, e.g. TNF, interleukins, interferons, pyrogens, elastase and plasminogen activator.

The anti-inflammatory action of glucocorticoids is largely through two main mechanisms: (i) suppression of prostaglandin and leukotriene synthesis through inactivation of the enzyme phospholipase A_2. In addition, they promote synthesis of a family of proteins called lipocortins, which reduce availability of the substrates of phospholipase A_2. (ii) Glucocorticoids suppress expression of COX-2.

Other effects of large doses include promotion of pepsin and acid secretion in the stomach and interference with normal renal function. They interfere with normal sleep patterns and may cause euphoria.

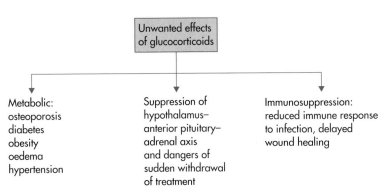

Metabolic:	Suppression of	Immunosuppression:
osteoporosis	hypothalamus–	reduced immune response
diabetes	anterior pituitary–	to infection, delayed
obesity	adrenal axis	wound healing
oedema	and dangers of	
hypertension	sudden withdrawal	
	of treatment	

Mechanism of unwanted effects

Clinical scenario: Glucocorticoids are still heavily prescribed in conditions including rheumatoid arthritis, asthma, chronic obstructive airway disease, inflammatory bowel disease and polymyalgia rheumatica. Approximately 0.5% of the adult population of the UK are taking glucocorticoids. Through their actions on the immune system and on inflammatory reactions, they have proved very effective, but the long-term side-effects include morbidity and mortality by, for example, accelerating atherosclerotic activity. Glucocorticoids are associated with bone loss, which occurs fastest during the first 12 months of therapy. Clearly, acceleration may be worsened in postmenopausal patients. Dose and length of treatment determine the severity of bone loss. Prescribers should consider the use of anti-osteoporotic medication if a dose of more than 7.5 mg glucocorticoid is to be taken for 6 months or more, and calcium and vitamin D should be prescribed.

Osteoporosis carries a high risk of fractures, with attendant risk of mortality in the elderly. Studies indicate that about 30% of patients on long-term glucocorticoid treatment may suffer osteoporotic vertebral fractures, and the risk of hip fractures is also greatly increased. Despite this, relatively few (~15%) patients on long-term glucocorticoid therapy are prescribed adequate treatments to minimise osteoporotic reactions and consequent fractures.

49 Rheumatoid arthritis I: Overview

Rheumatoid arthritis is an autoimmune disease causing inflammation and destruction of connective tissues around the joints, with attendant pain and the symptoms of inflammation, usually erythema, swelling, heat and impairment of function. Initially affecting small joints, e.g. fingers and toes, progress is often insidious, and if left untreated will spread to other, larger joints. Over time, irreversible joint damage will develop, resulting in deformity and long-term disability, including failure of weight-bearing joints. It is the commonest connective tissue disease, affecting at least 1–2% of the population. In young people, the disease is weighted towards women (F:M 3:1), although this gender difference is not seen in older affected people. The aetiology is not well understood, although there seems to be a genetic disposition to RA. HLA-DR4 is significantly more common in white sufferers, and susceptibility to RA is associated with a shared epitope on the HLA molecule. Many of the pathological changes of RA appear to be associated with increased activity of pro-inflammatory cytokines, particularly TNF-α and the interleukins IL-1β and IL-6. These discoveries have resulted in the introduction of the so-called biologic treatments (see below).

RA may manifest itself in other tissues, and extra-articular signs of RA include skin lesions, e.g. palmar erythema, bony nodules, vasculitis, pulmonary effusion and mitral valve disease, among others. Patients may become prone to infections, develop osteoporosis and become depressed. In addition, the presence of RA often complicates surgical and medical treatments.

Treatment: Traditionally, RA was treated symptomatically for pain and inflammation, using NSAIDs such as aspirin and later preparations. The advent of glucocorticoids was initially heralded as the discovery of a cure until the disastrous side-effects became apparent. Steroids are now used in much smaller doses and only for short-term treatment of flare-ups. The whole philosophy of the approach to RA treatment is now to tackle the disease head-on with vigorous treatment to slow disease progression and reduce the rate of tissue damage and deformity. Attempts are made to slow the progression of the disease with drugs that suppress the inflammatory reactions and suppress the immune system. These are the so-called **DMARDs**. Drugs used include antimalarials such as chloroquine and hydroxychloroquine, and other compounds including gold, sulfasalazine, penicillamine, azathioprine, ciclosporin and methotrexate. All are associated with occasionally serious side-effects and, because of their sometimes marked cytotoxic actions, patients on them need regular blood tests. Patients on antimalarials require regular eye tests.

Methotrexate, originally introduced as a cytotoxic drug for cancer treatment, has been found extremely useful in relatively low doses as a DMARD in RA. Its mode of action in RA is not well understood; in low doses its immunosuppressant activity may not be a significant component of its pharmacological action. It does reduce folic acid, which is given as a supple–ment to the once-weekly doses of methotrexate. It may cause nausea and occasionally alveolitis and bone marrow toxicity.

The **biologic drugs** are macromolecular drugs designed to neutralise the activity of the inflammatory cytokines and are dealt with more fully in the next spread.

Clinical scenario: A 44-year-old married woman was referred urgently to the department of rheumatology. Following a flu-like illness 21 months previously she had developed pain in both her hands, elbows, shoulders, knees and feet. This was associated with generalised stiffness throughout the morning, lethary and loss of appetite. Her GP had commenced her on high doses of an NSAID but to little avail. The symptoms had impaired her ability to work as computer programmer. On examination she had widespread symmetrical synovitis of her small and large joints outlined below. Investigations revealed an inflammatory response, a normochromic normocytic anaemia and a strongly positive rheumatoid factor. X-rays showed periarticular erosions of three metacarpals. A diagnosis of RA was made and its implications explained. She received an intramuscular depot injection of methylprednisolone (120 mg) and commenced weekly methotrexate starting at 7.5 mg. Folic acid was prescribed for the 2 days preceeding the methotrexate and she was advised to continue with the NSAID.

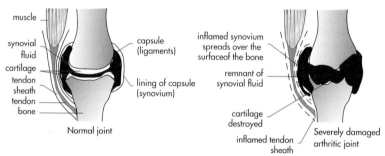

Damage to joint caused by RA

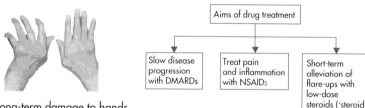

Long-term damage to hands caused by RA

Aims of drug treatment

50 Rheumatoid arthritis II: Specific drugs

Disease-modifying anti-rheumatic drugs are the most important drugs for RA and may be started early after diagnosis and continued for the rest of the patient's life.

Oral **sulfasalazine** is often the first choice for treatment and patients report symptomatic relief after approximately 6–8 weeks. Monitoring of liver function and blood counts immediately after starting treatment is essential, as hepatitis and bone marrow toxicity usually present within the first 6 months of treatment. Less serious side-effects include nausea, GIT upsets and headache. Soft contact lenses and urine may be discoloured yellow and reversible oligospermia has been reported.

Gold is injected intramuscularly as sodium aurothiomalate or given orally as auranofin. It causes remission, but tends also to cause skin rashes and diarrhoea, which discourages many patients. Serious renal reactions may be heralded by an initial proteinuria. Blood monitoring is essential as potentially lethal blood dyscrasias do occur.

Azathioprine is taken for systemic complications associated with RA and for synovitis. As with sulfasalazine, there is a danger of liver and bone marrow toxicity and regular monitoring is essential. Nausea is frequently the reason for discontinuation of treatment. **Penicillamine** has similar side effects and patients complain of nausea and a metallic taste which both resolve with time. **Antimalarials** such as **hydroxychloroquine** are safer than most other DMARDs but are less potent. They require ophthalmic monitoring due to the risk of retinopathy. **Ciclosporin** is immunosuppressant and is used orally for severe active arthritis that does not respond to other drugs. It is contraindicated in renal impairment, malignancy or uncontrolled hypertension, or if infections are present.

Methotrexate is immunosuppressive and is taken either orally or as a once-weekly subcutaneous injection. Unwanted effects include indigestion and nausea, which often resolve with time. More serious potential complications are alveolitis and bone marrow toxicity, and regular monitoring is essential. It is prescribed together with folic acid. Families should not be planned while on methotrexate and women on methotrexate should consider oral contraception, since the drug could cause fetal abnormalities.

Biologic agents, e.g. **infliximab** and **adalimumab,** are monoclonal antibodies directed against TNF-α. **Infliximab** is administered as an intravenous infusion every 6–8 weeks under hospital supervision and is prescribed together with methotrexate, which suppresses the body's immune response to infliximab. **Adalimumab** is given once or twice weekly as a subcutaneous injection. Infliximab has been associated with a worsening of demyelinating disease. **Etanercept** is a fusion protein p75 TNF-α receptor immunoglobulin which binds to circulating TNF-α, thus inactivating it. It has been associated with a suppression of bone marrow. **Anakinra** is a recombinant IL-Rα-receptor antagonist which patients self-administer subcutaneously daily. It may be prescribed together with methotrexate. A newer class of biologic anti-rheumatic drugs, called selective co-stimulation modulators, have been introduced. **Abatacept,** the first in this class, selectively modulates the CD80- or CD86-28 co-stimulatory signal required for full T-cell modulation. Regular blood monitoring is advisable. All these preparations suppress the immune response and patients at risk of sepsis or with diabetes are excluded from treatment. There is also the risk of exacerbation of latent TB after infections.

Clinical scenario: A 37-year-old woman was referred to the regional rheumatology unit of the local teaching hospital with DMARD-resistant RA. She had presented 6 years previously with a widespread erosive symmetrical seropositive illness. This had initially been treated with oral steroids and sulfasalazine to good effect. Two years into treatment, however, she relapsed and was given a short oral dose of steroids. This had not helped and sulfasalazine was replaced by weekly intramuscular injections of gold. This, although initially helpful, caused proteinuria. She had also tried methotrexate, which caused nausea at higher doses, and hydroxychloroquine, which was not helpful. On assessment she was disabled by her symptoms, anaemic and pessimistic. After discussion it was decided to commence treatment with methotrexate and infliximab, administered as an intravenous infusion every 8 weeks. This proved to be a success and after 4 months the interval between infusions was shortened to 6 weeks.

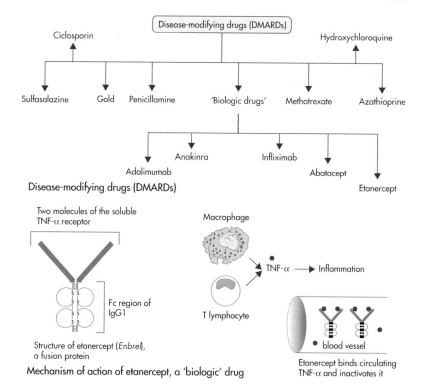

Disease-modifying drugs (DMARDs)

Mechanism of action of etanercept, a 'biologic' drug

Structure of etanercept (*Enbrel*), a fusion protein

Etanercept binds circulating TNF-α and inactivates it

51 Inflammatory polyarthritides I: Introduction

The group of inflammatory arthritides includes **RA, psoriatic arthropathy, inflammatory bowel disease, adult-onset Still's disease, scleroderma, juvenile idiopathic arthritis** and **SLE**. The various conditions are clinically distinguished by extra-articular features. For example, Patients with arthritic pain may also present with a malar rash, fever, ulcers and alopecia, suggestive of SLE, whereas psoriatic skin lesions coupled with arthritic pain may point to psoriatic arthropathy. Joint pains coupled with Raynaud's phenomenon might indicate the presence of scleroderma. The persistence (more than 6 weeks) bilateral, symmetrical inflammation of small and larger joints is a clear pointer to RA, even if the patient is rheumatoid factor (RF) negative. Joint pains and diarrhoea with blood in stools may point to enteropathic arthritis.

Inflammatory arthritis is characterised by early morning stiffness, lasting more than 30 minutes, pain that resolves quickly when the joint is moved, and elevated serum ESR and CRP. **Non-inflammatory arthritis** is characterised by early morning stiffness that lasts less than 30 minutes and joint pain that is exacerbated by movement. Important examples are hypothyroidism and osteoarthritis (see opposite).

Seronegative spondyloarthropathies (SpA) are a group of disorders with the following common features: (i) seronegative RF; (ii) the backbone (spondylo- is a prefix denoting the spine); and (iii) arthritic symptoms. The group includes **ankylosing spondylitis, inflammatory bowel disease,** including, among others, Crohn's disease and ulcerative colitis, **juvenile spondyloarthropathy,** psoriatic **spondyloarthropathy** and **Reiter's syndrome,** which is characterised by arthritis, urethral inflammation, sometimes horny skin lesions and conjunctivitis.

Treatment aims at reducing pain and inflammation and reducing the activity of the immune system. Corticosteroids are generally heavily relied upon, as are cytotoxic drugs.

Scleroderma (systemic sclerosis) is an umbrella term for a spectrum of disorders and derived its name through the skin thickening often associated with it. It is an autoimmune disease that may affect skin, the lungs, blood vessels, kidney and oesophagus. Raynaud's phenomenon is damage to the digits of the hands through atrophic changes resulting from ischaemia due to microcirculatory damage, or from factors such as working outdoors or with vibrating machinery. It is treated principally with calcium channel blockers and fish oils. Scleroderma typically develops in two phases, initially within the first 5 years with arthritis, weight loss, weariness and myositis. Fibrosis, especially of the lungs, follows, sometimes with skin hyperpigmentation and GIT, pulmonary and cardiac disease through fibrosis.

Treatments include those for Raynaud's phenomenon and the use of immunosuppressive drugs such as corticosteroids and cytotoxic drugs such as cyclophosphamide, methotrexate and azathioprine.

Reactive arthritis: This is a form of arthritis linked to infection, often of sexual organ or enteric association. See opposite for some of the pathogens associated with reactive arthritis.

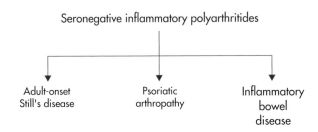

Seronegative inflammatory polyarthritides

- Adult-onset Still's disease
- Psoriatic arthropathy
- Inflammatory bowel disease

Treatment of spondyloarthropathies

Indication	Treatment
Persistent sexually-associated reactive arthritis Acute infection of the genital tract	Antibiotics
Inflamed bursae, entheses and joints	Local steroid injection
Acute flares, uveitis	Systemic steroids
Aggressive, persistent symptoms	Sulfasalazine, methotrexate
Enthesopathy, persistent synovitis, pain, spinal stiffness	NSAIDs
Maintaining muscle tone, spinal mobilisation	Physiotherapy

Some gut diseases associated with spondyloarthropathies

Acute bacterial infections
Amoebiasis, giardiasis
Crohn's disease
Coeliac disease
Ulcerative colitis
Whipple's disease

Some microorganisms associated with reactive arthritis

GIT

E. coli
Giardia lamblia
Salmonella spp.

Genitourinary

Chlamydia trachomatis
Neisseria gonorrhoeae
Ureaplasma urealyticum

52 Inflammatory polyarthritides II: Systemic lupus erythematosus

Systemic lupus erythematosus is a relatively rare autoimmune disease that affects women more than men (F:M = 9:1). This disparity may be even higher during pubertal and child-bearing years. African-Caribbean and Asian women are about 10 times more likely to develop SLE than their white counterparts. The disease presents in several different forms, depending on the patient, with different serological patterns of autoantibodies. Historically, diagnosis of SLE has been difficult and, to resolve this, a list of criteria has been agreed upon for diagnosis of SLE (see opposite).

Symptoms and diagnosis: Apart from generalised arthralgia, fatigue, alopecia and the classic mucocutaneous manifestations such as the malar rash and mouth ulcers, patients may develop more serious major organ involvement, e.g. kidney, cardiopulmonary or cerebral forms of SLE. Diagnosis includes blood tests for antinuclear and antiphospholipid antibodies, ESR and a complete blood count. It is generally agreed that absence of antinuclear antibodies makes a diagnosis of SLE unlikely. Diagnosis should include screening with antibodies to soluble cellular antigens, including Jo-1, LJI-RNP, Lo and Ra, to identify the SLE subset. The antiphospholipid antibody syndrome is an SLE subset associated with fetal death and is identified by the presence in the plasma of antiphospholipid antibodies, including lupus anticoagulant and anticardiolipin antibodies.

Cerebral lupus is problematic in that headache is associated with several different underlying causes, e.g. psychosocial stress, migraine and even toothache. Nevertheless, migraine is significantly more prevalent in patients with SLE than among the general population.

Treatment of SLE: There are no hard and fast rules for patient management due to the diversity of SLE. As with several other autoimmune problems, the disease goes through phases of quiescence and flare, and treatment often reflects this. Treatment involves patient support, lifestyle management and drugs. Patients should avoid direct sunlight and use sunscreens. Estrogens are asso–ciated with SLE and patients should take either progestogen-only or low-dose oral contraceptives. Patients contemplating HRT should be offered low-dose estrogen preparations and advised of the current uncertainty as to safety and risk. Patients with cardiopulmonary or renal disease must be monitored regularly for hypertension and target organ damage. Patients on corticosteroids or immunosuppressive drugs are at risk of potential fatal infections, and flu-like symptoms in these patients may be associated with these treatments.

Drug treatment of SLE: NSAIDs are prescribed for symptomatic pain relief of arthralgia, chest pain and headache. DMARDs include the corticosteroids, antimalarials and immunosuppressive drugs. Corticosteroids are important in controlling a flare, but need to be reduced in dose and frequency after treating a flare; a low dose of 2.5–5 mg prednisolone is considered acceptable for maintenance. Topical corticosteroids are often prescribed for cutaneous flares. The antimalarial drugs chloroquine and hydroxychloroquine are important for treatment of joint and skin manifestations of SLE, and doses are chosen to minimise the risk of ocular complications, although patients should be monitored for this adverse effect of these drugs. Immunosuppressive drugs, e.g. azathioprine, cyclophosphamide and methotrexate, are used for severe cases, e.g. kidney disease.

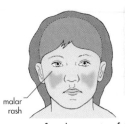

Eleven criteria for diagnosis of SLE – at least four must be present

- Antinuclear antibodies
- Arthritis
- Discoid rash
- Haematological disorder
- Immunological disorder
- Malar rash

- Neurological disorder
- Oral ulcers
- Photosensitivity
- Renal disorder
- Serositis

malar rash

Criteria for diagnosis of SLE

Manifestations of lupus
- Arthralgia
- Cardiopulmonary disease
- Cerebral lupus
- Fatigue
- Major organ disease – heart, lungs, kidneys
- Mucocutaneous symptoms

Manifestations of SLE

Management of lupus
- Lifestyle management
- Drugs
- Patient support

Management of lupus

Drugs

NSAIDs	Symptomatic relief of inflammation and pain. Use with caution in patients with kidney involvement
Corticosteroids Prednisolone	Used to treat flare-up of SLE and dose reduced for maintenance. Low doses are not generally useful to treat arthralgia. Used topically for cutaneous symptoms
Antimalarials Chloroquine Hydroxychloroquine	Used to treat joint and skin symptoms. Hydroxychloroquine is generally considered safer than chloroquine for the eyes, but routine ophthalmic screening is advisable
Immunosuppressive drugs Azathioprine Cyclophosphamide Methotrexate	Reserved for progressive, severe multi-organ disease, e.g. in the kidney. They are used under specialist supervision and are associated with side-effects linked to their cytotoxic actions

Drugs used to treat SLE

53 Inflammatory polyarthritides III: Raynaud's phenomenon and scleroderma

Raynaud's phenomenon (RP) involves spasm of the blood vessels supplying the fingers due to atherosclerosis and is often part of a more generalised auto-immune problem such as scleroderma. RP may also result from: (i) occupational causes, e.g. use of vibrating tools, exposure to vinyl chloride or working outdoors under conditions of extreme cold; (ii) drugs such as bleomycin, ergot, β-blockers and oral contraceptives; and (iii) autoimmune disease. The fingers become blanched and icy cold and gangrene occasionally results.

The presence of RP is generally considered part of the diagnosis of scleroderma. It may occur in patients with other autoimmune diseases (see opposite). RP occurs predominantly in women under 30 years of age. RP may occur months or years before the onset of symptoms of scleroderma. Scleroderma, also called systemic sclerosis, is an autoimmune disease characterised by skin thickening due to dermal fibrosis after inflammation, leaving an ivory-coloured, shiny appearance. Cutaneous scleroderma may be localised (termed **morphoea**) or generalised (diffuse cutaneous scleroderma). Scleroderma may affect internal organs, particularly the lungs, GIT, heart and kidneys, sometimes without cutaneous involvement (sometimes termed 'scleroderma sine scleroderma'). In the early stages, within the first 10 years of the disease, symptoms are generally confined to RP, minimal cutaneous fibrosis and some symptoms of oesophageal damage. In later stages, usually after 10 years, in addition to RP, patients develop skin thickening and problems such as pulmonary hypertension, oesophageal stricture and small bowel malabsorption. In the last stages of scleroderma, patients may develop widespread calcinosis, which is the abnormal deposit of calcium in the tissues, ulcers, anal incontinence and severe pulmonary hypertension.

Treatment: RP is treated mainly to increase blood flow to the fingers with vasodilators such as the calcium channel blockers diltiazem, nicardipine, felodipine or nifedipine. The carbonic anhydrase inhibitor captopril may be prescribed, and patients may be advised to use concentrated fish oils or gamolenic acid capsules as dietary supplements. Vasodilator drugs for RP may be prescribed for oral or parenteral use and in the later stages of scleroderma: surgical intervention may be decided upon in the form of digital sympathectomy.

Scleroderma treatment in the earlier stages is usually limited to treatment of RP and any oesophageal problems that may arise. Patients with the diffuse cutaneous form of scleroderma, which in the earlier phase generally presents in its oedematous form, may be prescribed immunosuppressive drugs such as antithymocyte globulin, cyclophosphamide or methotrexate. As the disease progresses into the later stages, skin changes stabilise and other organs may become affected, when scleroderma may become life threatening. Fibrosis of the lungs produces pulmonary vascular disease; in the heart arrhythmias arise; patients may suffer oesophageal reflux, for which the proton pump inhibitor **omeprazole** may be prescribed. Hypertensive renal crises and bacterial overgrowth may develop. Patients may be prescribed the anti-fibrotic drugs, interferon and penicillamine.

Patient management: Apart from the use of drugs, patients need to be discouraged from smoking, change their working conditions if possible and wear gloves, especially those that can be electrically warmed. Patients and their families need much support, especially in the later stages of the disease.

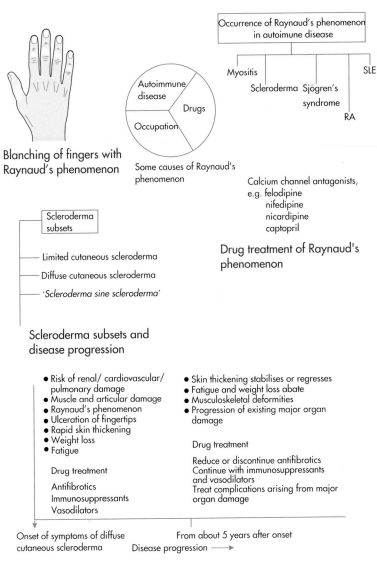

Blanching of fingers with
Raynaud's phenomenon

Some causes of Raynaud's
phenomenon

Autoimmune
disease

Drugs

Occupation

Occurrence of Raynaud's phenomenon
in autoimmune disease

Myositis

Scleroderma   Sjögren's
syndrome

SLE

RA

Calcium channel antagonists,
e.g. felodipine
       nifedipine
       nicardipine
       captopril

Drug treatment of Raynaud's
phenomenon

Scleroderma
subsets

— Limited cutaneous scleroderma

— Diffuse cutaneous scleroderma

— 'Scleroderma sine scleroderma'

Scleroderma subsets and
disease progression

- Risk of renal/ cardiovascular/
  pulmonary damage
- Muscle and articular damage
- Raynaud's phenomenon
- Ulceration of fingertips
- Rapid skin thickening
- Weight loss
- Fatigue

Drug treatment

Antifibrotics
Immunosuppressants
Vasodilators

- Skin thickening stabilises or regresses
- Fatigue and weight loss abate
- Musculoskeletal deformities
- Progression of existing major organ
  damage

Drug treatment

Reduce or discontinue antifibrotics
Continue with immunosuppressants
and vasodilators
Treat complications arising from major
organ damage

Onset of symptoms of diffuse
cutaneous scleroderma

From about 5 years after onset

Disease progression ⟶

Diffuse cutaneous scleroderma

54 Inflammatory polyarthritides IV: Gout

Gout is traditionally associated with the foot, and in particular the first metatarsophalangeal joint (big toe), when it is known as **podagra**. Gout describes any condition where pain and inflammation are caused by uric acid crystal deposition in any tissue. Other joints commonly affected include the shoulder, knee and hand. Causes may include dietary excesses, such as alcohol, hypertension, ketosis, diuretics, stress and surgery. Men are more prone to gout, which does run in families.

Symptoms: Onset is usually sudden and symptoms often appear overnight. The skin is red and painful to the touch. **Diagnosis** is most reliably made through identification of urate crystals in tissues; blood urate may be normal during an acute attack. Patients may have other indices common to inflammation, including raised CRP, ESR and plasma viscosity.

Treatment: Acute treatment is directed against pain and inflammation, whereas chronic treatment aims to prevent attacks by better lifestyle management and with drugs that either improve the renal excretion of urate or reduce its synthesis in purine metabolism. Drugs used in the long-term management of gout must not be used during an acute attack as they will exacerbate pain and inflammation. Treatment **of acute pain** involves the use of high doses of NSAIDs including **diclofenac, indometacin, naproxen** and **ketoprofen. Azapropazone** may be tried in patients in whom less toxic NSAIDs have failed, but the CSM contraindicates its use in patients with a history of peptic ulcer, and recommends reduced dosages in patients over 60 with ankylosing spondylitis, gout or RA. If they are prescribed, then proton pump inhibitors should be prescribed as well. Aspirin is contraindicated in the treatment of acute gout. **Colchicine,** a drug extracted from the meadow saffron (*Colchicum autumnale*), may be used orally in patients in whom NSAIDs are ineffective. In gout, it may work by inhibiting the migration of neutrophils into the joint. Colchicine binds to the protein tubulin and interferes with microtubule formation and hence cellular motility. It is contraindicated in pregnancy and should be used with caution in elderly patients and those with cardiac, GIT or renal impairment. Its most common **adverse effects** include diarrhoea, nausea, vomiting and abdominal pain. More severe reactions include GIT haemorrhage and hepatic and renal impairment.

Long-term management of gout with drugs aims to enhance urate excretion with uricosuric agents, notably **probenecid** and **sulfinpyrazone**, and to inhibit uric acid synthesis from purine metabolism with the xanthine oxidase inhibitor **allupurinol**. These drugs should never be used during an acute attack, as they could worsen the symptoms, e.g. by mobilising urate from sites of crystalline deposition. Allupurinol is frequently prescribed, especially in patients with urate stones and renal impairment, in whom uricosuric drugs are sometimes contraindicated. It is may be combined with sulfinpyrazone in some resistant cases. In the UK, probenecid is used on a named-patient basis to prevent nephrotoxicity associated with the antiviral drug cidofovir.

Adverse effects: Allupurinol may produce hypersensitivity reactions, and should be withdrawn if a rash appears. Probenecid has several adverse effects (see opposite).

Clinical scenario: A 60-year-old man presented to his general practitioner with an acutely painful big toe. He was known to his doctor as he had a 5-year history of hypertension for which he was taking enalapril and bendrofluazide. Weight and alcohol were issues that had also been discussed during previous consultations. On examination there was synovitis of the first metatarsophalangeal joint and surrounding soft tissue erythema. Podagra secondary to gout was diagnosed and supported by measurement of the patient's serum urate, which was raised. Diclofenac was prescribed for the acute episode and bendrofluazide was stopped. Symptoms resolved after 2 days and 3 weeks later the patient returned to the practice for review. Amlodipine was instituted in place of bendrofluazide. Again, weight and alcohol reduction was stressed. Allopurinol as a prophylactic agent was discussed, but after hearing about the potential side-effects the patient felt inclined to modify his lifestyle first.

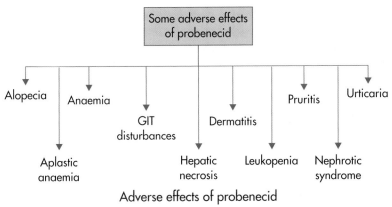

Adverse effects of probenecid

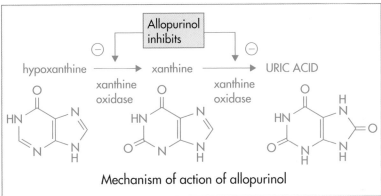

Mechanism of action of allopurinol

55 The perception of pain – the gate theory

Drugs that relieve pain may act at one of three sites: the first is at the site of pain generation, e.g. NSAIDs. The pain of inflammation is treated at the site where pain is generated, e.g. in the joint, mainly to inhibit the production of pain-producing chemicals such as the prostaglandins. Aspirin is an important drug that acts in this way (page 84). In the second site, pain may be blocked by local anaesthetics, which block the conduction of impulses along pain-mediating nerves. Pain is, however, *appreciated* in the CNS, and there are drugs that block the ability of the CNS to register that a painful stimulus has occurred. The endogenous opioids, e.g. met-enkephalin, and the opiates, e.g. morphine, act in this way (see below).

Sensory inputs to the CNS may carry information about mechanical, chemical or thermal stimulation from corresponding mechano-, chemical or pain receptors (also called nociceptors). Fibres from nociceptors carry information about painful stimuli to the spinal cord, where it is filtered before being allowed to travel to the brain; this filter is a target for the opioids and opiates. An understanding of opioid action at the spinal level is facilitated through knowledge of the **gate theory of pain.**

This theory was first proposed by Melzack and Wall in the 1960s[8] and is still the most popular theory to explain how painful stimuli are processed by the CNS. It also explains how opioids reduce pain. The mechanism is summarised opposite. Briefly, in the posterior horn of the spinal cord there is a relay gate, which receives signals via nerves that carry information about pain and touch from the rest of the body. High-intensity pain signals are allowed through the gate and ascend to higher centres in the thalamus, where pain is appreciated, and from there to the cerebral cortex, where interpretation and discriminatory processes occur. The gate is also regulated by low-intensity signals carrying information about touch, which travel to the brain in the dorsal columns. These pathways send branches to the gate and their inputs tend to close the gate and inhibit the transmission of pain impulses. This mechanism explains how strategies such as transcutaneous stimulation and counter-irritants such as Deep Heat cream may work to reduce the appreciation of pain: they may dampen the painful inputs at the 'gate'.

The gate mechanism is also regulated by inhibitory opioid-mediated inputs from the substantia gelatinosa, which is adjacent to the gate mechanism. These work to block transmission of pain signals through the gate. Furthermore, descending impulses from the cortex due to distractions (e.g. a book or hospital visitors) may be able to reduce pain at the gate by blocking transmission of incoming painful stimuli. Several brain areas, including the periaqueductal grey (PAG), nucleus raphe magnus (NRM) and other brain areas, are involved in the descending pathways that reduce appreciation of pain (**A**).

Role of opioids in the gate theory: Opium and morphine have been used for centuries to treat pain and their mechanism of action is now generally believed to be through their action on receptors for the endogenous opioid peptides β-endorphin and met-enkephalin. These opioids are highly concentrated in the spinal substantia gelatinosa and in the PAG, NRM and other brain areas involved in the appreciation of pain. Thus, the opioids may act widely in the CNS to inhibit the gate.

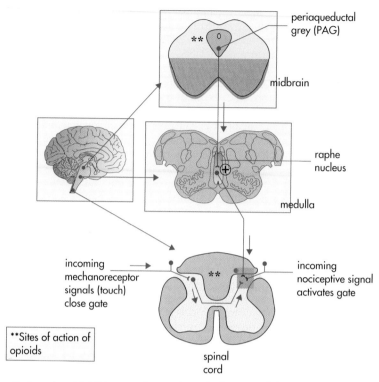

periaqueductal grey (PAG)

midbrain

raphe nucleus

medulla

incoming mechanoreceptor signals (touch) close gate

**

incoming nociceptive signal activates gate

**Sites of action of opioids

spinal cord

A. Postulated inhibitory pathways from the brain and the periphery to the pain gate mechanism in the spinal cord posterior horn

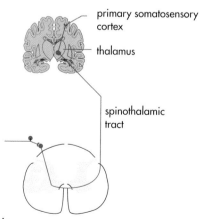

primary somatosensory cortex

thalamus

spinothalamic tract

B. Pain pathway to the brain

56 Palliative care

The term 'palliative' refers to a treatment that temporarily relieves a disease symptom, in this case mainly pain, but also encompasses other distress-producing modalities such as constipation, nausea and coughing. Palliative care does not treat or cure the underlying disease. Other uses of drugs as palliative measures include the treatment of CNS, cardiovascular, GI and respiratory complications of diseases such as cancer, or the treatment of adverse effects of relatively non-specific drugs used to treat diseases such as cancer or autoimmune inflammatory diseases. In essence, the aim of pain management nowadays is to free the patient from pain completely if possible and remove anxieties that accompany the disease. Palliative care is an integral and essential component of the treatment of patients during the terminal stages of disease, e.g. cancer, and drugs play an important part.

Pain modalities: Pain relief encompasses several different modalities associated with pain. These encompass not only the physical sensation of pain but also the patient's state of mind; factors such as fear, morale and mood are now taken into account when treating the patient with severe pain. Although cancer, even when advanced, is not always associated with pain, fear exacerbates whatever pain the patient may experience.

Pain management has several aims depending on the problem; in general terms, the aim is to provide relief at rest during the day, during movement and at night to give the patient some sleep. Apart from the use of drugs to treat pain directly by blocking mechanisms of pain (e.g. opioids), **adjuvant** drugs may block the underlying disease process (e.g. corticosteroids or DMARDs in RA; page 98). Cancer patients may be given bisphosphonates, which inhibit osteoclasts, to relieve metastatic bone pain. Patients with cancer of the GIT may require adjuvant therapy to relieve bowel obstruction, nausea, dehydration and vomiting (see opposite). Patients may receive psychological therapy, surgical intervention to interrupt pain pathways or immobilise a joint, and mechanical aids such as cooling or heating pads and walking aids.

Types of pain: Different types of pain require different drug regimens. For example, pain of neuropathic origin such as stroke or spinal cord compression and peripheral nerve injuries may require one or more of the following: opioids, spinal analgesics, N-methyl-D-aspartate (NMDA) receptor channel blockers (page 112), NSAIDs, antidepressants, anti-epileptics and local anaesthetics. Transcutaneous electrical nerve stimulation (TENS) may also be used. Pain originating at nerve endings, e.g. RA and other soft tissue damage, bone pain and pain through liver capsule damage are treated with NSAIDs alone or with opioids.

Monitoring effectiveness of treatment: Modern palliative care with respect to the use of drugs to treat pain demands that the patient know precisely the drug dose and frequency of administration, and be reassured that medical support teams are approachable if pain cover is not adequate. Patients must be made aware of possible adverse effects of drugs and advised to contact their support team if these occur; monitoring and follow-up by the team are essential to ensure that the patient is given adequate cover and is not experiencing potentially dangerous adverse effects. This is more easily done with in-patients, but out-patients on drugs must also be monitored and drug treatments modified before serious consequences of adverse effects occur. The carer and prescriber must maintain a curiosity about the effectiveness of the drugs and any untoward symptom.

Clinical scenario: A 74-year-old woman was admitted onto a surgical ward with large bowel obstruction. Two weeks previously she had been diagnosed with sigmoid colon cancer and was awaiting a decision regarding further investigation and treatment. On presentation to the hospital she was vomiting and in pain. She was dehydrated, had abdominal distension and scant bowel sounds. Blood tests revealed pre-renal failure and X-rays showed dilatation of the large bowel. A nasogastric tube was inserted and intravenous crystalloids and antibiotics were commenced. A CT scan the following day confirmed a sigmoid tumour with retroperitoneal involvement and distant metastases. The patient was booked for a sigmoidoscopy to attempt debulking and relief of the obstruction but declined this procedure. The prognosis was explained to her and she indicated that she would decline any further treatment. A referral to the palliative care team was made. Following consultation with the patient and her family, a syringe driver was prescribed. It included diamorphine, levomepromazine, midazolam and hyoscine. The nasogastric tube was left in place. Breakthrough analgesia was given as oromorph solution and titrated into the syringe driver. All other medications were stopped and the patient continued on fluids given subcutaneously.

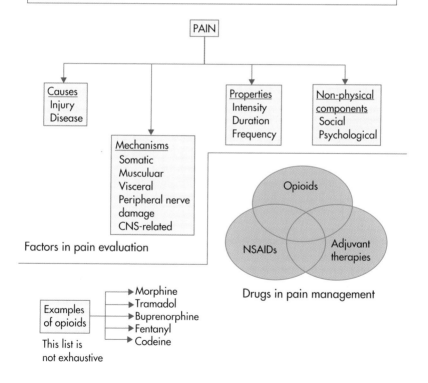

PAIN

Causes
Injury
Disease

Mechanisms
Somatic
Musculuar
Visceral
Peripheral nerve
damage
CNS-related

Properties
Intensity
Duration
Frequency

Non-physical
components
Social
Psychological

Factors in pain evaluation

Opioids

NSAIDs

Adjuvant
therapies

Drugs in pain management

Examples
of opioids

This list is
not exhaustive

Morphine
Tramadol
Buprenorphine
Fentanyl
Codeine

57 Opioids I: Introduction

Morphine and **codeine** are alkaloids extracted from opium, which is the dried exudate from the unripe seed capsule of the poppy *Papaver somniferum*. Codeine has about a seventh of the analgesic activity of morphine. Synthetic opioids include dextromoramide, dihydrocodeine, diamorphine (heroin), dipipanone, fentanyl, levorphanol, meperidine (pethidine), methadone, oxycodone and phenazocine. Naloxone and naltrexone are opioid antagonists and buprenorphine, meptazinol, nalbuphine and nalorphine are partial agonists, which at lower concentrations may be agonists at receptors, but are antagonists at higher concentrations. Most of the opioids are potentially drugs of abuse due to their central actions. Met-enkephalin and β-endorphin are endogenous peptide opioids.

Effects of the opioids: The **CNS effects** of opioids are mainly: (i) analgesia by depression of pain appreciation by the brain; (ii) euphoria; (iii) mild hypnosis, and can induce sleep; (iv) depression of respiration; (v) depression of the cough reflex; (vi) vomiting through stimulation of the chemoreceptor trigger zone (CTZ) in the brain stem; and (vii) tolerance and dependence. Dependence on opioids may initially be psychological, when the user exhibits compulsive drug-seeking behaviour, and this is followed with continued use by physical dependence, when the user suffers physical withdrawal symptoms when the drug is withdrawn, and drug-seeking behaviour is motivated not only by desire for euphoria, but also by fear of withdrawal symptoms. Tolerance may be defined as a condition when more of the drug is needed to achieve the same effect. Physical exercise, e.g. jogging, causes the release of β-endorphin in the brain and may be responsible for the euphoria associated with exercise. Other central effects include an action on the nucleus of the third nerve, resulting in constriction of the pupil, and stimulation of the vagus nerve, resulting in lowering of blood pressure and slowing of the pulse, which complicates its use to treat the pain of coronary thrombosis.

Peripheral effects include: (i) constipation by decreasing bowel peristalsis while increasing the tone; (ii) spasm of sphincters, including the sphincter of Oddi, which lies at the lower end of the bile duct, resulting in raised biliary pressure; (iii) urinary retention by interfering with bladder function; and (iv) histamine release, which could cause bronchoconstriction.

Note: Tolerance does not develop to the peripheral actions of morphine, and morphine addicts, who take abnormally high doses to achieve euphoria, are often chronically constipated.

Mechanism of opioid action: Opioids act on specific receptors in the nervous system, notably in the posterior horn of the spinal cord and in the midbrain, where met-enkephalin and β-endorphin occur as neuromodulators and form part of the pain gating system. Stimulation of these receptors inhibits transmission of pain signals to higher centres where pain is appreciated. Several different opioid receptor subtypes have been identified; the most important subtypes that mediate euphoria, analgesia and respiratory depression are termed μ and κ opioid receptors. There is evidence that opioids may mediate their analgesic action not only in the CNS but also through an action on opioid receptors on peripheral nerves.

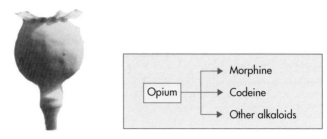

Poppy seed capsule

Opium → Morphine
       → Codeine
       → Other alkaloids

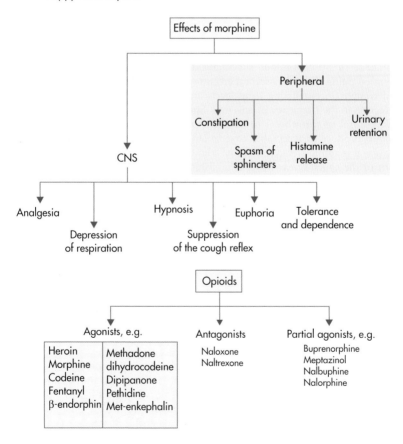

Effects of morphine

Peripheral
- Constipation
- Spasm of sphincters
- Histamine release
- Urinary retention

CNS
- Analgesia
- Depression of respiration
- Hypnosis
- Suppression of the cough reflex
- Euphoria
- Tolerance and dependence

Opioids

Agonists, e.g.

Heroin	Methadone
Morphine	dihydrocodeine
Codeine	Dipipanone
Fentanyl	Pethidine
β-endorphin	Met-enkephalin

Antagonists
Naloxone
Naltrexone

Partial agonists, e.g.
Buprenorphine
Meptazinol
Nalbuphine
Nalorphine

58 Opioids II: Clinical use

Opioids are used clinically for a number of conditions, notably: (i) analgesia; (ii) acute pulmonary oedema; (iii) diarrhoea; (iv) cough; and (v) medication before, during and after surgery. The most frequent use is for the treatment of pain, especially as part of palliative care in cancer.

Routes of administration. (i) **Oral**: morphine, codeine, meptazinol, oxycodone and methadone are examples of opioids that can be taken orally, in tablet, capsule or liquid form. (ii) **Buccal or sublingual**: morphine is absorbed slowly through the buccal mucosa and has in the past been used in this way. Buprenorphine is also absorbed through the buccal mucosa. A preparation of oral transmucosal fentanyl citrate, which has the acronym OTFC, is used for breakthrough pain. The oral route may lessen the addictive property of an opioid. For example, methadone, when taken orally, produces little euphoria, whereas injection produces euphoria – hence its use to wean opioid-dependent patients off the drugs. (iii) **Parenteral**: morphine, diamorphine (heroin), methadone and nalbuphine are some examples of opioids that are administered by injection. The oral route of administration may not be possible. For example, cancer patients on cytotoxic drugs may not be able to take or keep down analgesics administered orally. In some patients opioids may be administered by **continuous subcutaneous infusion** (CSCI), using a battery-operated pump. CSCI has several advantages, notably the elimination of peaks and troughs in circulating drug levels and hence better pain control, and a reduction in the frequency of injection. **Spinal morphine**: morphine is given via the epidural or intrathecal route when pain is intractable or when systemic opioids produce unacceptable adverse effects. It is a particularly potent route because it is administered in close proximity to opioid receptors in the posterior horn of the spinal cord. When administered this way, morphine is sometimes given with clonidine or bupivacaine. (iv) **Topical morphine**: morphine can be administered intra-articularly after joint surgery, where it acts on opioid receptors on nociceptive nerve fibres. The receptors are silent until activated by inflammation. Topical morphine is also useful for pain associated with cutaneous ulceration, or that is intractable to other routes of drug administration. It has also been used for rectal ulceration, oral mucositis and vaginal inflammation involving a fistula. It is administered as a gel.

Patient-controlled analgesia (PCA) is the use by the patient of an injection device that administers, usually subcutaneously or intravenously, a dose of opioid, usually morphine, to control pain.

Rectal: Morphine suppositories are used when oral and parenteral routes are not indicated.

Transdermal patches: Buprenorphine and fentanyl may be administered as transdermal patches, which produce stable blood levels with good control of pain.

Pain management is now a clinical discipline in its own right, with the aim of freeing the patient from pain at all times if possible. Opioids are indicated when pain is severe and constant, e.g. after injury, during the post-operative period, after a coronary thrombosis and for patients with cancer. The drugs, especially morphine, not only provide analgesia but also allay fear and induce sleep. In patients with terminal cancer, considerations of tolerance and dependence are not generally taken into account.

Opioids have arbitrarily been classified as 'weak' or 'strong' by comparing their analgesic potency with that of morphine.

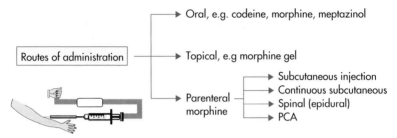

Routes of administration

Oral, e.g. codeine, morphine, meptazinol

Topical, e.g morphine gel

Parenteral morphine
→ Subcutaneous injection
→ Continuous subcutaneous
→ Spinal (epidural)
→ PCA

Patient-controlled analgesia (PCA; subcutaneous or intravenous)

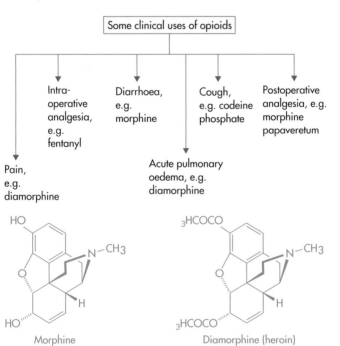

Some clinical uses of opioids

Intra-operative analgesia, e.g. fentanyl

Diarrhoea, e.g. morphine

Cough, e.g. codeine phosphate

Postoperative analgesia, e.g. morphine papaveretum

Pain, e.g. diamorphine

Acute pulmonary oedema, e.g. diamorphine

Morphine

Diamorphine (heroin)

59 Idiopathic Parkinson's disease I: Introduction

Idiopathic Parkinson's disease is a neurodegenerative disease of the brain. It occurs with equal incidence in men and women and the mean age of onset of symptoms is about 65 years, although in a small percentage (5–10%) of patients symptoms may first present after 40 years of age. Motor symptoms are rigidity, oculomotor disturbances (e.g. loss of blinking), hypokinesia, asymmetrical bradykinesia and loss of postural reflexes. These are often referred to as extrapyramidal symptoms because they reflect a malfunction of the central extrapyramidal system which controls fine movements. Cognition is generally unimpaired in the earlier stages, but may be affected by emotional reaction to distressing symptoms and the side-effects of the drugs used.

Aetiology: The cause of Parkinson's disease is unknown, although environmental and lifestyle factors such as pollution, toxins and smoking have been suggested. There may a genetic component, since first-degree relatives of patients with Parkinson's disease have approximately twice the chance of developing the disease. Genes on chromosomes 6 and 17 have been tentatively implicated in the aetiology of Parkinson's disease. Parkinson's disease is currently incurable and the life expectancy for patients is significantly reduced. The mean duration from disease onset (in patients younger than 75 years) was experimentally found to be approximately 9–10 years. Disturbances to motor function are caused by the progressive loss of a specific pathway in the basal ganglia of the brain, the so-called **nigrostriatal pathway (B)**. This is a dopaminergic pathway ascending from the substantia nigra to the corpus striatum. The substantia nigra has two important nuclei: the pars reticularis and the pars compacta. The inhibitory dopaminergic pathway arises in the pars compacta and sends ascending dopaminergic pathways to at least three nuclei in the corpus striatum. Through its inhibitory influence on those three nuclei in the striatum, the ascending dopaminergic pathway exerts an inhibitory tone on the extrapyramidal motor system. The extrapyramidal system 'fine tunes' voluntary movement, and the reduced function or absence of the nigrostriatal pathway unmasks the untempered efferent drive of the extrapyramidal system.

Dopamine, a catecholamine, is an important CNS neurotransmitter. It is the neurotransmitter of the nigrostriatal pathway, and this knowledge has resulted in the development of drugs used to restore an inhibitory influence on the extrapyramidal system. Theoretically, drugs can be developed that: (i) enhance dopamine synthesis and release from its nerve endings in the corpus striatum; (ii) mimic the action of dopamine through their binding to dopamine receptors on cells in the striatum (dopamine agonists); (iii) inhibit the breakdown of dopamine after it has been released from nerve endings; and (iv) inhibit the action of excitatory neurotransmitters of the extrapyramidal system. One such excitatory neurotransmitter is acetylcholine (B). The most frequently used drug is a dopamine agonist (see next spread).

Other approaches to treatment: Surgery is attempted to reduce extrapyramidal effects. Pallidotomy, which is removal of the globus pallidus in the basal ganglia, and electrical stimulation of both thalamic and subthalamic centres in the brain have been attempted, but the effectiveness of these surgical procedures, if any, remains unknown.

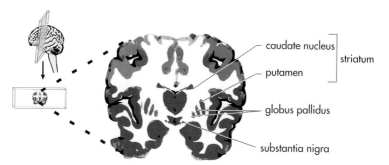

- caudate nucleus ⎤
  ⎬ striatum
- putamen ⎦
- globus pallidus
- substantia nigra

A. Some central components of the extrapyramidal system

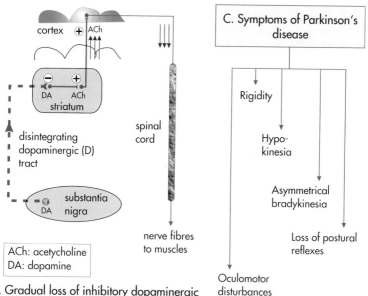

cortex ⊕ ACh

⊖ ⊕
DA   ACh
striatum

disintegrating
dopaminergic (D)
tract

substantia
DA   nigra

ACh: acetycholine
DA: dopamine

spinal
cord

nerve fibres
to muscles

B. Gradual loss of inhibitory dopaminergic
pathway in Parkinson's disease

C. Symptoms of Parkinson's
disease

Rigidity

Hypo-
kinesia

Asymmetrical
bradykinesia

Loss of postural
reflexes

Oculomotor
disturbances

60 Idiopathic Parkinson's disease II: Treatment I

Introduction: Current pharmacological approaches are: (i) dopaminergic drugs to replace or mimic dopamine in the brain and protect brain dopamine from enzymic degradation; and/or (ii) anticholinergic drugs such as **benzatropine** to reduce muscarinic cholinergic influence in the extrapyramidal system. Adjuvant therapy includes drugs to counteract the side-effects of the principal drug treatments. The most important drugs to achieve aim (i) are administration of **levodopa**, a precursor of dopamine, or of dopamine agonists such as **lisuride** or ropinirole, which act directly on striatal dopamine receptors. A supplementary strategy is the use of a monoamine oxidase B inhibitor (MAOI-B), notably **selegiline**, which blocks the enzymes that metabolise dopamine. **Entacapone** is an inhibitor of catechol-O-methyltransferase (COMT), which occurs in post-synaptic nerve terminals and breaks down dopamine. Drugs are not automatically prescribed when the disease is first identified, but only when symptoms interfere with the patient's everyday life. About 90–95% of patients respond well to treatment with drugs.

Levodopa is an amino acid that is the precursor of dopamine in the biosynthetic pathway. Levodopa is prescribed together with an extracerebral dopa-decarboxylase inhibitor (see opposite), which blocks the peripheral but not the central conversion of levodopa to dopamine, thus reducing the peripheral side-effects of dopamine, which include cardiovascular effects, and nausea and vomiting. The dopa-decarboxylase inhibitors used are **benserazide** and **carbidopa** and these are incorporated into oral tablets called **co-beneldopa** and **co-careldopa**, respectively. This combination is very useful in the treatment of older and frailer patients and those with other diseases. Treatment with levodopa is started with low doses and the dosage is ramped up very gradually; the aim is to keep doses as low as possible to limit side-effects, especially disorientation and confusion in older patients. Rigidity and tremor may be abolished completely at first by the drug.

Side-effects of levodopa: Unwanted effects on *first* taking the drug include nausea and anorexia, which can be treated with **domperidone**, a drug that blocks the peripheral actions of dopamine. Patients may experience central disturbances including nightmares, hallucinations, headaches, drowsiness and disorientation. Levodopa/dopa-decarboxylase inhibitor combinations have been reported to cause sudden sleep onset, which has serious implications for those who take the drugs and drive. *Longer-term effects*: more seriously, levodopa effectiveness and predictability of effect decrease with prolonged usage, and so-called on–off effects occur, when the patient suddenly loses the ability to move voluntarily in the middle of a movement and 'freezes'. Most patients on levodopa also develop dyskinesia; this involves unpleasant writhing movements of the face and limbs and can be severe. The dose of levodopa is reduced but this brings the reoccurrence of rigidity. Implicit in this is the fact that with time the effectiveness of a dose of levodopa decreases. In advanced Parkinson's disease, so-called 'end-of-dose' deterioration occurs when the duration of action of a given dose of levodopa is significantly reduced. This may be due not only to the loss of dopaminergic nerve endings in the striatum but also to extensive down-regulation of dopamine receptors. Attempts are made to counter end-of-dose deterioration by using prolonged-action preparations and selegiline with levodopa.

Contraindications to levodopa include breastfeeding, pregnancy and closed-angle glaucoma.

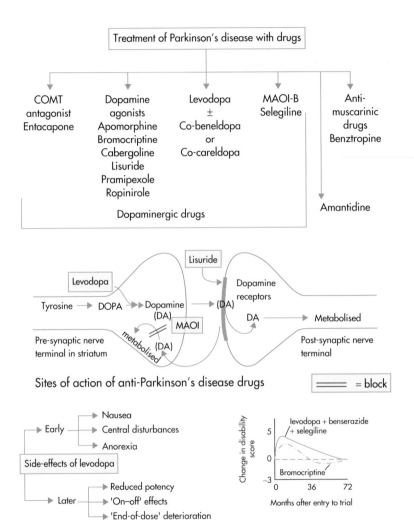

Treatment of Parkinson's disease with drugs

COMT antagonist
Entacapone

Dopamine agonists
Apomorphine
Bromocriptine
Cabergoline
Lisuride
Pramipexole
Ropinirole

Levodopa
±
Co-beneldopa
or
Co-careldopa

MAOI-B
Selegiline

Anti-muscarinic drugs
Benztropine

Dopaminergic drugs

Amantidine

Sites of action of anti-Parkinson's disease drugs

Tyrosine → DOPA ⇒ Dopamine (DA) → (DA)

Levodopa

Lisuride

Dopamine receptors

DA → Metabolised

MAOI

metabolised (DA)

Pre-synaptic nerve terminal in striatum

Post-synaptic nerve terminal

====== = block

Side-effects of levodopa

Early
- Nausea
- Central disturbances
- Anorexia

Later
- Reduced potency
- 'On–off' effects
- 'End-of-dose' deterioration

Change in disability score

levodopa + benserazide + selegiline

Bromocriptine

Months after entry to trial

Loss of drug potency with time (Adapted from Parkinson's Disease Research Group (*BMJ* 1993; **307**: 472))

61 Idiopathic Parkinson's disease III: Treatment II

Dopamine agonists bind to DA receptors in the basal ganglia, thus mimicking the action of endogenously released DA. They may be prescribed as alternative therapy to levodopa in newly diagnosed patients or together with levodopa; in some patients the combination may reduce the incidence of complications with treatment over the first 2–5 years. At least three different subtypes of DA receptors have been identified, namely D_1, D_2 and D_3. The more potent agonists and those with the longest duration of action, e.g. **pergolide**, bind to both D_1 and D_2 subtypes. **Lisuride**, with a shorter duration of action, binds mainly to D_1 receptors. **Bromocriptine** and **cabergoline** have similar therapeutic profiles. **Pramipexole** binds to D_2 and D_3 receptors. **Ropinirole**, a D_2 agonist, is useful in younger patients who are intolerant to levodopa. DA agonists may also be neuroprotective as antioxidants; there is increased oxidative stress in early Parkinson's disease, and if this is so then DA agonists would be logical choices in the early stages of the disease. **Apomorphine**, a very powerful DA agonist, is used during 'off' periods that occur after prolonged use of levodopa. It is an emetic, is difficult to use, demands much patient education regarding its effects and, ideally, should be used under close medical supervision. The biggest problem for the patient is nausea, which may be controlled with domperidone.

Side effects and contraindications of DA agonists: The CSM has advised that patients should be screened for electrolytes, urea and ESR, and should have chest X-rays and lung function tests before taking ergot-based DA agonists. This is because these drugs are associated with pulmonary, pericardial and retroperitoneal fibrotic reactions. As with levodopa/dopa-decarboxylase inhibitors, DA agonists cause sudden sleep reactions and daytime sleepiness. They are also associated with psychotic reactions, including hallucinations. Several of these drugs are contraindicated in pregnancy, breastfeeding and patients with coronary insufficiency, a history of fibrotic reactions or psychotic disorders, and in those with a history of pituitary tumour.

Selegiline is an MAO inhibitor specific for MAOI-B. When used as monotherapy, selegiline may delay the need to start patients on levodopa. It does, however, provide limited symptomatic relief. It is often prescribed together with levodopa either with or without a dopa-decarboxylase inhibitor, which allows the dose of levodopa to be reduced.

Adverse effects, precautions and contraindications: There are reports of unexplained, increased mortality in patients on combined levodopa/selegiline therapy. Orthostatic hypotension has been tentatively suggested as a cause, and selegiline is contraindicated in patients with orthostatic hypotension because of the risk of falls.

> **Prescriber's note:** These adverse effects of selegiline may be related to dose, and a newer, buccally absorbed preparation of selegiline has enabled the dosage to be reduced considerably.

Entacapone inhibits DA breakdown through the peripheral inhibition of COMT. It is prescribed together with levodopa. Entacapone may increase the 'on' periods with levodopa, and decrease the 'off' times; the dose of levodopa could thus be reduced with entacapone. **Adverse effects** include discoloured urine, dyskinesias, dizziness, GIT upsets and, rarely, hepatitis. **Contraindications** include pregnancy, breastfeeding and phaeochromocytoma (epinephrine-secreting tumour).

Clinical scenario: A 63-year-old woman was referred by her GP to a consultant neurologist, complaining of tremor in both hands, especially the right hand, and that she felt 'slower'. On examination she had no evidence of postural instability, but had a typical parkinsonian tremor of the right hand, a positive glabellar tap (persistent reflex blinking when tapping the glabellar bone between the eyebrows), and cogwheel rigidity in the right upper limb and neck muscles. The consultant diagnosed early Parkinson's disease and prescribed a dopamine agonist, ropinirole, starting with 0.25 mg three times a day for 1 week, thereafter increasing the dose gradually over succeeding weeks. The consultant saw the patient about 18 months later, and noted that she was responding well to the ropinirole, and that she was somewhat more bradykinetic. The tremor was worse and he recommended that the patient remain on ropinirole and start Madopar, a proprietary combination of levodopa and the decarboxylase inhibitor benserazide. He also arranged consultation with the specialist Parkinson's nurse.

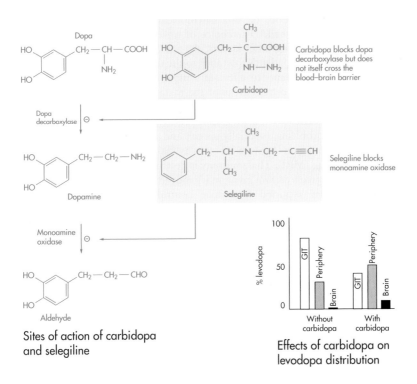

Sites of action of carbidopa and selegiline

Effects of carbidopa on levodopa distribution

62 Idiopathic Parkinson's disease IV: Treatment III

Amantadine was originally developed as a treatment for influenza but is now used to treat Parkinson's disease. It may work by stimulating DA release from the nerve terminal and possibly also by preventing re-uptake of DA into the nerve terminal after its release. Thus, the efficacy of amantidine will decrease with progressive loss of dopaminergic nerve terminals in the striatum. There is still uncertainty about its usefulness. It has been used as monotherapy in the early stages in patients who cannot tolerate levodopa, and it may counteract the levodopa-induced dyskinesias in some patients with advanced disease.

Adverse effects and contraindications: Amantadine is associated with dizziness, blurred vision, GIT upsets, oedema and livedo reticularis (discoloured skin). It is contraindicated in patients with epilepsy, a history of gastric ulceration, renal disease and in women who are pregnant or breastfeeding.

Anticholinergic drugs: These block the action of acetylcholine (ACh) at its receptors in the cholinergic systems, particularly in the striatum of the extrapyramidal system, thus reducing its tremorigenic influence. Examples include **benzatropine, orphenadrine** and **procyclidine**. Given the widespread distribution of ACh systems in the body, these drugs are associated with many adverse effects, including the exacerbation of psychiatric problems in patients, and are now rarely used.

A treatment guideline for the pharmacological management of Parkinson's disease has been published.[9] The choice of treatment, however, will need to take into account, among other factors, the age of the patient, the severity of the symptoms and the patient's tolerance to the drugs.

Surgery: Earlier attempts to alleviate symptoms of Parkinson's disease by surgical destruction of certain areas of the thalamus and the globus pallidus with liquid nitrogen, or deep brain electrical stimulation of these areas, were hit-and-miss operations with worsening of existing symptoms, and introduction of new problems, especially speech and gait difficulties, but they are now being used again because of the availability of CT and magnetic resonance imaging (MRI). **Thalamotomy** is destruction of a precise area of the thalamus that controls certain involuntary movements. In one study, unilateral thalamotomy was reported to reduce contralateral tremor and rigidity significantly for at least 8 years.[10] **Thalamic stimulation** appears to be effective and relatively safe in reducing drug-resistant tremor and may have fewer adverse effects than thalamotomy.[11] **Pallidotomy** is destruction of the globus pallidus internus (GPi; B), the neurons of which discharge abnormally in patients with Parkinson's disease, and is the most frequently used surgical procedure. The main long-lasting beneficial effect reported is the removal of contralateral dyskinesias. Unilateral **GPi stimulation** is reported to improve motor performance in some patients, but data are still relatively scarce.[12] Modern unilateral **subthalamic nucleus stimulation** has been reported to be safer than when originally introduced, and is of comparable efficacy to GPi stimulation in the management of advanced Parkinson's disease.

The advances in imaging and surgical techniques have restored the hope that these operations will give patients relief from symptoms, greatly reducing the incidence of adverse effects, and may eventually lead to more sophisticated treatments, e.g. the use of stem cell therapy.

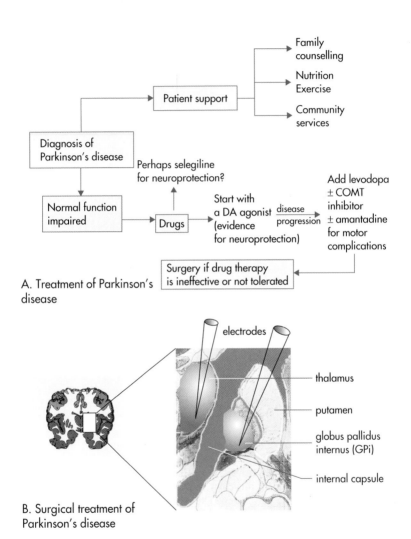

A. Treatment of Parkinson's disease

B. Surgical treatment of Parkinson's disease

63 Epilepsy I: Introduction

Epilepsy is characterised by recurrent seizures. It may be idiopathic or caused by structural brain damage. It is important to distinguish seizure occurrence and epilepsy. Seizures are clinical manifestations of inappropriate and abnormally high stimulation of an area of cortical neurons and may be 'one-off' attacks. Epilepsy is a **chronic** disorder. Two main patterns of epileptic electrical discharges occur: (i) discharges arising from focal cortical disturbances, called **partial seizures**, and (ii) synchronous electrical discharges over both hemispheres, called **generalised seizures**. Partial seizures have been further sub-classified as **simple** and **complex**. Many different forms of epilepsy exist and attempts have been made to classify these (see opposite).

Partial seizures: EEG patterns generated during **simple partial seizures** commonly begin in the frontal or temporal lobes of the cortex. Immediately before the seizure there may be an aura reflecting the functional role of that part of the cortex. Patients may experience unpleasant smells and tastes, rising epigastric sensations and psychotic episodes. The patient remains conscious and cognitive ability may be unimpaired. Partial seizures may spread and become generalised. **Complex partial seizures** are distinguished from simple seizures by varying degrees of loss of consciousness. They may start as simple partial seizures, usually originating in the temporal lobe, but progress to more severe symptoms, including complete loss of consciousness. During these attacks, conscious patients may display so-called ictal automatisms, which include stereotyped behaviour such as compulsive fidgeting, lip-smacking or facial contortion. Patients may inadvertently get themselves into trouble in public places through antisocial behaviour. It is believed that ictal automatism (automatic movements during a brain seizure) and impaired consciousness may be due to electrical discharges arising in the limbic system. During the post-ictal period patients are often confused.

The electrical waves that cause a **generalised seizure** are thought to arise as a primary discharge in the brain-stem reticular formation that rises to the thalamus, from where it is relayed to the cortex. The EEG during a generalised seizure is characterised by a spike–wave discharge that may be generated by over-activity of slow calcium currents in the thalamus.

At the onset of a **major generalised seizure** the patient collapses to the ground unconscious, with muscle spasms. During the tonic phase, lips and skin become blue (cyanosed) through lack of respiration. There may be reflex bowel and bladder emptying. The clonic or convulsive phase follows, when the unconscious patient exhibits generalised rhythmic spasms and may bite the tongue severely. This is followed by a period of coma during which the patient gradually rises to full consciousness, but is confused, and experiences headache and the painful aftermath of muscular spasm and a bitten tongue. The patient will be lethargic and may fall asleep. The patient usually regains consciousness within 1 hour of onset of the seizure.

Absence seizures are suffered by children, and may be **typical** or **atypical**. Atypical seizures are relatively prolonged and occur usually because of pre-existing brain damage. The child loses contact with the world around him or her and ceases any activity. Typical absence seizures are less common and less prolonged than atypical seizures, and usually consist of frequent, momentary loss of contact with the surroundings.

Status epilepticus is the occurrence of successive seizures without recovery of consciousness. It has to be treated as an emergency because it could be fatal or cause permanent damage.

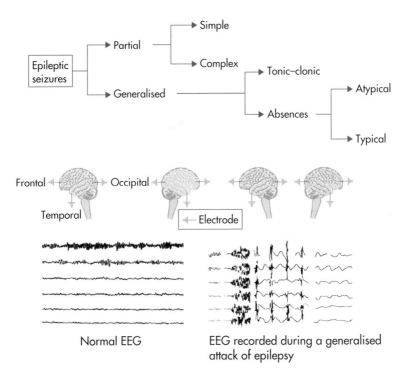

Normal EEG

EEG recorded during a generalised attack of epilepsy

Clinical scenario: A typical absence may present with daily, brief and intermittent reduced or absent awareness, blinking or twitching of eyelids, activity arrested, automatic facial movements, e.g. chewing, lip-smacking, and mycoclonic jerks. Patients may drop with an atonic seizure, and a prone patient may appear 'blank'. A complex partial seizure may feature only loss of awareness. Other prodromes (initial symptoms before the attack) may include cardiovascular symptoms such as tachycardia or arrhythmias. There may be chest pain or transient complete heart block. Sleep disorders may present, such as obstructive sleep apnoea and narcolepsy. The patient may experience a panic attack, and feel anxiety and fear with consequent lightheadedness and orofacial paraesthesiae ('pins and needles'). It may be difficult to distinguish an epileptic fit from symptoms produced by, for example, head injury or by a non-epileptic attack disorder ('pseudoseizures').

64 Epilepsy II: Occurrence and implications of epilepsy

Worldwide, epilepsy is the second most prevalent neurological disorder after stroke, and affects approximately 1% of the world's population.[13] Epilepsy affects a significant proportion of the population in the UK. It has been found that at least 30 000 people develop epilepsy every year, and about 1 in 25 people will experience a form of seizure at least once during his or her lifetime. There is some evidence for epidemiological studies showing that men are slightly more prone to epilepsy than women.

Seizures may occur in neonates, children and adolescents, and adults. Causes of **neonatal onset** of seizures include: (i) asphyxia, hypoxia or intracranial trauma or haemorrhage during delivery; (ii) congenital brain malformation; (iii) electrolyte or metabolic disturbances; and (iv) infection. During **childhood** and **adolescence**, seizures may be precipitated by, in addition to the above: (i) brain tumours; (ii) cerebral degenerative diseases or cerebral palsy; (iii) chemical toxicity, e.g. lead or drugs; (iv) febrile convulsions; (v) hydrocephalus; (vi) idiopathic (unknown) brain changes; (vii) other diseases, e.g. kidney disease; or (viii) Lennox–Gastaut syndrome, which is a severe form of childhood epilepsy where the patient suffers several different seizure types – this usually manifests itself between the ages of 3 and 5, and rarely occurs before the age of 2 and after the age of 8 years. In **adults**, epilepsy may be caused by a number of the causes listed above, as well as by: (i) cerebral degenerative disease; (ii) cerebral vascular disease, e.g. infarction; (iii) drug abuse and withdrawal, including alcohol; and (iv) idiopathic (unknown) origin.

Drugs may precipitate seizures (**A**). Some general anaesthetics, antibiotics, anti-depressants and endocrine agents (e.g. insulin) may be epileptogenic in some patients.

Prognosis: The prognosis in epilepsy is considered to be good, in that between 70 and 80% of treated patients will eventually become free of seizures. Treatment is usually stopped if patients remain seizure free for 3–5 years. Relapses are more likely to occur within the first year after cessation of drug treatment. There is evidence that the more serious the case of epilepsy was, or the longer it had been left untreated before the initiation of drug treatment, the greater the risk of a relapse after remission. The risk of a relapse is also greater in cases of juvenile myoclonic epilepsy or in patients in whom there are brain lesions that cause the seizures. A minority of patients may be resistant to treatment and develop chronic active epilepsy. In these patients, the prognosis is generally poor, and they may develop other neurological or psychological problems.

The **social implications** of epilepsy are potentially serious for adults who suffer recurrent seizures, especially if they decide to discontinue treatment. For example, patients who drive and experience a relapse after discontinuing drug treatment risk losing their driving licence, which could have serious consequences if driving is an important part of employment. A history of epilepsy makes a young person's chances of gaining employment difficult; some employers prefer an employee to be on medication, whereas others will offer employment only if the prospective employee is off all medication. Social interactions are inevitably affected by epilepsy. Activities such as driving, working with hazardous machinery or chemicals, or pastimes such as rock climbing, which involve a degree of personal risk, are sometimes 'off-limits', especially if the person is not on medication. These strictures are often frustrating for people who are otherwise active and eager to play a normal part in society.

Clinical scenario: In about 40% of cases, epilepsy and epileptic-like seizures have an identifiable cause. These causes include brain damage during intrauterine life or perinatally, infection, brain tumours, postnatal trauma to the head and inadvertent surgical causes. Seizures may appear as part of the aetiology of diseases such as hepatic disease, chronic alcoholism and hypoglycaemia. They may be induced iatrogenically during treatment with, for example, psychotropic drugs during the progression of neurodegenerative diseases. The correct choice of treatment depends on an accurate diagnosis. Accurate identification of seizure cause is essential since it will determine the choice of treatment, and EEG and neuroimaging are important tools, as well as a thorough patient history.

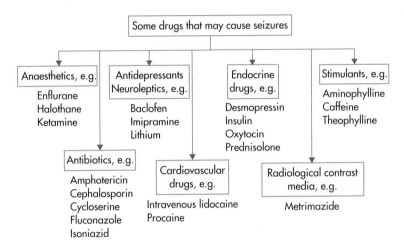

A. Some drugs that may cause seizures

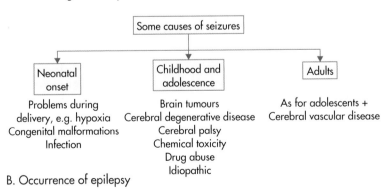

B. Occurrence of epilepsy

65 Epilepsy III: Theories of brain mechanisms underlying seizures: the basis of drug action

Partial seizures arise mainly in the amygdala and hippocampus of the limbic system, and in the neocortex. An upset in the neuronal systems using glutamate, the principal excitatory brain neurotransmitter, and γ-aminobutyric acid (GABA), the principal inhibitory brain neurotransmitter, may be important in the generation and propagation of seizure activity. Also important is synchronous neuronal discharge among synaptically connected neurons of, for example, pyramidal neurons of the cortex; such a network must be of sufficient critical mass to propagate an electrical wave over a wider area.

The anatomical localisation of susceptible neuronal networks is still being worked out and many data point to (i) the neocortical pyramidal cells, which project to distant neuronal systems, and (ii) interneurons, e.g. basket cells, which play an important role in the feedback inhibition of pyramidal cell activity.

Receptor mechanisms underlying this synchronous electrical discharge almost certainly include glutamate and GABAergic receptors. Widespread inhibition of GABA-mediated inhibitory synapses coupled with paradoxical switching of GABAergic inhibitory synapses, which operate through the $GABA_A$ receptor, to excitatory ones may facilitate the epileptogenic spread of activity. The post-synaptic $GABA_A$ receptor has binding sites for GABA itself, barbiturates, benzodiazepines, Zn^{2+} ions and convulsant drugs such as picrotoxin. $GABA_A$ receptors hyperpolarise the membrane through Cl^- ion influx. The pre-synaptic $GABA_B$ receptor is linked to second messenger systems through which it presumably inhibits further neurotransmitter release. $GABA_B$ agonists such as baclofen have been reported to exacerbate seizures, presumably by blocking GABA release.

There are at least two main inotropic subtypes of the glutamate receptor, which mediate fast synaptic transmission, ionotropic receptors and meta-botropic, which mediate slower synaptic transmission. These were identified through the ions that mediate their depolarisation and the substances that bind them. Thus, ionotropic receptor subclasses use Na^+ inflow and K^+ outflow for membrane depolarisation and bind NMDA, kainate and α-amino-2, 3-dihydro-5-methyl-3-oxo-4-isoxazolepropanoic acid (AMPA). NMDA receptors also possess a Ca^{2+} channel that may mediate Ca^{2+}-mediated neuronal damage in status epilepticus. Metabotropic receptors modulate synaptic activity through the activation of intracellular cyclic AMP and inositol phosphate second messenger systems. These receptor types, as well as GABA and glutamate transporters on neuronal and glial cells, are possible targets for drug development. A fundamental ionic event appears to be an early, abnormally large rise in extracellular potassium, which would lower the threshold for firing; the rise is, however, relatively slow and other ionic mechanisms presumably contribute to the spread of **electrical activity to other** brain areas. It has been suggested that so-called 're-entrant' and localised loops of electrical circuits may cause partial seizures.

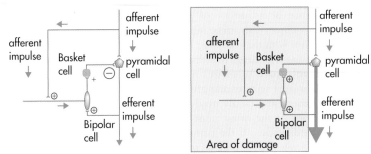

Effect of brain damage on pyramidal cell discharges

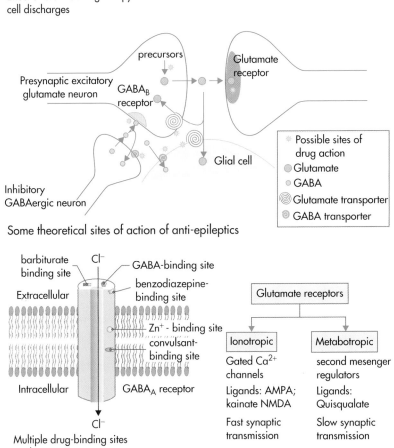

Some theoretical sites of action of anti-epileptics

Possible sites of drug action
- Glutamate
- GABA
- Glutamate transporter
- GABA transporter

Multiple drug-binding sites on the $GABA_A$ receptor

Glutamate receptors	
Ionotropic	**Metabotropic**
Gated Ca^{2+} channels	second mesenger regulators
Ligands: AMPA; kainate NMDA	Ligands: Quisqualate
Fast synaptic transmission	Slow synaptic transmission

Drugs are not commonly prescribed for a single, apparently unprovoked seizure, except when a grossly abnormal EEG accompanies the seizure, or if there is evidence or a history of structural brain damage. Seizures have occurred, for example, with stress, febrile states and sleep deprivation, and after excessive sessions with the computer. The issue is controversial, and some now treat a first seizure with drugs to reduce the probability of a subsequent seizure.

Treatment with drugs: When treatment, is started, monotherapy is advisable. The aim is to prevent seizures and provide the patient with as normal a lifestyle as possible. Patient and family needs must be addressed. Adverse effects and contraindications of the drugs must be explained. The choice of drugs will depend on the diagnosis. If the patient reacts badly to the first drug chosen, another appropriate drug should be prescribed. If the first drug prescribed does not prevent a second seizure despite increasing the dose, it is unlikely that another will work. In that case, the patient should be reassessed.

Partial seizures: Commonly used starting drugs include carbamazepine (often as a controlled-release preparation), lamotrigine, sodium valproate and topiramate. All of these drugs may be prescribed once or twice daily. Newer drugs for partial seizures include levetiracetam, oxcarbazepine, which can also be used for tonic–clonic seizures, and tiagabine. Gabapentin may be prescribed as adjunct therapy for both partial and secondary generalised seizures.

Adverse effects: Carbamazepine and lamotrigine are both associated with headaches, nausea and skin rashes, and are teratogenic. Carbamazepine may cause diplopia (double vision) and dizziness, and lamotrigine may cause insomnia. Sodium valproate is associated with hair loss, tremor and weight gain, and topiramate with cognitive slowing, kidney stones, sedation and weight loss. Both sodium valproate and topiramate are teratogenic. Gabapentin, levetiracetam, oxcarbazepine and tiagabine all cause neurological problems. Gabapentin may cause weight gain and altered liver function. (See the BNF for a more comprehensive list of adverse effects.)

Precautions and contraindications: Carbamazepine is contraindicated in patients with a history of bone marrow depression, porphyria and if there are AV conduction abnormalities, unless the patient is paced. Precautions are needed if there is a history of haematological reactions to drugs, or of liver or skin disorders. Patients must not be withdrawn suddenly from carbamazepine (or from anti-epileptics generally, unless unavoidable) due to the danger of seizures. As with many other anti-epileptics, precautions are necessary in the event of pregnancy and breastfeeding. Patients on lamotrigine should be monitored for clotting, hepatic and renal parameters. Topiramate is definitely contraindicated in breastfeeding, and patients on topiramate should be adequately hydrated, especially if there is a history of renal disease. Topiramate is associated with acute myopia and secondary angle-closure glaucoma. If raised intraocular pressure is detected, the drug should be withdrawn as quickly as possible without precipitating a seizure and steps taken to reduce intraocular pressure. Sodium valproate is contraindicated in patients with active liver disease, a family history of liver disease and porphyria. It is associated with occasional fatal hepatic failure in young children. It should be used with caution, if at all, in patients with SLE, or who are breastfeeding.

Case scenario: A 17-year-old schoolboy experienced, for the first time, a generalised tonic–clonic seizure while studying for examinations; his GP put it down to sleep deprivation and suggested that it might be an isolated event. Three years later, after starting a degree course in medicine, the patient suffered another tonic–clonic seizure. A 30-minute EEG was normal and metabolic tests were also normal, and so carbamazepine was prescribed. The seizures recurred and the patient was referred to a local epilepsy unit where a 3-hour EEG revealed a brief generalised 3–4 Hz spike-and-wave discharge, which is characteristic of juvenile myoclonic epilepsy. The carbamazepine was stopped and sodium valproate prescribed instead. The patient has suffered no further seizures since then and has tolerated the valproic acid well.

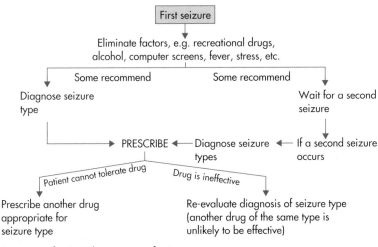

Strategies for initial treatment of seizures

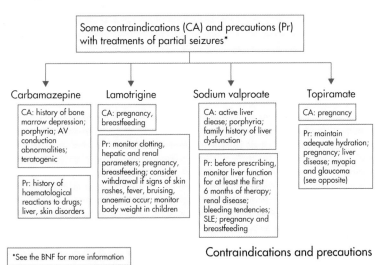

*See the BNF for more information

Contraindications and precautions

Several drugs used to prevent partial seizures are also used for **tonic–clonic (generalised) seizures**. These include **carbamazepine, lamotrigine** and **sodium valproate**.

Phenytoin has for many years been the most widely prescribed drug for epilepsy, but its popularity is waning due to the introduction of newer, safer drugs and because of its unpleasant adverse effects (see opposite). Phenytoin has zero-order kinetics, which means that the rate of metabolism of the drug is independent of its concentration. In other words, a toxic blood concentration is metabolised at the same rate as a very low concentration. Furthermore, there is not a linear response between daily dose and steady-state plasma concentrations (see opposite). Phenytoin is strongly bound to plasma proteins and will displace other drugs such as aspirin from their binding sites. It also induces the liver enzymes that metabolise other drugs, e.g. hydrocortisone, oral contraceptives, theophylline, tricyclic antidepressants and thyroxine, among others. Well-known **adverse effects** of phenytoin include gum hypertrophy, greasy skin and hirsutism, skin rashes, macrocytic anaemia through folic acid deficiency and lymph node enlargement. Phenytoin is still used intravenously for status epilepticus (page 138).

Phenobarbital, a barbiturate, was the first drug available for epilepsy, but is rarely used because of its neurotoxicity. A major discouragement to its use is its deleterious effects on cognition, alertness and mood. It is still widely used in developing countries because of its relatively low cost. Phenobarbital enhances the action of GABA by binding to the $GABA_A$ receptor (page 131).

Benzodiazepines such as **clobazam, clonazepam** and **diazepam** are effective in controlling all forms of seizures, and are believed to act via the $GABA_A$ receptor (page 131). They cause sedation and are associated with a severe withdrawal syndrome, which may include the precipitation of epileptic seizures. **Lorazepam** is used to treat status asthmaticus.

Newer anti-epileptic drugs for tonic–clonic seizures include **oxcarbazepine** (page 132).

Management of chronic epilepsy: The minority of patients who do not become seizure free after drug treatment but continue to suffer seizures are usually difficult to treat. The patients are demoralised and need the active involvement of organisational services. With drugs, monotherapy should be aimed for but some patients will need combinations of two drugs. It may be difficult to find the optimal combinations and dose regimens. Good control with drug combinations may be difficult due to poor patient compliance, adverse reactions and longer-term toxicity. When tackling the chronic epileptic: (i) it is essential at first to review thoroughly the previous history of diagnosis, drug treatment, compliance and seizure occurrence; (ii) all previous adverse effects and known drug interactions for this patient must be known before treatment; (iii) drug and dose will be chosen on the basis of this history, e.g. a drug may have been previously prescribed too low a dose; (iv) ensure that patients do not continue to draw on existing home stocks of previously used anti-epileptic drugs; (v) do not withdraw patients too quickly from currently used anti-epileptic drugs, especially barbiturates, benzodiazepines or carbamazepine; (vi) if seizures continue to occur despite the use of maximal doses compatible with patient tolerance, then there should be an investigation of compliance, including serum drug measurements, tablet counts, and patient and family counselling, and possibly the switching to another, previously untried drug; and (vii) if none of the above helps, surgery may be considered.

Clinical scenario: A 50-year-old man with a history of alcohol abuse, already well known to Accident and Emergency, was admitted with tremor, anxiety, palpitations and sweating. He had recently binged on alcohol, but due to circumstance had not drunk alcohol in the previous 36 hours. During his initial assessment he became very abusive and attempted to assault the charge nurse. Shortly afterwards he sustained two seizures, the second of which was terminated by administration of intravenous diazepam (Diazemuls). Following this, he slept soundly for 6 hours, snoring loudly. His airways were however, deemed patent and normal oxygen saturations were maintained on air. Blood tests were relatively normal and he was given maintenance fluids and intravenous Pabrinex (ascorbic acid, anhydrous glucose, nicotinamide, pyridoxine HCl, riboflavin and thiamine HCl). He was also started on a reducing regimen of chlodiazepoxide.

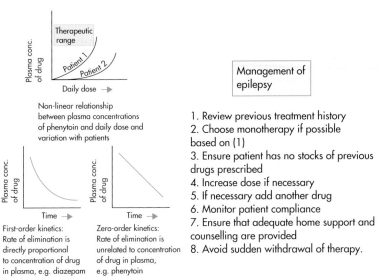

Non-linear relationship between plasma concentrations of phenytoin and daily dose and variation with patients

First-order kinetics: Rate of elimination is directly proportional to concentration of drug in plasma, e.g. diazepam

Zero-order kinetics: Rate of elimination is unrelated to concentration of drug in plasma, e.g. phenytoin

Phenytoin pharmacokinetics, make dose management difficult

Management of epilepsy

1. Review previous treatment history
2. Choose monotherapy if possible based on (1)
3. Ensure patient has no stocks of previous drugs prescribed
4. Increase dose if necessary
5. If necessary add another drug
6. Monitor patient compliance
7. Ensure that adequate home support and counselling are provided
8. Avoid sudden withdrawal of therapy.

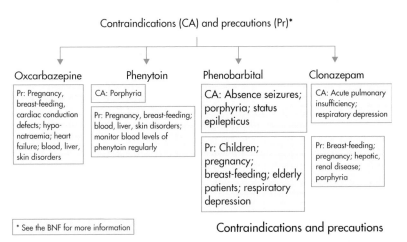

Contraindications (CA) and precautions (Pr)*

Oxcarbazepine

Pr: Pregnancy, breast-feeding, cardiac conduction defects; hypo-natraemia; heart failure; blood, liver, skin disorders

Phenytoin

CA: Porphyria

Pr: Pregnancy, breast-feeding; blood, liver, skin disorders; monitor blood levels of phenytoin regularly

Phenobarbital

CA: Absence seizures; porphyria; status epilepticus

Pr: Children; pregnancy; breast-feeding; elderly patients; respiratory depression

Clonazepam

CA: Acute pulmonary insufficiency; respiratory depression

Pr: Breast-feeding; pregnancy; hepatic, renal disease; porphyria

* See the BNF for more information

Contraindications and precautions

Treatment of paediatric epilepsy: Children may suffer absence seizures, previously termed 'petit mal'. Here, ethosuximide is the main drug for treatment of absence seizures and has displaced trimethadone, which is associated with hypersensitivity reactions and sedation. Zonisamide, a newer drug, is also effective for treatment of absence seizures. Ethosuximide and zonisamide may exert their anti-epileptic effects by blocking T-type Ca^{2+} channels, and ethosuximide may also affect both Na^+ and K^+ currents.

Adverse effects of ethosuximide include various neurological disorders such as psychoses, night terrors, sleep disturbances, aggressiveness, hyperactivity, ataxia, dizziness, depression and mild euphoria. Rare haematological disorders include agranulocytosis and aplastic anaemia. Precautions with ethosuximide include liver and kidney disorders, porphyria and breastfeeding. Other drugs that may be tried for absence seizures include lamotrigine for atypical seizures and sodium valproate. Acetazolamide, a carbonic anhydrase inhibitor, may help absence seizures.

Note: Drugs that should not be used for absence seizures include phenobarbital, phenytoin, and primidone. The NICE have published guidelines for prescribing newer anti-epileptic drugs in children (see opposite).

Treatment of the elderly: Most cases first presenting in old age are partial, with or without secondary generalisation. Most have been treated with sodium valproate. Physiological changes with ageing affect drug action, especially pharmacokinetics. **Absorption:** reduced GIT motility delays gastric emptying, and acid output from gastric parietal cells is reduced, which enhances absorption of more basic drugs and impairs absorption of more acidic drugs. Diminished cardiac output reduces splanchnic blood flow, which could decrease the functional absorptive area of the alimentary tract. **Distribution:** drug distribution is a function of the drug's physicochemical properties. With ageing, lean body mass declines and fatty tissue increases, resulting in a higher apparent volume of distribution of lipophilic drugs, e.g. carbamazepine, diazepam and phenytoin, with attendant dangers of toxicity. Hydrophilic drugs such as gabapentin will have a lower volume of distribution. Another factor is the reduction of plasma proteins such as albumin, which bind drugs and keep them circulating and inactive. By the age of 80 years, plasma albumin is 20% lower and, because albumin binds, for example, phenobarbital, phenytoin and sodium valproate, the unbound and therefore pharmacologically active circulating concentrations of these drugs could be toxic at doses considered safe in younger patients, given their zero-order kinetics of elimination. Renal mass is reduced in the elderly, and this will affect the clearance of drugs such as gabapentin and vigabatrin, which are excreted mainly by the kidneys.

Treatment of elderly patients usually requires lowering of the dose of an anti-epileptic drug, although this is not a hard-and-fast rule. Although sodium valproate is often prescribed for elderly patients, there are insufficient data to support this general rule, although some analyses suggest that the drug is as effective as carbamazepine, phenobarbital and phenytoin in preventing both partial and generalised seizures.

Metabolism and elimination: Hepatic clearance of drugs and liver enzyme activity are both reduced in elderly patients. This will reduce the rate of clearance of drugs such as phenytoin, which could have serious consequences.

Clinical scenario: A 69-year-old man was admitted to hospital following a seizure at home. One year before, he had sustained a stroke that had affected his right arm, right leg and speech. He made a good functional recovery and continued on aspirin, atenolol and simvastatin. Over the 6 weeks preceding admission he had noticed self-terminating episodes when his right arm started shaking. This progressed to attacks where, instead of self-terminating, the shaking was followed by tonic–clonic seizures. On assessment at hospital he was drowsy and post-ictal but there were no other localising neurological symptoms. A CT scan revealed an area of infarction in his left cerebral cortex and he was diagnosed with post-stroke epilepsy. He was prescribed 300 mg sodium valproate twice a day and was discharged. Three months later he still complained of periodic right arm shaking and the dose was increased.

NICE guidance on anti-epileptic drugs for children (abridged)[14]

1. Gabapentin, lamotrigine, oxcarbazepine, tiagabine, topiramate and vigabatrin are recommended for children who have not benefitted from older drugs, who cannot tolerate them or who are near to or at child-bearing age

2. Vigabatrin is recommended as first-line therapy for management of infantile spasms (West's syndrome)

3. Monotherapy if possible, trying different drugs, taking precautions during change overs

4. Combination therapy only if monotherapy fails to control seizure activity; if unsuccessful, revert to monotherapy or combination therapy previously known to help the child

5. In girls of child-bearing potential, risks to unborn child and with concomitant oral contraceptives must be discussed with girl and/or carer

6. Occurrence of the first non-febrile seizure requires early examination by a specialist to ensure precise and early diagnosis and appropriate treatment

7. Treatment should be reviewed regularly to prevent maintenance for long periods on ineffective or poorly tolerated drugs and to ensure compliance

8. Recommendations on treatment choice and importance of regular monitoring is the same for children with specific needs, e.g. learning problems, as for the general population of epileptic children

NICE guidance on anti-epileptics in children

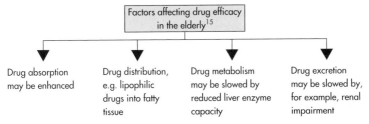

Effects of ageing on pharmacokinetics

69 Epilepsy VII: Treatment IV

Status epilepticus is the persistence of recurrent or prolonged tonic–clonic seizures for 30 minutes or more. A tonic–clonic seizure that persists for 5 minutes or more should be taken as status epilepticus and treated as such immediately, since it is more amenable to treatment in the earlier stages. Tonic–clonic status epilepticus occurs most frequently in: (i) children; (ii) patients with structural damage in the frontal lobe; and (iii) mentally ill patients. It can be precipitated in epileptic patients by, for example: (i) metabolic disorders; (ii) drug withdrawal; (iii) underlying disease progression; and (iv) intercurrent illness. The incidence of tonic–clonic status epilepticus in the UK is estimated at about 18–30 cases per 100 000 people, and about 9000–14 000 new cases are diagnosed each year. Approximately 5% of adult epileptic patients will suffer at least one episode of tonic–clonic status epilepticus, and the probability of an episode in children is at least double that in adults.

Patient treatment in tonic–clonic status must be initiated rapidly because of the danger of cerebral damage through excitoxicity (neural damage through excessive excitatory neurotransmitter release), hypoxia and ischaemia, and is tackled in stages:

Stage 1 (within the first 10 minutes): the airways are secured, oxygen administered because hypoxia is common and cardiopulmonary resuscitation performed if necessary.

Stage 2 (within the first 30 minutes): intravenous lines should be established for emergency anticonvulsant therapy and fluid replacement. Larger veins are chosen to avoid thrombosis and phlebitis, caused by several anti-epileptic drugs at the site of injection. Drugs must not be mixed but administered at different sites. Blood pressure, pulse rate, ECG, biochemical parameters, pH, clotting and other haematological parameters are monitored as well as liver and kidney function. Glucose is administered only if there is hypoglycaemia. Glucose must be used with caution as it may precipitate Wernicke's encephalopathy in patients with alcoholism. Glucose administered to normoglycaemic patients may aggravate nerve damage. A benzodiazepine such as lorazepam is usually administered intravenously and the dose repeated if the first dose does not stop the seizure. Ventilation will be required in patients with respiratory failure.

Stage 3 (established status epilepticus from 30 to 90 minutes): this stage is defined as that when tonic–clonic status epilepticus persists despite early treatment, and the patient should be transferred to intensive care. Three main drug regimens may be followed: intravenous loading doses of phenytoin, fosphenytoin or sub-anaesthetic doses of phenobarbital, followed by repeated intravenous or oral administration. Combination therapy with diazepam for fast onset and phenytoin for prolonged action may be attempted by some practitioners. Patients suffering postoperative or severe complicated status epilepticus should be given general anaesthesia.

Stage 4 (after 60–90 minutes – refractory status epilepticus): this stage is associated with high morbidity and a generally poor prognosis. Ventilation is usually necessary, and intravenous propofol or thiopental is commonly used, as is continuous infusion of midazolam.

Non-pharmacological therapy in epilepsy includes patient education on relaxation, avoidance of seizure-precipitating stimuli, e.g. computer games, biofeedback, which is the positive reinforcement by patients of 12–15 Hz EEG activity in the cortical sensory motor regions, exercise and diet, e.g. the ketogenic diet (high fat, low carbohydrate).

Clinical scenario: A 42-year-old woman was brought into casualty after suffering a generalised tonic–clonic seizure. The patient was unresponsive. Her husband reported that she had a long history of post-traumatic seizures that were managed with phenobarbital and phenytoin. In casualty the patient suffered another seizure and intravenous lorazepam was administered to a total of 7.5 mg but the seizure continued. The airways were patent and vital signs were normal. The patient was given a rapid infusion of fosphenytoin (1 g over 10 minutes) and another infusion of 500 mg fosphenytoin over 5 minutes. This stopped the seizure and the patient was stable but unresponsive. The patient was transferred to the intensive care unit where metabolic, cardiopulmonary and toxicology tests were negative, and the patient was found to have low blood levels of both phenytoin and phenobarbital. The patient regained consciousness within 4 hours without any evidence of ill-effects from the seizure. She was advised to comply with prescribed dose regimens for her medication and discharged the following day.

Stage 1* (0 – 10 minutes)	Stage 2* (within 30 minutes patient hospitalised)	Stage 3* (0 – 60/90 minutes – established SE)	Stage 4* (30 – 90 minutes – refractory SE)
Secure airways Administer oxygen Cardiopulmonary resuscitation	Intravenous lines established for drug administration of, for example, lorazepam or lidocaine if attack persists General anaesthesia for patients with post-operative or severe complicated SE	Determine aetiology Transfer to intensive care if attack persists and administer sub-anaesthetic phenobarbital or phenytoin or fosphenytoin Initiate pressor therapy if indicated	Transfer to intensive care Intracranial pressure monitoring Continuous midazolam infusion or intravenous propofol or thiopental Put patient on to long-term maintenance therapy

Stages of status epilepticus (SE)

*Note: treatments chosen will depend on the condition of the patient

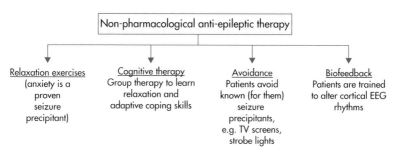

Non-pharmacological anti-epileptic therapy

Relaxation exercises (anxiety is a proven seizure precipitant)

Cognitive therapy Group therapy to learn relaxation and adaptive coping skills

Avoidance Patients avoid known (for them) seizure precipitants, e.g. TV screens, strobe lights

Biofeedback Patients are trained to alter cortical EEG rhythms

Non-pharmacological anti-epileptic therapy

70 Headache I: Non-migraine headache[16]

It has been estimated that about 70% of the adult population suffer headache at least once every month, although in most cases the underlying aetiology is probably benign. Headaches have been classified broadly as (i) **chronic** or **acute** and (ii) **continuous** or **intermittent**, and occur as various combinations of (i) and (ii). Most headaches suffered are **acute/intermittent**, and these in turn are classified into two major types, **migraine** and **acute muscle contraction headache** (MCH; also called acute tension headache). Some rare forms of acute headache fall outside this classification, e.g. the so-called 'ice-pick' or 'ice-cream' headache, which is caused by cold. **Chronic** headaches are those suffered daily or almost daily. These headaches are further subclassified on the basis of headache duration into those lasting less than 4 hours (**cluster headaches**), and those lasting 4 hours or longer, when the patient is most probably suffering from a condition termed **chronic daily headache (CDH)**.

Acute muscle contraction headache does not usually interfere with normal daily activities, is usually managed by the patient and responds well to over-the-counter (OTC) drugs such as aspirin, paracetamol and ibuprofen. Acute MCH, unlike migraine may persist for longer periods and is not aggravated by normal daily activities. Unlike the case with migraine, acute MCH is not usually associated with phonophobia, photophobia or other heightened sensory sensitivities. The cause is unknown but may involve soft tissue inflammation.

Ice-pick (ice-cream) headache is an intense, piercing and very short-lasting pain (lasting usually 15–30 seconds and occasionally up to a minute). The aetiology is unknown. It may be triggered by ice-cold foods. It often presents on one eye and may recur several times during the day. The short duration of the attack complicates treatment, which is more often preventive in the form of daily treatment with, for example, anti-inflammatory drugs such as indometacin or sustained-release preparations of diclofenac, provided that there are no contraindications, e.g. gastric problems.

Cluster headache is a comparatively rare (approximately 0.25% of the population) but very severe attack of intermittent headache that may last anything up to 3 hours. It may occur several times daily and is accompanied by several exacerbating symptoms, mainly affecting the eye and nose, including rhinorrhoea, ptosis, miosis, facial perspiring, nasal congestion and lacrimation. Cluster headache may be episodic (80–90% of cases) or chronic; episodic cluster headache may last weeks or months with extended periods of remission, whereas chronic attacks may persist for more than a year. **Treatment** is mainly prophylactic, using sodium valproate or verapamil, a cardioactive calcium channel inhibitor. Attacks are treated with oxygen if possible, and with 5-HT_{1D} receptor agonists such as sumatriptan. Little epidemiological information about treatment is available.

Chronic daily headache is one of the more prevalent headache forms and occurs more in men. Neck injury, e.g. whiplash, may be a causative or contributory factor. CDH may be diagnosed through its persistence (6 months or longer), associated muscular neck pain and migraine-like symptoms. Some patients develop analgesic dependence, notably to codeine phosphate and migraine treatments, which can actually exacerbate headache. Treatment involves: (i) weaning patients off analgesics; (ii) physiotherapy for neck spasm; and (iii) appropriate medication. Acceptable drugs include tricyclic antidepressants, e.g. prothiaden, and anti-epileptics, e.g. sodium valproate, topiramate and gabapentin.

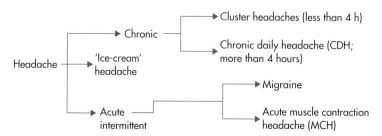

Headache classification

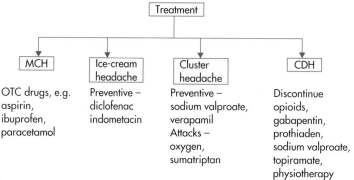

Treatment

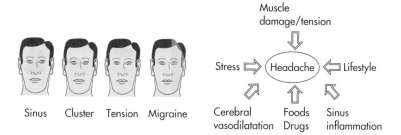

71 Headache II: Migraine[17]

Migraine is defined by the International Headache Society (IHS) as a recurrent headache occurring with or without aura and lasting 4–72 hours. It is usually unilateral, pulsating and moderate or severe, and may be aggravated by routine physical activity. Common accompanying symptoms include nausea, vomiting, phonophobia and photophobia. It is more prevalent in middle-aged women. It appears to be 50% more likely with a familial history of migraine. Sufferers may experience one or two attacks each month and usually fewer than 40 each year. The attack lasts around a day. Trigger factors may alone, or in combination with others, trigger an attack. The attack occurs in phases: a prodromal period before the attack, when the patient may experience lethargy and unusual cravings – prophylactic treatment during this period may prevent the attack; the final phase is the postdrome, when the patient is 'washed out' or euphoric.

Management involves patient education, especially avoiding trigger factors. Drug treatment may be acute, to treat the symptoms, or prophylactic. Two broad categories of treatment have been described: (i) analgesic and analgesic combinations, and (ii) migraine-specific therapies.

Analgesia involves the use of simple OTC analgesics such as paracetamol, sometimes alone or combined with caffeine or codeine, NSAIDs e.g. aspirin, ibuprofen and tolfenamic acid, which is licensed in the UK to treat an acute attack of migraine. Patients over-using codeine-containing preparations may develop CDH and need professional help. Drugs may be administered rectally to avoid nausea and vomiting. Alternatively, gastric motility agents such as domperidone or metoclopramide may be prescribed with an analgesic.

Migraine-specific therapies: 5-HT_{1B} and 5-HT_{1D} **receptor agonists (triptans)** are currently the mainstay of acute treatment. 5-HT_{1D} receptors mediate vasoconstriction of cerebral vessels. Triptans available in the UK are **almotriptan, eletriptan, frovatriptan, naratriptan, rizatriptan, sumatriptan** (the most frequently used) and **zolmitriptan**. Sumatriptan and zolmitriptan are formulated for oral, nasal or subcutaneous administration. Drugs should be taken immediately after attack onset.

Adverse effects and contraindications of 5-HT agonists are due mainly to their vasoconstrictor effects, and include tingling, pressure and tightness of throat and chest, as a result of possibly an anaphylactic reaction. Nausea, dizziness and tiredness are common adverse effects. Contraindications include TIA sufferers, severe or uncontrolled hypertension, and coronary vasospasm. 5-HT antagonists should not be used prophylactically.

Other drugs used include isometheptene mucate, ergotamine and dihydro-ergotamine, although the 5-HT_1 agonists have largely supplanted these. Ergotamine has a low relief rate, especially when administered orally, and causes abdominal cramp and nausea. Dihydroergotamine produces less severe side-effects than does ergotamine, but is not as efficacious as the triptans.

Drug prophylaxis may be considered for patients who suffer frequent, disabling attacks. β-Blockers, e.g. **propranolol** (except in asthmatics), **pizotifen**, a 5-HT antagonist and antihistamine, **sodium valproate** or **cyproheptadine**, an antihistamine with calcium channel-blocking and 5-HT receptor-blocking actions, may be tried. **Methysergide** is an effective prophylactic, but has serious side-effects, e.g. retroperitoneal fibrosis, and should be reserved for patients in whom alternative prophylactics have failed.

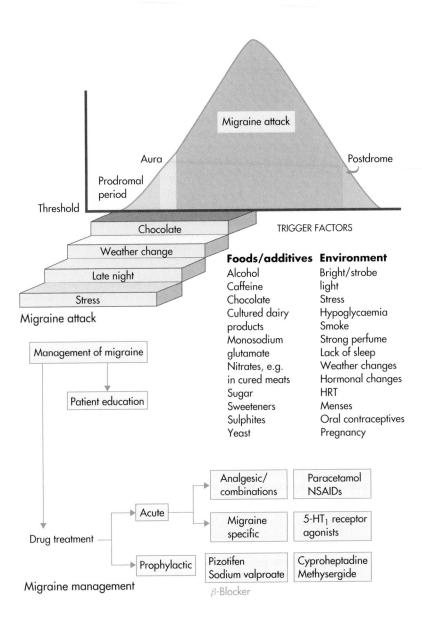

Migraine attack

Aura

Postdrome

Prodromal
period

Threshold

Migraine attack

Chocolate

Weather change

Late night

Stress

TRIGGER FACTORS

Foods/additives
Alcohol
Caffeine
Chocolate
Cultured dairy
products
Monosodium
glutamate
Nitrates, e.g.
in cured meats
Sugar
Sweeteners
Sulphites
Yeast

Environment
Bright/strobe
light
Stress
Hypoglycaemia
Smoke
Strong perfume
Lack of sleep
Weather changes
Hormonal changes
HRT
Menses
Oral contraceptives
Pregnancy

Management of migraine

Patient education

Drug treatment

Acute

Analgesic/
combinations

Paracetamol
NSAIDs

Migraine
specific

5-HT$_1$ receptor
agonists

Prophylactic

Pizotifen
Sodium valproate
β-Blocker

Cyproheptadine
Methysergide

Migraine management

72 Headache III: Facial pain

Facial pain can occur directly through facial structures or by referral from neighbouring structures, e.g. the neck. Three important causes are acute sinusitis, trigeminal neuralgia and post-herpetic neuralgia. The paranasal sinuses are air-filled cavities lined with mucous membranes, which open into the nasal cavity. The trigeminal (fifth cranial) nerve splits into the ophthalmic, maxillary and mandibular nerves.

Acute sinusitis is inflammation of one or more of the paranasal sinuses. It is often associated with rhinitis and usually develops from viral infections such as colds or flu. Bacterial infection may complicate the inflammation, with potentially serious consequences if the sphenoidal sinuses, which are in close proximity to the CNS, are infected. Sinusitis is often wrongly diagnosed or suspected and treated without prior investigation

Treatment for sinusitis is often an antibiotic and symptomatic treatment, e.g. vasoconstrictors and steam inhalation. The BNF recommends **amoxicillin, doxycycline** or **erythromycin** if pain and a purulent discharge have persisted for at least 7 days; treatment should be given for 3–7 days. Most viral infections will clear up spontaneously. Pain is treated with **ibuprofen** or **paracetamol,** and opioids such as **codeine** if severe. Sympathomimetic nasal decongestants should not be used for more than 5–7 days at a time because they may cause 'rebound' nasal congestion. Persistent severe pain and other symptoms may require specialist intervention, including endoscopic surgery to re-open sinus drainage and aggressive management, especially if sphenoidal sinusitis is diagnosed.

Trigeminal neuralgia is nerve pain affecting the facial structures. It is assumed to be caused by irritation or compression of the trigeminal (fifth cranial) nerve, the three main branches of which serve the ophthalmic, maxillary and mandibular regions. The most common compressing tissue is the superior cerebellar artery where the nerve leaves the brain stem. The pain is sudden, lancinating and shock like. Trigger modalities include light, hot, cold, touch, vibration and proprioceptors in the masticatory muscles. **Diagnosis** involves the use of MRI to exclude cranial tumours or demyelination associated with multiple sclerosis (MS). Possible compression of the trigeminal nerve root close to the brain stem can be investigated using MR angiography.

Treatment for idiopathic trigeminal neuralgia usually begins with a choice from **carbamazepine, oxcarbazepine, baclofen, gabapentin** and **sodium valproate.** Some patients respond to phenytoin. Higher doses of carbamazepine require monitoring of plasma levels. A combination of amitriptyline and either gabapentin or carbamazepine is sometimes used. Surgery, when needed, includes microvascular decompression of the trigeminal nerve. Injections are sometimes employed partially to ablate the trigeminal ganglion.

Post-herpetic neuralgia is facial pain following the viral herpes zoster (shingles), particularly in older patients, and often affects the ophthalmic branch of the trigeminal nerve. Attacks cease spontaneously about 3 years after initial onset in approximately 50% of patients. Treatment is with antiviral drugs as soon as possible after onset of herpes infection. Rashes are treated with calamine lotion with simple analgesics and, once cleared, tricyclic antidepressants or gabapentin is prescribed to manage the pain.

Diagnostic criteria for acute sinus headache

A. Purulent discharge in the nasal passage, either spontaneous or by suction

B. Pathological findings in one or more of the following tests:
- Radiographic examination
- CT or MRI
- Transillumination

C. Simultaneous onset of headache and sinusitis

D. Headache location:
- Acute frontal sinusitis with pain directly over the sinus,

with possible radiation to vertex or behind the eyes
- **Acute maxillary sinusitis,** with pain over antral area (cheekbones) and possible radiation to forehead and upper teeth
- **Acute ethmoidal sinusitis,** with pain between the eyes and possible radiation to the temples (temporal area)
- **Acute sphenoidal sinusitis,** with pain in the back of the head (occipital region), vertex, frontal region and behind the eyes

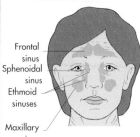

Frontal sinus
Sphenoidal sinus
Ethmoid sinuses
Maxillary sinus

Location of the facial sinuses

Treatment

Bacterial infection
Amoxicillin
Doxycycline
Erythromycin

Decongestants,
e.g. pseudoephedrine

Surgical intervention
Sinus drainage
Packing the sinus spaces

Acute sinusitis

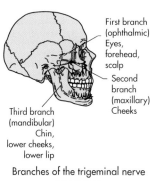

First branch (ophthalmic)
Eyes, forehead, scalp

Second branch (maxillary)
Cheeks

Third branch (mandibular)
Chin, lower cheeks, lower lip

Branches of the trigeminal nerve

Diagnostic criteria for trigeminal neuralgia

A. Paroxysmal attacks of facial and frontal pain lasting from a few seconds to less than 2 minutes

B. The pain has at least five of the following features:
- Intensely severe
- Attack is precipitated by daily activities, e.g.
  - brushing teeth
  - eating
  - talking
  - washing face
- Pain is distributed along one or more branches of the trigeminal nerve
- Pain is sudden, lancinating or burning and superficial
- Complete absence of pain between attacks

C. There is no neurological deficit

D. Attacks are stereotyped to the individual patient

E. Exclusion of other possible causes of the facial pain after patient interview, examination and any relevant investigations

Treatment

Drug treatment
Amitriptyline
Carbamazepine
Oxcarbazepine
Baclofen
Gabapentin
Sodium valproate

Surgery
Microvascular decompression
Partial ablation of the trigeminal ganglion

Trigeminal neuralgia

73 Meningitis and encephalitis

Meningitis is inflammation of the meninges. Acute meningitis may be **septic bacterial** or **aseptic viral**. Viral meningitis usually resolves within a few weeks without any specific treatment. **Bacterial meningitis** is relatively rare but much more serious and may result in brain damage and death unless rapidly diagnosed and treated with antibiotics. The main symptoms of bacterial meningitis in infants are raised temperature and irritability, and sometimes a tense fontanelle (opening in infant's skull where bones have not yet fused). CSF contains neutrophils and CSF pressure is markedly raised. Symptoms such as headache and neck pain, which adults report, are not easy to detect in infants. Meningitis is relatively rare and thus early symptoms may be ignored or misdiagnosed. The infecting bacteria include *Haemophilus influenzae* type b (Hib), *Neisseria meningitidis* (causes meningococcal meningitis) and *Streptococcus pneumoniae* (causes pneumococcal meningitis). In the UK, *N. meningitidis* serogroups B and C are the most common infecting agents in childhood meningitis.

Treatment: Early diagnosis and treatment with antibiotics and fluid resuscitation are imperative and, especially if meningococcal meningitis (B) is suspected, benzylpenicillin or cefotaxime (in case of penicillin allergy) is administered; the patient must be admitted to hospital immediately. In cases of penicillin and cephalosporin sensitivity, chloramphenicol (initially) and vancomycin or rifampicin may be considered (see BNF for more details and dosages). In any event, organ resistance to antibiotics should be tested. Patients should be treated with antibiotics for at least 5 days.

Vaccination: Meningococcal group C conjugate vaccine is now administered as standard practice to children from 2 months and is also recommended for anyone with a dysfunctional or absent spleen. Vaccination is also either essential or recommended for travel, depending on which country is being visited. See the BNF for detailed information.

Encephalitis is inflammation of the brain tissue caused by viral infection and is generally considered to be a far more serious clinical condition than viral meningitis. The patient initially suffers a sudden and acute onset of headache, fever, often disturbed consciousness and possibly seizures. Spinal fluid contains white and sometimes red blood cells. The infecting viruses include several of the herpes type, arvoviruses, retroviruses including HIV-1 (human immunodeficiency virus 1) and HTLV-1 (human T-lymphocytic virus 1), arenaviruses, including lymphocytic choriomeningitis and Lassa fever virus, and also rabies. Herpes simplex is probably the most virulent and dangerous encephalitic virus; it causes focal destruction in the anterior temporal lobes and in the orbital frontal brain, resulting in bizarre personality and behavioural changes, hallucinations and seizures.

Treatment is with the antiviral drug aciclovir, a cyclic analogue of the nucleoside guanosine. Aciclovir is a prodrug in that the virus takes it up and phosphorylates it to produce a suicide inactivator of viral DNA synthesis by inhibiting the viral enzyme DNA polymerase, resulting in premature termination of the growing DNA chain. There are reports that aciclovir-resistant strains of herpes simplex have developed, resulting in encephalitis, pneumonia and some mucocutaneous infections in immunocompromised patients. **Precautions** with aciclovir include pregnancy, breastfeeding and renal impairment, because aciclovir crystallises out in the tubules; adequate hydration should be maintained.

146

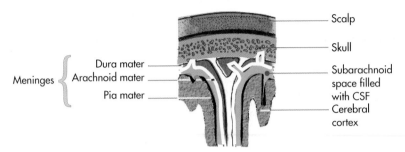

A. The meninges

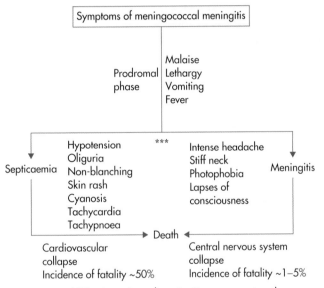

***Septicaemia and meningitis may occur together

Treatment: intravenous or intrasseous benzylpenicillin in children if possible; alternatively intramuscular benzylpenicillin into a warm limb; If penicillin allergic give third-generation cephalosporin; hospitalise fast

B. Meningococcal meningitis

74 General anaesthetics I: Premedication

Pre-surgical medication: The anaesthetist must be informed if patients are on pre-existing medication before surgery. Existing medication may need to be stopped, or it may be necessary to continue medication during the peri-surgical period. Drugs that should not normally be stopped include drugs for anxiety, asthma, cardiovascular disease, epilepsy or glaucoma, Parkinson's disease or thyroid problems, and drugs of dependence or immunosuppressants. The anaesthetist must be informed if patients are on drugs that cause adrenal atrophy, such as corticosteroids, because patients without corticosteroid cover during an operation may suffer a profound drop in blood pressure. Decisions regarding patients on drugs for HIV or who are on anticoagulant therapy require expert advice as to whether anticoagulants should be used. Drugs that should normally be stopped for the operation include MAOIs (at least 2 weeks before surgery). Tricyclic antidepressant therapy may be maintained, but the anaesthetist must be informed because of the increased risk of potentially serious drug interactions with vasopressor drugs, and of cardiac arrhythmias. Lithium can be continued for minor surgery, but should be stopped 24 hours before major surgery. Combined oral contraceptives and HRT should be stopped at least 4 weeks before major surgery because of the risk of deep venous thrombosis, and should be resumed only after full mobilisation is achieved. In cases of non-elective surgery, prophylactic heparin should be used as well as graduated compression hosiery.

Medication before or during surgery includes the administration of drugs to: (i) allay fear; (ii) suppress secretions; and (iii) increase pH and reduce volume of gastric contents. Premedication is not used as frequently nowadays.

(i) **Anxiety:** Frequently stated fears include fear of dying, mistakes during surgery, waking up during surgery, being seen naked and post-surgical pain. Anxiolytic drugs used include **temazepam**, or the longer-acting **lorazepam** or **diazepam**, all given orally.

(ii) **Secretion suppressants** may be needed, especially to reduce salivary secretion, which may interfere with airway management during induction and surgery. It is useful for procedures such as an awake fibreoptic intubation, before the use of ketamine, and before examination of the upper airways in children. Antimuscarinic drugs used include **atropine** given intramuscularly or orally (preferred route in children). **Glycopyrronium bromide** (glycopyrrolate) is an antimuscarinic drug that is given intramuscularly or intravenously during surgery to decrease secretions. It is more potent and long lasting than atropine, and produces less tachycardia.

(iii) **Gastric volume reduction and pH increase:** This may be necessary under certain circumstances to prevent acid aspiration (Mendelson's syndrome), which is the regurgitation and aspiration of the gastric contents during surgery, especially emergency surgery or during labour. Non-particulate antacids, e.g. **sodium citrate,** may be used for existing stomach contents, and proton pump inhibitors, e.g. omeprazole, or H_2-receptor antagonists, e.g. ranitidine. It may be administered the night before and the morning of delivery. Metoclopramide speeds up gastric emptying and may be given a few hours before delivery in obstetric patients.

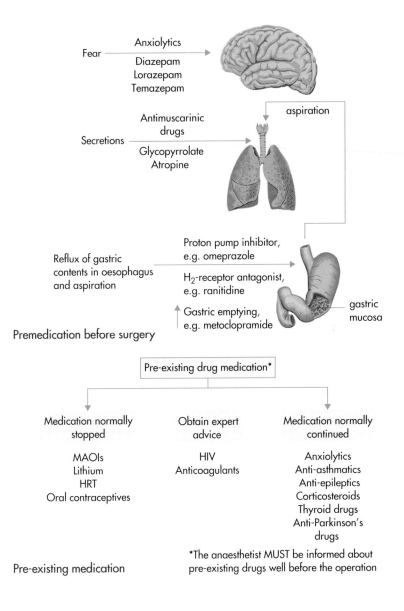

Fear ——— Anxiolytics
Diazepam
Lorazepam
Temazepam

Secretions ——— Antimuscarinic drugs
Glycopyrrolate
Atropine

aspiration

Reflux of gastric contents in oesophagus and aspiration

Proton pump inhibitor, e.g. omeprazole

H$_2$-receptor antagonist, e.g. ranitidine

↑ Gastric emptying, e.g. metoclopramide

gastric mucosa

Premedication before surgery

Pre-existing drug medication*

Medication normally stopped	Obtain expert advice	Medication normally continued
MAOIs	HIV	Anxiolytics
Lithium	Anticoagulants	Anti-asthmatics
HRT		Anti-epileptics
Oral contraceptives		Corticosteroids
		Thyroid drugs
		Anti-Parkinson's drugs

*The anaesthetist MUST be informed about pre-existing drugs well before the operation

Pre-existing medication

75 General anaesthetics II: Induction of anaesthesia

General anaesthesia for surgery taking appreciably more than 15 minutes is induced with intravenous general anaesthesia and maintained with a gaseous anaesthetic. Intravenous induction agents include **thiopental sodium, propofol, ketamine** and **etomidate**. They are preferred because loss of consciousness is achieved with one arm–brain circulation. Also, intravenous injection is less intimidating than a face-mask. All are associated with hypotension and apnoea, and may be contraindicated in patients with lesions that may obstruct the airways. Resuscitative apparatus must be on hand when they are used.

Thiopental sodium is a short-acting barbiturate, and like other barbiturates depresses the respiratory centre, resulting in hypoventilation and sometimes apnoea. There is rapid loss of normal muscle tone, causing a transient further depression of respiration. **Administration** is via the dorsum of the hand, avoiding the danger of extravasation in the arm and accidental intra-arterial injection; it is dissolved in an alkaline medium that through extravasation and intra-arterial injection will cause serious pain and perhaps permanent ischaemic damage distal to the injection site. Unconsciousness is achieved within about 20 seconds and is maintained for 5–10 minutes. Redistribution away from the brain to fat and muscle terminates its anaesthetic action, and metabolism is prolonged over several hours, ruling out use as a continuous intravenous infusion. **Side-effects** include arrhythmias, laryngeal spasm and hypersensitivity reactions.

Propofol is a rapidly metabolised intravenous induction agent with a rapid recovery phase; this renders it suitable for use with short procedures. It is injected as an emulsion as it is oil soluble, and blood lipids should be monitored with continuous infusion to avoid fat overload. Propofol causes pain on injection and some practitioners mix it with lidocaine. Other uses include sedation of patients over long periods in intensive care units. **Side-effects** include pulmonary oedema and transient apnoea and hypotension. **Contraindications:** adolescents under 17 years because of the risk of potentially fatal consequences including cardiovascular collapse, hyperlipidaemia, rhabdomyolysis (disintegration of striated muscle fibres) and metabolic acidosis.

Ketamine may be administered for induction either intramuscularly or by intravenous injection or infusion. Unlike other agents, it is also a powerful analgesic. In sub-anaesthetic doses it produces dissociative analgesia, when the patient is conscious but pain free, may answer questions and move around, but is unaware of the surroundings. Respiratory depression is rare, and ketamine causes a rise in blood pressure, rendering it useful in children with cardiac disease. Recovery is slow. **Side-effects:** hallucinations and nightmares are common during recovery, which limits its use for induction. Concomitant diazepam may prevent nightmares. **Contraindications** include hypertension and predisposition to hallucinations.

Etomidate is preferable to thiopental for some practitioners, because of the larger safety margin between the dose needed for anaesthesia and the dose that produces cardiovascular and respiratory depression, and more rapid metabolism and elimination, which reduces the 'hangover' effect. Etomidate, incidentally, is not a barbiturate. **Side-effects and contraindications:** extraneous muscle movements may occur during induction, which are counteracted by administering a short-acting benzodiazepine or an analgesic opioid just before induction. The opioid also minimises pain on injection. Etomidate suppresses adrenocortical function with prolonged use and should be avoided with severely ill patients.

Induction of anaesthesia

Induction agents are usually administered Intravenously. They are highly lipid soluble; this gets them to the brain fast. Intravenous administration is less intimidating than an inhalation mask. Induction agents have a relatively rapid recovery if not infused. Induction agents may be associated with apnoea and cardiovascular effects, e.g. arrhythmias and hypotension.

Induction agents

Thiopental sodium
Propofol
Ketamine
Etomidate

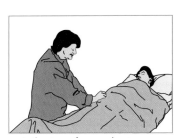

Induction of anaesthesia
outside the operating theatre

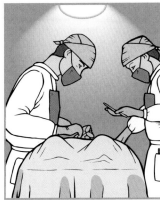

Gaseous anaesthesia inside
the operating theatre

Induction and maintenance of anaesthesia

Choice of induction agent			
Thiopental sodium	Propofol	Ketamine	Etomidate
Short-acting barbiturate	May cause pain on injection	Given either intravenously or intramuscularly	Good safety margin
Can be hypotensive in hypovolaemic patients	May cause transient apnoea	Powerful analgesic	Rapid metabolism and elimination
Depresses myocardial tissue	and pulmonary oedema	effect Causes rise in blood pressure	Muscle movements during induction
May cause laryngeal spasm	Rapid recovery	Recovery slow	Suppresses adrenal function
Concerns with extravasation	Contraindicated in young adolescents	Causes nightmare hallucinations	
Causes hangover			

Choice of induction agent

76 General anaesthetics III: Maintenance of anaesthesia

Inhalational anaesthesia is maintained using gases and volatile liquids such as **desflurane, enflurane, halothane, isoflurane** and **sevoflurane**, which are halogenated hydrocarbons (**A**), and nitrous oxide. Anaesthetic potency correlates with the oil/gas partition coefficient (**B**). Inhalational anaesthetics are administered using specialised systems, e.g. see (**C**). The ideal conditions of anaesthesia are given in (**D**) and ideally, a general anaesthetic should: (i) have a low minimum alveolar concentration (MAC); (ii) rapidly bring the patient to stage 3 (surgical stage of anaesthesia; [**E**]); (iii) have a good margin of safety between stages 3 and 4; (iv) be non-flammable; and inexpensive; (v) be analgesic; (vi) be non-toxic to liver and other organs; (vii) be rapidly eliminated with no after-effects; and (viii) have no odour. No anaesthetic completely fulfils all these criteria.

Desflurane and **sevoflurane** are preferred to isoflurane because of their more rapid onset and offset. Both are volatile liquids at room temperature and desflurane requires a special vaporiser. Desflurane has a pungent odour and has relatively low potency. It is administered with nitrous oxide, or oxygen-enriched air. Sevoflurane is often administered with nitrous oxide and oxygen. Isoflurane is administered with a nitrous oxide–oxygen mixture. Enflurane and halothane are similar in action, although halothane is more powerful and enflurane is less hepatotoxic. Both are cardiovascular and respiratory depressants. Enflurane's major adverse effect is the possibility of seizures.

Precautions and contraindications with enflurane and halothane include porphyria and epilepsy. Sevoflurane is best avoided with renal impairment. Absolute contraindications for all include susceptibility to malignant hyperthermia.

Halothane is used mainly for veterinary anaesthesia. Its use has declined because of hepatotoxicity. Halothane is oxidised to trifluoroacetic acid, which reacts covalently with several liver enzymes, generating an immune response.

Nitrous oxide (N_2O) is a non-flammable, colourless gas at room temperature with a sweet odour. It is both anaesthetic and analgesic and is used in both general surgery and dentistry. **Entonox** is a mixture of N_2O: oxygen (50% of each), which produces analgesia without anaesthesia. N_2O is not potent enough to use alone in general surgery and is used together with other agents to reduce dosages. It is often used for its analgesic properties during childbirth.

Safety note: Continual exposure to N_2O can depress white cell formation because it inactivates several enzymes involved in DNA and protein synthesis. It can also cause megaloblastic anaemia because it interferes with vitamin B_{12} action. This caution applies to both patients and staff, among whom N_2O is suspected of causing cases of fetal malformation and spontaneous abortion.

Adverse effects of inhalational anaesthetic agents to a greater or lesser extent are: **cardiovascular:** (i) arrhythmias; (ii) decreased myocardial contractility; (iii) decreased cardiac output; (iv) hypotension; (v) increased sensitivity of the myocardium to catecholamines; and (vi) decreased renal blood flow.

CNS: (i) increased intracranial pressure; (ii) reduced cerebral metabolic rate; (iii) increased cerebral blood flow; and (iv) greater risk of epilepsy.

Respiration: (i) bronchodilatation; (ii) reduced respiratory response to hypercapnia (abnormally high blood levels of CO_2) and hypoxia; (iii) ventilation is depressed; and (iv) airway obstruction and laryngospasm.

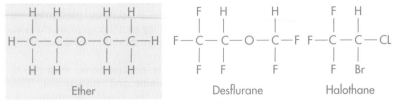

A. Structure of some inhalational anaesthetics

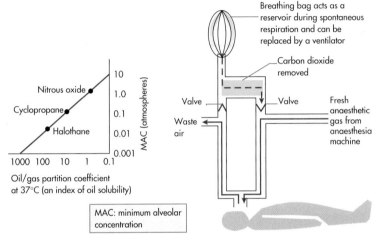

MAC: minimum alveolar concentration

B. Oil solubility and anaesthetic potency

C. Circle breathing system

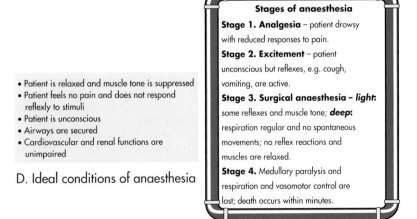

- Patient is relaxed and muscle tone is suppressed
- Patient feels no pain and does not respond reflexly to stimuli
- Patient is unconscious
- Airways are secured
- Cardiovascular and renal functions are unimpaired

D. Ideal conditions of anaesthesia

Stages of anaesthesia

Stage 1. Analgesia – patient drowsy with reduced responses to pain.

Stage 2. Excitement – patient unconscious but reflexes, e.g. cough, vomiting, are active.

Stage 3. Surgical anaesthesia – *light*: some reflexes and muscle tone; ***deep*:** respiration regular and no spontaneous movements; no reflex reactions and muscles are relaxed.

Stage 4. Medullary paralysis and respiration and vasomotor control are lost; death occurs within minutes.

E. Stages of anaesthesia

77 General anaesthetics IV: Muscle relaxants

Muscle relaxants paralyse skeletal muscle reversibly by blocking neurotransmission at the motor endplate (A); they do this by preventing the neurotransmitter acetylcholine (ACh) from binding to its receptor on the postsynaptic muscle membrane. Two types of drugs are used: (i) non-depolarising, competitive and (ii) depolarising, non-competitive drugs.

Non-depolarising, competitive drugs include **pancuronium**, **rocuronium**, **vecuronium**, **atracurium**, **cisatracurium**, **gallamine** and **mivacurium**. They block ACh from binding to its receptors on the muscle membrane (A), resulting in a flaccid paralysis. These drugs may be classified as short acting (15–30 minutes), medium acting (30–40 minutes) or long acting (60–120 minutes). None is analgesic or sedative, and none is known to trigger malignant hyperthermia. Choice depends, for example, upon the length of the procedure, renal status and susceptibility of the patient to histamine release. **Atracurium** and **vecuronium**, which are short- to intermediate-acting drugs, are preferred to the longer-acting pancuronium. Atracurium is useful with hepatic or renal problems because it is inactivated by body temperature and pH, thus bypassing the liver and kidneys. **Rocuronium**, a short-acting drug with rapid onset (2 minutes), is useful for quick procedures, e.g. tracheal intubation. Administration is by intravenous injection or infusion.

Precautions: Benzylisoquinolinium drugs, notably **mivacurium** (but with the exception of **cisatracurium**), are associated with histamine release; this may result in bronchospasm, hypotension, tachycardia and, rarely, anaphylaxis. None of the aminosteroid group mentioned here is associated with clinically significant histamine release. Other precautions include hypothermia and myasthenia gravis, when lower doses may be needed.

> **Treatment note**: The effects of the competitive, non-depolarising muscle relaxants can be reversed by anticholinesterases, e.g. neostigmine.

Depolarising muscle relaxants: Of these, only suxamethonium is used. Its chemical structure is based on that of ACh (B). Onset is rapid (about 60 seconds) and duration of action is short (5–10 minutes) due to rapid hydrolysis by plasma pseudocholinesterase. It causes a transient muscular response (twitching or fasciculation) and thereafter holds the muscle membrane in a transient depolarisation whereby ion channels are in an inactive state (C) and no further depolarisation is possible.

Uses and administration of suxamethonium: In general anaesthesia, such as for short-term relaxation, e.g. tracheal intubation, by intravenous injection or infusion or by intramuscular injection. It is also used to modify epileptic seizures. Administration should be after induction and not before, because there may be painful muscle fasciculation before paralysis.

Adverse reactions include: (i) bradycardia and salivation, which may be blocked by prior treatment with atropine; (ii) postoperative muscle pain; (iii) cardiovascular effects, e.g. tachycardia, arrhythmias, hyper- or hypotension and cardiac arrest; (iii) hyperkalaemia, myoglobinaemia and myoglobinuria; (iv) bronchospasm, prolonged respiratory depression, apnoea; and (v) increased gastric pressure. About 1 in 3000 of the population metabolises suxamethonium more slowly, resulting in paralysis for 2–3 hours. The condition is called suxamethonium apnoea.

Contraindications include: (i) history of malignant hyperthermia; (ii) hyperkalaemia (raised blood levels of K⁺); (iii) muscle trauma; (iv) recent burns; and (v) slow suxamethonium metabolisers.

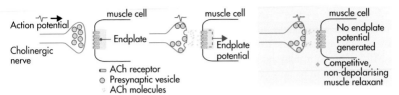

A. Competitive muscle relaxant action

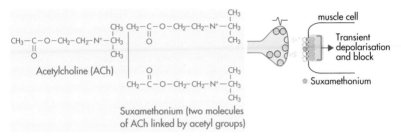

Acetylcholine (ACh)

Suxamethonium (two molecules of ACh linked by acetyl groups)

B. Suxamethonium: structure

C. Suxamethonium: action

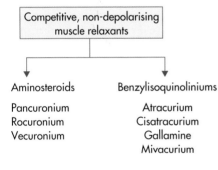

Adverse effects of suxamethonium
- Bradycardia, salivation
- Cardiovascular disturbances
- Bronchospasm
- Histamine release
- Pain resulting from fasciculation
- Hyperkalaemia (raised plasma potassium)
- Suxamethonium apnoea
- Malignant hyperpyrexia
- Increased intraocular pressure
- Increased gastric pressure

Drug	Duration of action	Histamine release	Comments
Atracurium	20–30 minutes	Slight	Most used
Cisatracurium	20–30 minutes	None	
*Gallamine	45–90 minutes	None	Causes tachcardia
Mivacurium	10–15 minutes	Moderate–severe	
*Pancuronium	45–90 minutes	None	
Rocuronium	2–30 minutes	None	Fastest onset
Vecuronium	20–30 minutes	None	Commonly used

*Contraindicated in patients with kidney failure.

78 Antidepressants: Treatment of depression with drugs

Depressive disorders are conditions of persistent low mood, loss of enjoyment, interest and energy, and in more serious cases patients may take to their beds and contemplate suicide. Depression may be accompanied by anxiety and loss of sleep. The aetiology is unknown, but appears to involve disorders of mono-amine neurotransmitter turnover, especially norepinephrine and serotonin.

Mild depression may be treated without drugs, but persistent moderate-to-severe depression usually requires drugs (**A**). Historically, MAOIs and tricyclic antidepressants were routinely prescribed, but are being superseded by the selective serotonin re-uptake inhibitors (SSRIs).

Selective serotonin re-uptake inhibitors block the re-uptake of serotonin into the nerve terminal, thus prolonging its action (**B**). Those in use in the UK include **citalopram, escitalopram, fluoxetine, fluvoxamine, paroxetine** and **sertraline**. They are now favoured over other antidepressants, e.g. tricyclics, because of fewer muscarinic actions and fewer cardiotoxic effects, and they lack the food-related complications of the MAOIs. They are also used to treat panic attacks. There are concerns, however, about the incidence of suicide and in the UK they are not prescribed to new patients under the age of 18. There may also be an increased risk with fluoxetine and paroxetine.

Monoamine oxidase inhibitors (**MAOIs**) are less frequently used nowadays. The most commonly used are **isocarboxazid** and **phenelzine**. They are sometimes recommended for patients who are refractory to other anti-depressants and those with hysterical, hypochondriacal and atypical features. They are also best prescribed if tricyclics (see below) have failed rather than the other way round. The most dangerous MAOI is probably **tranylcypromine** because of a stimulant effect and a powerful drug interaction with clomipramine. All are taken orally as tablets. All have delayed onset of action and withdrawal after discontinuation. **Moclobemide** is a reversible MAO-A enzyme inhibitor (RIMA) indicated for social phobia and major depression. It may cause less interaction with dietary amines but cannot be used with other MAOIs. **Drug and food interactions:** MAOIs block the breakdown of pressor neurotransmitters such as norepinephrine and of dietary tyramine (e.g. in herrings, broad bean pods, chocolate, mature cheese, yeast and beef extracts). Tyramine potentiates pressor actions of norepinephrine by potentiating its release from sympathetic nerve terminals. This may cause a dangerous rise in blood pressure, called a hypertensive crisis.

Tricyclic antidepressants block the re-uptake of norepinephrine into the nerve terminal, thus potentiating its endogenous actions (**C**). Uses: They are generally reserved for patients with endogenous depression associated with sleep disturbances and appetite loss, and with panic disorders. Sedative tricyclics, which are more useful in agitated patients, include amitriptyline, clomipramine, dosulepin, doxepin, maprotiline, mianserin, trazodone and trimipramine. Less sedative tricyclics, e.g. **amoxapine, imipramine, lofepramine and nortriptyline,** are used for apathetic and withdrawn patients. **Adverse effects,** especially cardiovascular effects, reflect the mechanism of action of tricyclics, and include arrhythmias, heart block and hypertension. Antimuscarinic effects include blurred vision, dry mouth, constipation and urinary retention. **Contraindications** include patients on or still withdrawing from MAOIs. See the BNF for more details.

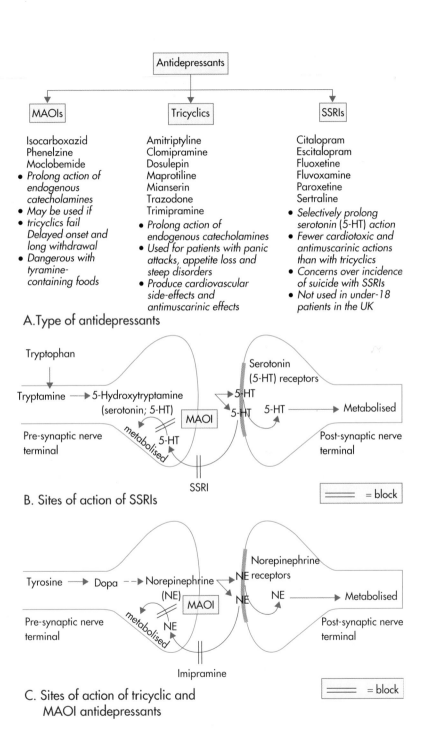

A. Type of antidepressants

Antidepressants

MAOIs

Isocarboxazid
Phenelzine
Moclobemide
- *Prolong action of endogenous catecholamines*
- *May be used if*
- *tricyclics fail Delayed onset and long withdrawal*
- *Dangerous with tyramine-containing foods*

Tricyclics

Amitriptyline
Clomipramine
Dosulepin
Maprotiline
Mianserin
Trazodone
Trimipramine
- *Prolong action of endogenous catecholamines*
- *Used for patients with panic attacks, appetite loss and steep disorders*
- *Produce cardiovascular side-effects and antimuscarinic effects*

SSRIs

Citalopram
Escitalopram
Fluoxetine
Fluvoxamine
Paroxetine
Sertraline
- *Selectively prolong serotonin (5-HT) action*
- *Fewer cardiotoxic and antimuscarinic actions than with tricyclics*
- *Concerns over incidence of suicide with SSRIs*
- *Not used in under-18 patients in the UK*

B. Sites of action of SSRIs

Tryptophan

Tryptamine → 5-Hydroxytryptamine (serotonin; 5-HT)

Serotonin (5-HT) receptors

Pre-synaptic nerve terminal

Post-synaptic nerve terminal

5-HT → Metabolised

metabolised 5-HT

MAOI

SSRI

$\overline{\overline{}}$ = block

C. Sites of action of tricyclic and MAOI antidepressants

Tyrosine → Dopa --→ Norepinephrine (NE)

Norepinephrine receptors

Pre-synaptic nerve terminal

Post-synaptic nerve terminal

NE → Metabolised

metabolised NE

MAOI

Imipramine

$\overline{\overline{}}$ = block

79 Treatment of anxiety (anxiolytic drugs)

Clinical anxiety is a blanket term for a poorly understood syndrome characterised to a greater or lesser extent by panic attacks, apprehension, irritability, poor concentration and poor sleep patterns. A syndrome termed generalised anxiety disorder (GAD) is currently used, and the pharmacological treatments available for this and other forms of anxiety include benzodiazepines (not generally recommended for GAD), β-blockers and antidepressants such as tricyclics and SSRIs, especially for panic attacks (see previous spread). Benzodiazepines are not recommended for long-term use. Of equal or possibly even more importance is the non-pharmacological support, which is summarised in detail by the National Institute for Health and Clinical Excellence (NICE)[19] (B).

Orally active **benzodiazepines** such as **lorazepam** and **oxazepam** are used, but these have a relatively high risk of withdrawal symptoms. Longer-acting drugs used include **diazepam**, which has been used intravenously in panic attacks, although there is danger of respiratory depression. NICE[19] recommends that benzodiazepines should not be used for panic disorders. **Adverse effects** of diazepam (and other benzodiazepines) include paradoxical aggression and hostility reactions in some patients, visual disturbances, light-headedness, amnesia and ataxia in elderly people. There is also the danger of dependence. Benzodiazepines are not recommended for more than 4 weeks and are **contra-indicated** in patients with respiratory depression, acute pulmonary insufficiency, sleep apnoea syndrome, severe liver disease or any condition that includes depression. Generally, no sedating antipsychotic or benzodiazepine should be used to treat panic disorders.

Selective serotonin re-uptake inhibitors (see also previous spread) and **tricyclic antidepressants** have been reported to help in the management of panic disorders. Unless otherwise indicated, an SSRI licensed for use in panic disorder should be the first choice. Patients should be advised that there is a delay in the onset of experience of benefit, that abrupt withdrawal from these drugs or arbitrary dose reduction is inadvisable, and about the known **adverse effects**. The most commonly reported include sleep disturbances, GIT upsets, dizziness and skin reactions such as tingling or numbness. Patients should be supplied with written information about these drugs, if available.

Pharmacological treatment of GAD: Paroxetine, a SSRI, is licensed and often recommended for treatment of GAD, as are some other SSRIs. Paroxetine is indicated also for obsessive–compulsive disorders, social phobia, post-traumatic stress disorder and depression. Patients should be kept on a prescribed drug for at least 12 weeks unless there are untoward adverse effects, before trying another. Higher doses of the drug may be offered unless not tolerated, and if the drug proves effective the patient should be maintained on the optimal dose of the drug for at least 6 months, after which the dose may be gradually reduced.

Contraindications to the use of tricyclics include cardiac disorders and severe liver diseases. SSRIs should be used with caution, e.g. in epileptic patients, in diabetes, in patients with a history of bleeding disorders, and in breast-feeding and pregnancy. SSRIs impair cognitive and judgement skills, e.g. driving.

Patient compliance is often a problem in the treatment of depression and anxiety disorders, due in part to the delayed onset of action, the adverse effects of drugs and the state of mind of the patient, who often needs considerable support, encouragement and psychological therapy with specialist mental health professionals (see opposite).

Symptoms	Diagnosis	Pharmacological treatment*	Drugs
Mood low; interest low Energy low; sleep disturbance Guilt feelings; suicidal thoughts	Clinical depression	Antidepressants	See spread 78
Intermittent anxiety or panic attacks and avoidance behaviour to preventattacks	Panic disorder with or without agoraphobia	SSRI or tricyclic drug Benzodiazepines less effective	e.g. Fluoxetine Paroxetine Amitriptyline
Almost constant and inappropriate anxiety with poor sleep, irritability and over-arousal	Generalised anxiety disorder (GAD)	SSRI Benzodiazepine for not more than 2–4 weeks	e.g. Fluoxetine Paroxetine Perhaps diazepam for 2–4 weeks

A. Pharmacological treatment of anxiety

*In all cases, age, health, previous and concurrent drug treatments and other patient-specific status must be taken into account when prescribing, and patients given information about known adverse effects of drugs prescribed. Patient compliance must be monitored.

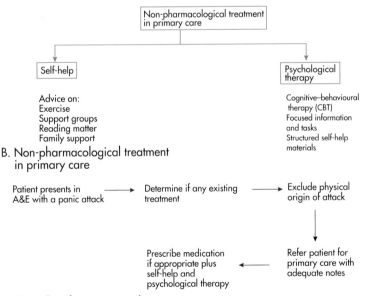

Non-pharmacological treatment in primary care

Self-help

Advice on:
Exercise
Support groups
Reading matter
Family support

Psychological therapy

Cognitive–behavioural therapy (CBT)
Focused information and tasks
Structured self-help materials

B. Non-pharmacological treatment in primary care

Patient presents in A&E with a panic attack → Determine if any existing treatment → Exclude physical origin of attack

Prescribe medication if appropriate plus self-help and psychological therapy ← Refer patient for primary care with adequate notes

C. Procedure for panic attack presentation in A&E

80 Treatment of insomnia

Insomnia is the inability to obtain sufficient and regular restful sleep, resulting in impaired function and irritability during waking hours. Criteria for the diagnosis of insomnia are: (i) failing to fall asleep within 30 minutes; (ii) interruption of sleep for more than 30-minute intervals; (iii) ratio of time asleep to time in bed less than 0.85; and (iv) occurrence of sleep disturbance more than three nights per week.[20] Insomnia is currently classified (**A**) as: (i) transient, lasting 2–3 days, from, for example, jet lag, noise, shift work; (ii) short-term, lasting up to 3 weeks, from, for example, physical illness, stress; and (iii) chronic, with poor or little sleep lasting 3 weeks or more, from, for example, excessive alcohol or drug misuse, or psychiatric problems. Chronic use of prescribed drugs, e.g. anticonvulsants, β-blockers and others (**B**), may cause insomnia.

Sleep apnoea is a sleeping disorder caused by intermittent insufficiency of ventilation, resulting in snoring and sleep interruption. Fat deposition in the neck may be a contributory factor. It is treated with mechanical aids, e.g. the continuous positive airway pressure (CPAP) machine or the mandibular advancement splint. Restless legs syndrome (Ekbom syndrome) is an urge to move the legs because of uncomfortable sensations described as 'itching', 'crawling' or 'electric', which can also cause insomnia.

Treatment of insomnia (**C**): **Lifestyle changes** include: (i) dietary, e.g. eliminating or reducing intake of alcohol, caffeine and other dietary stimulants, such as chocolate, especially during the evening; (ii) physical and relaxation exercises during the day and up to 4 hours before retiring; work scheduling may be changed; (iii) the establishment of regular bedtime and rising routines; (iv) avoiding stimulant activities such as TV or computing shortly before bedtime; and (v) smoking, which may interfere with sleep through nicotine withdrawal.

Pharmacological treatment is recommended only for transient and short-term insomnia.[20] Drugs should not be prescribed for insomnia for longer than absolutely necessary. For transient insomnia, short-acting benzodiazepines such as **temazepam** and **lorazepam** may be prescribed for one or two nights. The adverse effects and consequences of long-term use of benzodiazepines are described elsewhere (page 158). Alternatively, the so-called '**Z**' drugs, **zalepon**, **zolpidem** or **zopiclone**, are recommended for short-term use.[21] These drugs are contraindicated in obstructive sleep apnoea, in patients with liver disease, and in pregnant and breastfeeding mothers. See the BNF for more details. Longer-term use of hypnotics should be discouraged. These drugs do have, to a greater or lesser extent, hangover and psychomotor impairment effects. They may also induce psychological and physical tolerance and dependence. Hypnotics are generally contraindicated in elderly patients, who are more susceptible to the ataxic and confusional state induced by these drugs, and are therefore in danger of falling.

Other hypnotic drugs include **barbiturates**, more of historical interest, and chloral hydrate and other chloral compounds, which have previously been prescribed for children with night terrors and elderly people, but which are gastric irritants. **Chlormethiazole** is prescribed for elderly people because it is not significantly associated with hangover effects, but does cause gastric irritation. OTC sedative antihistamines **diphenhydramine** and **promethazine** may cause ataxia and confusion, especially in elderly patients. **Melatonin**, which inhibits cortisol, has been used for the treatment of insomnia in children and in the treatment of jet lag.

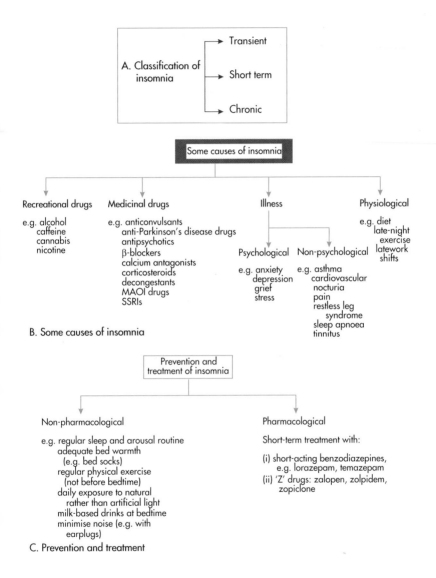

A. Classification of insomnia
- Transient
- Short term
- Chronic

Some causes of insomnia

Recreational drugs

e.g. alcohol
caffeine
cannabis
nicotine

Medicinal drugs

e.g. anticonvulsants
anti-Parkinson's disease drugs
antipsychotics
β-blockers
calcium antagonists
corticosteroids
decongestants
MAOI drugs
SSRIs

Illness

Psychological

e.g. anxiety
depression
grief
stress

Non-psychological

e.g. asthma
cardiovascular
nocturia
pain
restless leg
syndrome
sleep apnoea
tinnitus

Physiological

e.g. diet
late-night
exercise
latework
shifts

B. Some causes of insomnia

Prevention and treatment of insomnia

Non-pharmacological

e.g. regular sleep and arousal routine
adequate bed warmth
(e.g. bed socks)
regular physical exercise
(not before bedtime)
daily exposure to natural
rather than artificial light
milk-based drinks at bedtime
minimise noise (e.g. with
earplugs)

C. Prevention and treatment

Pharmacological

Short-term treatment with:

(i) short-acting benzodiazepines,
e.g. lorazepam, temazepam
(ii) 'Z' drugs: zalopen, zolpidem,
zopiclone

81 Anti-psychotic drugs

Psychosis is an umbrella term for a group of mental illnesses that cause loss of contact with reality, including paranoia, schizophrenia and bipolar disorder psychosis. **Symptoms** include delusions, hallucinations, grossly inappropriate behaviour, poverty of thought and violent mood swings. The aetiology is largely unknown, except when symptoms are triggered by brain damage or toxic substances. Anti-psychotic drugs (**A**) may temporarily restore normal behaviour, improve mood and render violent patients docile.

Anti-psychotic drugs[22] aim to restore normal behaviour without impairing consciousness. Older drugs licensed for use in the UK to treat psychoses include **benperidol, chlorpromazine hydrochloride, flupentixol, fluphenazine hydrochloride, haloperidol, levomepromazine, promazine, sulpiride** and **trifluoperazine**. Their mechanism of action is unknown, although many increase prolactin secretion, which suggests an inhibition of central dopamine D_2 receptors, although several other neurotransmitters may also be implicated (**B**). Several produce **adverse effects** including sedation and extrapyradimal symptoms (i.e. tremors and muscle twitching) (**C**). Other effects include anti-muscarinic effects such as dry mouth, blurred vision and interference with micturition. A poor psychological state combined with the nature and severity of adverse effects often results in poor patient compliance.

The low selectivity of anti-psychotics militates for a wide range of **contraindications and precautions,** including pregnancy and breastfeeding, depression, hepatic disease, jaundice, blood dyscrasias, epilepsy, a family history of open-angle glaucoma, Parkinson's disease and phaeochromocytoma. Newer, so-called atypical anti-psychotics – **amisulpiride, clozapine, olanzapine, quietapine, risperidone,** sertindole (but see the BNF) and **zotepine** – are often better tolerated and produce fewer extrapyramidal effects.

Lithium and its salts (carbonate and citrate) are used for prophylaxis and to treat: (i) aggression, (ii) mania, (iii) bipolar and recurrent depression and (iv) self-mutilating behaviour. Their use requires constant specialist supervision, including blood level monitoring, given the low therapeutic index of lithium and its adverse effects. **Symptoms** of lithium toxicity include ataxia, dysarthria (inability to articulate words properly) and convulsions, which may be fatal.

The term schizophrenia covers a set of severe mental disorders characterised by loss of contact with reality, hallucinations, often involving hearing voices, and delusions. Patients often believe that their thoughts and actions are known and controlled by others. The aetiology is unknown but believed to involve disturbances of brain amine function. Both genetic and environmental factors may precipitate schizophrenia.

The **NICE** has published guidelines for the treatment of schizophrenia,[23] including recommendations that the atypical anti-psychotics should be: (i) considered for first-line treatment of newly diagnosed schizophrenia; (ii) used during an acute attack when communication with the patient is impossible; (iii) used when older drugs produce unacceptable adverse effects; and (iv) used for relapsed patients previously poorly controlled with older drugs, but not for patients adequately controlled with older drugs that do not produce unacceptable adverse effects. In addition, clozapine should be prescribed if the schizophrenic patient is inadequately controlled for each of two sequentially used other anti-psychotics (including an atypical psychotic drug), each having been tried for 6–8 weeks.

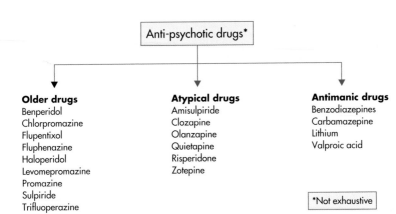

Older drugs
Benperidol
Chlorpromazine
Flupentixol
Fluphenazine
Haloperidol
Levomepromazine
Promazine
Sulpiride
Trifluoperazine

Atypical drugs
Amisulpiride
Clozapine
Olanzapine
Quietapine
Risperidone
Zotepine

Antimanic drugs
Benzodiazepines
Carbamazepine
Lithium
Valproic acid

*Not exhaustive

A. Types of anti-psychotic drugs

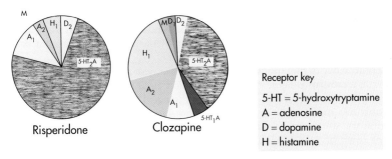

Risperidone

Clozapine

Receptor key

5-HT = 5-hydroxytryptamine
A = adenosine
D = dopamine
H = histamine

B. Relative receptor affinities of two anti-psychotic drugs

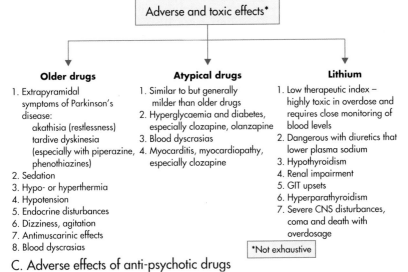

Adverse and toxic effects*

Older drugs
1. Extrapyramidal symptoms of Parkinson's disease:
   akathisia (restlessness)
   tardive dyskinesia (especially with piperazine, phenothiazines)
2. Sedation
3. Hypo- or hyperthermia
4. Hypotension
5. Endocrine disturbances
6. Dizziness, agitation
7. Antimuscarinic effects
8. Blood dyscrasias

Atypical drugs
1. Similar to but generally milder than older drugs
2. Hyperglycaemia and diabetes, especially clozapine, olanzapine
3. Blood dyscrasias
4. Myocarditis, myocardiopathy, especially clozapine

Lithium
1. Low therapeutic index – highly toxic in overdose and requires close monitoring of blood levels
2. Dangerous with diuretics that lower plasma sodium
3. Hypothyroidism
4. Renal impairment
5. GIT upsets
6. Hyperparathyroidism
7. Severe CNS disturbances, coma and death with overdosage

*Not exhaustive

C. Adverse effects of anti-psychotic drugs

82 Dementia: Alzheimer's disease

Dementia is irreversible loss of cerebral function characterised by cognitive and memory impairment, personality changes and ultimately loss of autonomic control. The most common are Alzheimer's disease, vascular dementia and dementia with Lewy bodies. Symptoms may be treated with antipsychotic drugs, but Alzheimer's disease and dementia with Lewy bodies are unique in being treated with drugs aimed at a specific neurotransmitter, i.e. acetylcholine (ACh).

The progression of Alzheimer's disease is inexorable, with progressive memory and cognitive loss, and development of confusion, aggression and personality change. At postmortem examination, cortical atrophy is found, with characteristic neurofibrillary tangles and senile plaques, indicating deposition of abnormal amyloid tissue. Disruption of cholinergic pathways may be important in the aetiology of Alzheimer's disease in view of the drugs used to treat it. Late onset disease occurs at 65 or older, and early onset occurs (rarely) in younger patients. The cause is unknown, but approximately 60% of patients carry the apolipoprotein E4 (Apo-E4) allele gene, which is associated with increased risk of disease development. Genotyping is not, however, a reliable predictor for the disease and diagnosis should be made only after other psychiatric, neurological or systemic causes of dementia have been excluded. In patients with early onset disease, there is evidence for an autosomal–dominant inheritance due to mutations on pre-senelin or amyloid precursor protein genes.

Drug treatment is based on a categorisation as (i) mild-to-moderate and (ii) moderate-to-severe forms of Alzheimer's disease. Drugs available (**A**) are the anxiolytics, to relieve fears and calm the patient, and the reversible ACh inhibitors **donepezil, galantamine** and **rivastigmine**. These inhibit the breakdown of ACh to choline and acetate (**B**). Galantamine is also an ACh nicotinic receptor agonist. **Memantine** is a voltage-dependent, non-competitive NMDA-receptor antagonist (**C**). The drug inhibits the action of glutamate, which has an elevated level of activity that could contribute to neuronal damage. All are available in tablet or capsule form for oral administration. Approximately 30–50% of patients given these drugs show a noticeable decrease in loss of cognitive ability after about 3 months. The NICE has, however, made a recent recommendation that anticholinesterase (AChE) antagonists donepezil, galantamine and rivastigmine not be used for mild-to-moderate Alzheimer's disease.[24]

Adverse effects largely reflect the augmentation of parasympathetic autonomic activity. These include nausea, vomiting, dyspepsia, diarrhoea, rhinitis, urinary incontinence, psychiatric disturbances and cardiovascular effects, such as arrhythmias, bradycardia and hypertension and, rarely, SA and AV block. **Precautions and contraindications** vary (see the BNF), but generally these drugs should be used with caution or not at all in hepatic or renal disease, asthma, supraventricular conduction abnormalities, peptic ulcers, chronic obstructive pulmonary disease, urinary retention or obstructive bowel disease. Pregnancy and breastfeeding are contraindications for these drugs. Parkinson's disease, in which there is excessive central cholinergic action in brain areas that normally suppress extrapyramidal movement (e.g. tremor), is a contraindication for the use of drugs that enhance cholinergic activity.

Other treatments that may be beneficial, but are of unproven or doubtful efficacy (**D**), include *Gingko biloba* and estrogens in women, although estrogens are implicated in postmenopausal breast cancer and cardiovascular accidents.

Clinical scenario: An 81-year-old widow was referred by her GP to the local memory clinic run by the Department of Psychiatry of Old Age. At the consultation she was accompanied by her daughter, a retired nurse. There was no significant past medical history and the patient had never smoked or drunk alcohol to excess. The patient acknowledged that her memory had become unreliable recently and once or twice she had felt confused and disorientated while shopping in a supermarket. Her daughter felt that the house was becoming untidy and that occasionally her mother had forgotten to wash herself or clean out food that had gone off in the fridge. The psychiatrist performed a Mini-mental State Examination and the patient scored 25/30, with deficits in calculation, recall and construction. No abnormalities were detected on routine blood tests and the CT scan of the brain was normal. After discussion with the patient, donepezil was started, with caution as to the side-effects of nausea, vomiting, diarrhoea and headaches.

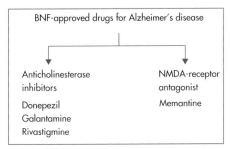

BNF-approved drugs for Alzheimer's disease

Anticholinesterase inhibitors

Donepezil
Galantamine
Rivastigmine

NMDA-receptor antagonist

Memantine

D. Treatments of unproven or doubtful efficacy

Amantadine
Estrogens
Gingko biloba
Physostigmine
Selegiline
Tacrine
Vitamin E

A. Drugs tried for Alzheimer's disease

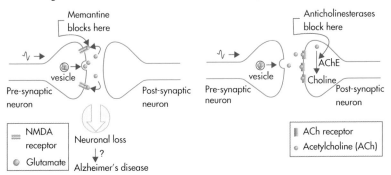

C. Mechanism of action of memantine

B. Mechanism of action of anticholinesterases

83 Drug addiction

Drug addiction is a **psychological compulsion** for and sometimes also **physical dependence** on drugs. Psychological compulsion is a craving coupled with compulsive drug-seeking behaviour, whereas physical dependence is an adjustment of homoeostatic mechanisms such that withdrawal of the drug produces physical symptoms. **Tolerance** is the phenomenon whereby a higher dose of the drug is needed to obtain the same effect. Substances not currently considered medicinal, e.g. alcohol, nicotine, ecstasy, cocaine and cannabis, which, like opioids, act in the so-called reward centres of the brain, are summarised in (**A**).

Morphine and **heroin** are opiate analgesics causing both psychological and physical dependence by binding to the μ, δ and κ opioid receptors in the brain; these receptors bind the endogenous peptides, the endorphins, enkephalins and dynorphin, through which they mediate analgesia, sedation, hunger and mood, particularly euphoria. Heroin is diacetylmorphine (diamorphine), which passes more rapidly into the brain where it is deacylated to morphine. Euphoria appears to be mediated by μ and δ receptors in the ventral tegmental area, where they reduce GABA release with consequent increase in dopaminergic activity (**B**). The κ receptors may mediate dysphoric actions of some synthetic opiates (nightmares). The aetiology of tolerance and physical dependence are not fully understood but may involve down-regulation of neurotransmitter receptors.

The symptoms of opiate withdrawal are greatly feared by opiate addicts, whose drug-seeking behaviour is often motivated more by fear than by a craving for the euphoric effect. The symptoms are largely magnifications of autonomic activity, including dilated pupils, cramps, shivering, dilated pupils, piloerection ('goose bumps'), lacrimation, nasal discharge, diarrhoea, vomiting and nausea. All of these symptoms are stopped by administration of an opiate, suggesting that opiate receptors play a major role in withdrawal aetiology.

Treatment aims: (i) management of withdrawal symptoms; (ii) prevention of withdrawal; (iii) weaning the addict off heroin; and (iv) keeping former addicts off opiates. **Lofexidine**, an α_2-adrenoceptor agonist, reduces sympathetic tone. It should be used with caution with cardiovascular disease. **Methadone**, an opiate, prevents withdrawal symptoms and is not a potent euphoric agent orally, although it is addictive. It is administered as an oral liquid and the dose is gradually reduced over time. It is a potent euphoric agent if administered intravenously. **Buprenorphine** is a partial agonist. Partial agonists have antagonist properties under some circumstances (e.g. dose). Buprenorphine is used to wean addicts moderately addicted to morphine or heroin. It has to be used with care because it may precipitate withdrawal symptoms in addicts on high doses of opiates through its partial antagonist activity. Buprenorphine does have potential for misuse and so should be used only on patients already addicted to opiates. Naltrexone is an opioid and opiate antagonist and is used only in patients already weaned off opiates to discourage a return to these drugs.

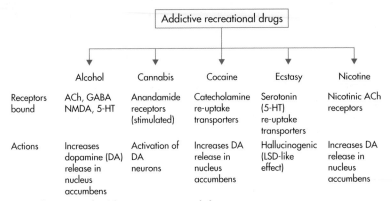

	Alcohol	Cannabis	Cocaine	Ecstasy	Nicotine
Receptors bound	ACh, GABA NMDA, 5-HT	Anandamide receptors (stimulated)	Catecholamine re-uptake transporters	Serotonin (5-HT) re-uptake transporters	Nicotinic ACh receptors
Actions	Increases dopamine (DA) release in nucleus accumbens	Activation of DA neurons	Increases DA release in nucleus accumbens	Hallucinogenic (LSD-like effect)	Increases DA release in nucleus accumbens

A. Mechanisms of addictive recreational drugs

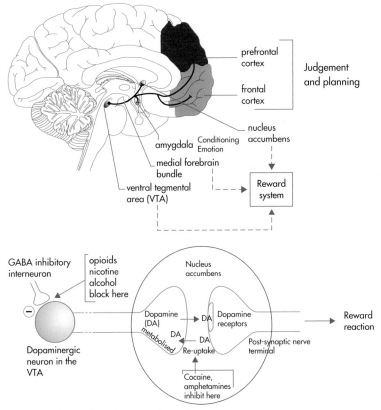

B. GABA-dopaminergic reward regulatory system

84 Local anaesthetics

Local anaesthesia may be defined as loss of all sensation within a circumscribed area. Analgesia is loss only of pain sensation. Local anaesthetics are usually applied either by injection or by topical application to a mucous membrane. Patients are conscious during procedures that employ local anaesthesia, e.g. in dentistry, and during some surgery to minimise the morbidity and mortality risks of general anaesthesia. Patient co-operation becomes possible and hospitalisation is sometimes unnecessary. Financial constraints within the NHS make the use of local anaesthsia highly attractive, but patient education needs to be taken into account. Local anaesthesia uses substances that block transmission of nerve impulses along the axon (**C**) and often vasoconstrictors to keep the local anaesthetic at the site of surgery and to aid haemostasis. Virtually all local anaesthetic agents with the exception of cocaine are vasodilators. Local anaesthesia is terminated by uptake of the drug into the systemic circulation and metabolism, with the attendant risk of toxicity.

Cocaine was first used as a local anaesthetic in the UK in 1886. **Novocaine** was synthesised in 1905 and **lidocaine** (**lignocaine**) was first used clinically in 1946. Chemically they are either amino esters, e.g. cocaine, procaine and benzocaine, or amino amides, e.g. lidocaine, bupivacaine (**A and B**). At a physiological pH they exist in the lipid-soluble unionised form in equilibrium with the ionised form. They penetrate the membrane in the unionised form and the ionised form binds to sodium channels and blocks them reversibly (**C**). Those currently listed in the BNF include **bupivicaine**, **levobupivacaine**, **lidocaine**, **procaine** and **ropivacaine** (**B**).

Lidocaine, the most commonly used, has a rapid onset and when mixed with epinephrine has a duration of action of 1–2 hours. It is formulated: (i) with epinephrine in **injectable form** for dental analgesia; (ii) as a **gel** together with chlorhexidine for urethral catheterisation; (iii) as an **ointment** for dental use, painful nipples, haemorrhoids, herpes labialis, herpes zoster and pruritis ani; (iv) as a **cream** for minor skin procedures; (v) as a **topical spray** for the larynx or pharynx; and (vi) with epinephrine as a **topical solution** for ear, nose and oropharyngeal use. It can also be used as a bolus intravenous injection to suppress ventricular arrhythmias, which may follow MI or cardiac arrest.

Adverse effects are representative of those for local anaesthetics generally and result from escape into the systemic circulation. They include cardiovascular effects, notably hypotension, bradycardia and possibly cardiac arrest. The margin of safety for local anaesthetics is relatively low. In general, toxicity depends not only on overdose, but also on the route of application, age and weight of the patient, vascularity of the tissues injected and the time over which the drug is administered. CNS effects include respiratory depression, confusion and convulsions. Hypersensitivity reactions have also been reported (**D**). **Precautions** should be taken with patients with cardiac, respiratory or hepatic disorders and elderly patients, and lidocaine is **contraindicated** in patients with complete heart block or hypovolaemia.

Bupivacaine has a slower onset of action (about 30 minutes) but a much longer duration of action (2–4 hours). It is therefore very popular for continuous epidural infusion during labour, for spinal anaesthesia generally and for post-operative pain relief. **Adverse effects** are notably cardiotoxicity, which is worse than with lidocaine, and bupivacaine should never be used for intravenous regional anaesthesia. Ropivacaine is structurally similar to bupivacaine, although with a slightly shorter duration of action, and it is less cardiotoxic. It produces less motor blockade than bupivacaine, which restores mobility more quickly.

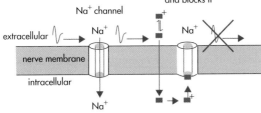

Lidocaine – an amino amide

Procaine – an amino ester

Drug	Relative potency	Duration of action (minutes)	% bound to plasma proteins	pK_a	Relative lipid solubility
Procaine	1	60–90	5	8.8	1
Lidocaine	2.5	90–200	70	7.6	4
Bupivacaine	7.5	180–600	95	8.0	28

- The pK_a is the pH at which the drug is 50% ionised. Physiological pH is 7.4. Most local anaesthetics have pK_a higher than physiological pH, therefore they exist mainly in the charged state.
- Plasma-bound drugs are unavailable to tissues and have to dissociate into the free state in order to be active.
- The more lipid soluble the drug the easier it is to cross the nerve cell membrane to the cytoplasmic side.

A. Chemical structures of local anesthetics

B. Actions and properties of local anaesthetics

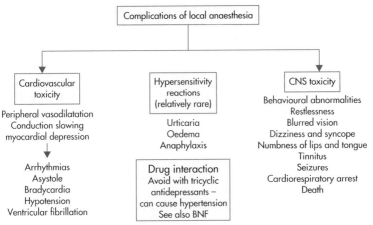

- ■ Uncharged local anaesthetic – can cross a lipid bilayer
- ■+ Charged local anaesthetic – binds to sodium channel and blocks it

C. Mechanism of action of local anaesthetics

Complications of local anaesthesia

Cardiovascular toxicity

Peripheral vasodilatation
Conduction slowing
myocardial depression
↓
Arrhythmias
Asystole
Bradycardia
Hypotension
Ventricular fibrillation

Hypersensitivity reactions (relatively rare)

Urticaria
Oedema
Anaphylaxis

Drug interaction
Avoid with tricyclic
antidepressants –
can cause hypertension
See also BNF

CNS toxicity

Behavioural abnormalities
Restlessness
Blurred vision
Dizziness and syncope
Numbness of lips and tongue
Tinnitus
Seizures
Cardiorespiratory arrest
Death

D. Complications of local anaesthetics

85 Peripheral neuropathies

'Peripheral neuropathies' is a blanket term to describe a set of (sometimes) progressive and incurable disorders of the peripheral nervous system, some of which are known to be of autoimmune origin (C). Nerves affected may be sensory/and or motor. Functionally, the consequences are loss of innervation resulting in loss of sensation and/or movement. Demyelination destroys the conducting ability and surrounding tissue damage and inflammation can also disrupt neuronal function (A and B). Neuropathies may be secondary to other diseases such as diabetes (C), and to other autoimmune diseases such as SLE and RA. Neuropathies may also result from alcoholism, hypothyroidism, vasculitis, paraproteinaemia (abnormal blood proteins), toxic chemicals, e.g. arsenic, lead and mercury, repetitive stress, cancer, kidney or liver disease, and from vitamin deficiencies, especially of the vitamin B group.

The longest nerves are the most vulnerable, so hands and feet are often affected more than shoulders or hips. This is **symmetrical neuropathy**. Mononeuro-pathies, where only one nerve is affected, often result from nerve compression or other form of physical damage. Polyneuropathies are often a consequence of diabetes, possibly due to the effect of raised glucose on raised osmotic pressure within the peripheral circulation, resulting in vessel rupture and tissue damage, particularly at the extremities. Previously, treatments for peripheral neuropathies aimed, for example, to suppress the immune system, but advances in the understanding of nerve regeneration are producing newer treatments. When nerve roots are affected as well this is a **polyradiculoneuropathy**.

Treatments for the various neuropathies vary but in principle aim, where possible, to target the cause of axonal and/or myelin damage, and to treat inflammation, pain and consequences of muscle paralysis such as breathing and digestive difficulties, and loss of mobility.

Guillain–Barré syndrome (GBS) is a temporary but severe autoimmune neuropathy of possibly viral or bacterial origin in which myelin sheaths are destroyed through lymphocyte attack. About two-thirds of all cases occur after surgery, infection or immunisation. Polyradiculoneuropathy is common in GBS and CIDP (see below). For patients the attack is often terrifying, because they may find themselves in intensive care units, in pain, completely paralysed and needing artificial ventilation. Recovery takes from weeks to months. Occasionally, the disease may become chronic. Variant forms of GBS are acute motor axonal neuropathy (AMAN) and acute motor and sensory axonal neuropathy (AMSAN), in which not only motor but also sensory axons are attacked; in these forms, recovery is slower and more often likely to become chronic. Investigative tests are summarised in (D).

Treatments for badly affected patients (E) include therapeutic plasma exchange (TPE) and intravenous immunoglobulin (IVIG), which is a cocktail of antibodies raised against the antibodies attacking the nerves. Patients who do not respond to IVIG may respond better to TPE, particularly if there is evidence of axonal involvement.[25] Treatment should be initiated promptly, because efficacy falls off with delay. Corticosteroids have been used but there is controversy over their efficacy. **Adverse effects and precautions**: IVIG may cause chills, fever and general malaise and, rarely, anaphylaxis. It is contraindicated in patients with known class-specific antibody to IgA. IVIG may interfere with immune responses to certain live virus vaccines.

Chronic inflammatory demyelinating polyradiculoneuropathy (CIDP) is a rare chronic and usually motor neuropathy which may resolve spontaneously or after treatment, and it may recur. Treatment is with immunosuppressants, e.g. azathioprine and steroids, and with TPE or IVIG.

Diabetic neuropathies often affect the extremities and the most effective and important pharmacological strategy is blood sugar control; ACE inhibitors are also effective.

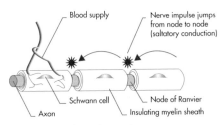

A. Peripheral myelinated nerve structure

Blood supply

Nerve impulse jumps from node to node (saltatory conduction)

Schwann cell

Axon

Node of Ranvier

Insulating myelin sheath

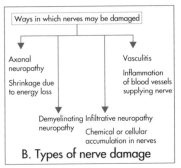

Ways in which nerves may be damaged

Axonal neuropathy

Shrinkage due to energy loss

Vasculitis

Inflammation of blood vessels supplying nerve

Demyelinating neuropathy

Infiltrative neuropathy

Chemical or cellular accumulation in nerves

B. Types of nerve damage

C. Some causes of peripheral neuropathy

- Alcoholism
- Chronic inflammatory demyelinating polyradiculoneuropathy
- Diabetes
- Guillane–Barré syndrome
- Hereditary sensorimotor neuropathy
- Thyroid underactive
- Idiopathic axonal neuropathy (unknown aetiology)
- Kidney failure
- Paraproteinaemia (abnormal blood proteins)
- Vitamin B deficiency

D. Investigative tests for peripheral neuropathy

- Medical, environmental history
- Genetic (DNA) tests
- Nerve conduction tests
- Lumbar puncture, nerve biopsy
- Blood, urine tests
- X-rays

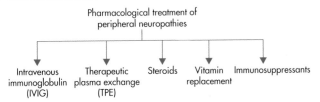

Pharmacological treatment of peripheral neuropathies

Intravenous immunoglobulin (IVIG)

Therapeutic plasma exchange (TPE)

Steroids

Vitamin replacement

Immunosuppressants

E. Pharmacological treatments

86 Myasthenia gravis and Lambert–Easton myasthenic syndrome

Myasthenia gravis (MG) is an autoimmune disease in which antibodies to ACh receptors bind to ACh receptors and block ACh at the neuromuscular junction. MG is often associated with thymus hyperplasia or thymoma. Clinical presentation varies (A). A diagnosis of MG is confirmed by observing a transient recovery after a single injection of **edrophonium**, a very short-acting anticholinesterase, and most patients will test positive for circulating ACh receptor antibodies. Ocular symptoms, notably ptosis, occur first, and patients experience muscular weakness, exacerbated by exercise; reflexes are, however, usually unaffected. There may be loss of facial expression, and difficulty with speech, chewing and swallowing. Respiratory symptoms include shortness of breath, especially when prone. MG may be exacerbated by aminoglycosides, lithium, penicillamine and phenytoin. The prognosis is variable and often improved with immunosuppressive drugs.

Treatment falls into four main classes:

(i) **Oral anticholinesterases**, including **neostigmine**, **pyridostigmine** and **distigmine**. **Adverse effects** are numerous, given the widespread involvement of ACh as a neurotransmitter in both the autonomic nervous system and at the neuromuscular junction (NMJ). With higher doses patients may experience toxic symptoms, including diarrhoea, miosis, nystagmus and excessive secretions, e.g. salivation, bronchial secretion, sweating and lacrimation. Cardiovascular effects include bradycardia, hypotension and heart block. CNS effects include agitation and excessive dreaming. **Precautions and contraindications**: asthma demands extreme precaution and intestinal or urinary obstruction is an absolute contraindication.

(ii) **Immunosuppressant corticosteroids** as immunosuppressants include **prednisolone** in small but gradually incremental doses daily or on alternate days until remission, when doses should be stepped down gradually. In generalised (as opposed to ocular) MG, **azathioprine** may be started together with prednisolone, thus allowing for lower doses of the steroid.

(iii) **Thymectomy** is usually done if a thymoma as present, and in some cases of generalised MG without thymoma.

(iv) **TPE** may be done in cases of respiratory weakness and life-threatening situations, together with protection of the airways, if required.

Lambert–Eaton myasthenic syndrome (LEMS) is a rare autoimmune disorder with reduced release of ACh from the nerve terminal (B); about 60% of patients have small cell lung carcinoma, with cells that possess voltage-gated Ca^{2+} channels. Antibodies to voltage-gated Ca^{2+} channels are detected in the circulation, suggesting that the antibodies result from an initial immune attack on the tumour. Spontaneous presynaptic ACh release is unaffected and repetitive stimulation increases the endplate potential before an action potential is eventually triggered; this explains why during a voluntary muscle contraction there is an initial augmentation of strength. Patients experience muscle weakness and loss of reflexes. The condition can be distinguished from MG by applying galvanic stimulation, when electromyography shows increased evoked potentials, whereas in MG evoked potentials are reduced.

Pharmacological treatment involves (i) tumour treatment and (ii) immunosuppressant drugs. In patients without cancer, prednisolone is sometimes used together with azathioprine. In severe cases, TPE may be used.

A. Clinical presentation in myasthenia gravis (MG)

Group I – ocular MG: eyes only
Group IIA and IIB – mild and moderate–severe generalised MG
Group III – acute MG with respiratory difficulties
Group IV – late chronic disease with involvement of pelvis and lower limbs

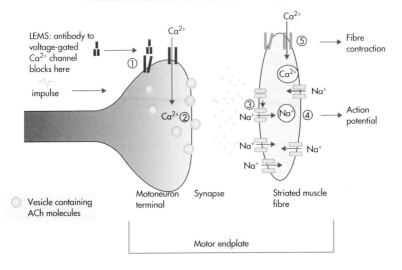

B. Signal transmission at the motor endplate

1. Impulse arrives at nerve terminal and depolarises plasma membrane
2. This transiently opens voltage-gated Ca^{2+} channels and Ca^{2+} enters the cell. This triggers exocytosis of ACh into the synaptic left
3. ACh binds to its receptors on the plasma membrane of the muscle cell and opens Na^+ channels transiently, in turn triggering more Na^+ channels, which results in:

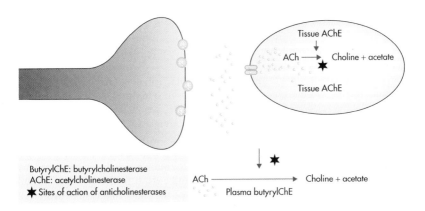

ButyrylChE: butyrylcholinesterase
AChE: acetylcholinesterase
★ Sites of action of anticholinesterases

87 Endocrine control systems

Endocrine hormone synthesis and release are tightly controlled by **feedback systems** to the hypothalamus and pituitary gland, and these systems are targets for drug treatments. For example, the hypothalamus produces **corticotrophin-releasing hormone (CRH)**, which travels to the anterior pituitary in the portal circulation (see opposite), where it releases **adrenocorticotrophic hormone (ACTH)**. ACTH is released into the general circulation and, in the adrenal gland, it promotes the synthesis and release of the adrenocortical steroids, including **cortisol**, into the circulation. Cortisol acts in the hypothalamus and the anterior pituitary to inhibit further release of CRH and ACTH, thus completing the loop or axis. Thus, when there is under- or over-activity of the adrenocortical system, drugs can be employed to test the integrity of the system. This knowledge is used also to protect patients who have been on long-term glucocorticoid (e.g. prednisolone) treatment, which may completely suppress the adrenal axis. Therefore prednisolone is withdrawn gradually to allow the axis to recover. In addition, drugs can be used to localise the site of a lesion within a particular endocrine system, e.g. a patient may present with symptoms of Cushing's disease, in which there is over-activity of the adrenal cortex. This could be due to excess secretion of ACTH, which stimulates excess cortisol secretion.

Other major feedback systems include the hypothalamic–anterior pituitary–gonadal axis, which controls sex hormone release (see opposite). Knowledge of this system has produced the **oral contraceptives** (page 184) and the use of analogues of the hypothalamic-releasing hormone **gonadotrophin-releasing hormone** (GnRH; page 182) to treat prostate cancer. The techniques of *in vitro* fertilisation and fertility treatments owe their existence to the discovery of the mechanisms underlying the control of the axis.

Similarly, the hypothalamic **thyrotrophin-releasing hormone (TRH)** releases **thyrotrophin (TSH)** from the anterior pituitary, and TSH controls **thyroid hormone** metabolism and release from the thyroid gland. Thyroid hormone feeds back to the hypothalamus and the pituitary to regulate its own blood levels.

Both basic and clinical pharmacology owe their existence in large part to the discovery of **receptor antagonists**, which have proved invaluable in endocrine-related disorders, e.g. the discovery of the estrogen receptor antagonist tamoxifen produced the first tissue-targeted drug for the treatment of breast cancer. Cyproterone acetate blocks the action of androgens at the androgen receptor in the prostate gland and is used in the treatment of prostate cancer. Spironolactone, a potassium-sparing diuretic, produces its effects by blocking the aldosterone receptor in the kidney tubule.

Knowledge of feedback mechanisms is vital for diagnostic testing, e.g. a tumour in the adrenal gland may release large quantities of cortisol, which suppresses the release of pituitary ACTH. Here, very high circulating cortisol together with very low or undetectable circulating ACTH is highly suggestive of an adrenal tumour. If, on the other hand, both cortisol and ACTH in plasma are abnormally high, this points to either a hypothalamic or a pituitary problem. Similarly, both hypo- and hyperthyroidism can be investigated by measuring circulating hormones of the thyroid axis. It is also worth mentioning here that the need to measure hormones of the endocrine system produced the technique of radioimmunoassay, which has proved invaluable for the measurement of infinitesimal amounts of chemicals in tissues of the body.

Clinical scenario: A 42-year-old woman was referred by her GP with hyperprolactinaemia. She complained of feeling excessively tired over the last few months, with a loss of libido. Her periods had stopped and she had noticed that she was expressing milk. Recently she had developed a headache. On examination her skin was pale and hairless and she had a bitemporal hemianopia. Blood tests were consistent with hyperprolactinaemia and hypopituitarism. An MRI scan was performed and showed a pituitary tumour extending from the pituitary fossa and compressing the optic chiasma. Treatment was initiated with bromocriptine, a dopamine agonist.

ACTH: adrenocorticotrophic hormone
CRH: corticotrophin-releasing hormone
DA: dopamine
FSH: follicle-stimulating hormone
GH: growth hormone
GHRH: growth hormone-releasing hormone
GnRH: gonadotrophin-releasing hormone
LH: luteinising hormone
TRH: thyrotrophin-releasing hormone
T_3: triiodothyronine
T_4: thyroxine

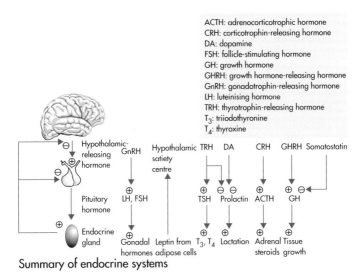

Summary of endocrine systems

88 Treatment of growth disorders

Growth hormone (GH), also referred to as **somatotropin**, is a polypeptide synthesised in somatotroph cells in the anterior pituitary gland and is a member of a family of polypeptide hormones, including prolactin. Its release is governed by two hypothalamic hormones, growth hormone-releasing hormone (GHRH) and somatostatin, which inhibits GH release. During growth, it has powerful effects on tissue growth and bone elongation. In adults it has important tissue regulatory activities.

Under-secretion of GH in children is usually a result of GHRH deficiency and results in dwarfism. In adults, GH deficiency is usually caused by a decrease in its production through: (i) pituitary lesions, caused by, for example, surgery or cranial irradiation; and (ii) peri-pituitary lesions, e.g. adenomas. Clinical features of GH deficiency in adults are summarised in the diagram. Serious consequences of metabolic changes in adults include increased risk of atheroma formation and cardiovascular accidents and mortality. Diagnosis of GH deficiency is made by measuring serum GH in response to the insulin tolerance test.

Treatment: In 2002, the NICE recommended GH for: children with proven deficiency; Prader–Willi syndrome, which is congenital obesity associated with small genitalia; mental handicap; diabetes mellitus; and chronic renal insufficiency before puberty. For adults, NICE recommends treatment only if three criteria are met, i.e. severe GH deficiency, impaired quality of life and if the patient is already receiving treatment for another pituitary hormone deficiency. Synthetic human GH is used, which avoids the risk of Creutzfeldt–Jakob disease (CJD) infection and cross-species reactions. It is usually supplied as a powder for reconstitution and subcutaneous or intramuscular injection, either using a needle or with a needle-free device. These injections are usually administered in the evening to mimic physiological conditions. Adverse reactions are usually relatively mild, but may include persistent headache, joint pains, and swelling of the feet and ankles. See the BNF for more details of the products available, precautions and adverse effects.

Excess secretion of GH in children and young adolescents, before fusion of the bony epiphyses, results in gigantism. In adults, over-secretion of GH results in acromegaly. Excess GH secretion is usually from a pituitary adenoma, although rare cases of ectopic GH-releasing tumours do occur. The symptoms of acromegaly include coarsening of the soft tissues of the feet, hands and facial features, and an enlarged mandible (lower jaw), together with hypertrophy of the liver, heart and kidney connective tissue. About 10% of acromegalic patients are diabetic because of lower glucose tolerance. Diagnosis is confirmed by increased serum insulin growth factor (IGF) and inability of raised GH levels to suppress serum IGF during an oral glucose tolerance test.

Treatment: Surgical removal of the pituitary adenoma is undertaken if possible, with or without radiotherapy. Careful surveillance of the tumour is required as significant expansion may occur during treatment. **Somatostatin** or one of the somatostatin analogues **octreotide** and **lanreotide** may be prescribed and is administered by subcutaneous injection according to the manufacturer's directions. **Adverse effects** include GIT upsets, such as steatorrhoea and diarrhoea. Chronic use of somatostatin analogues occasionally results in persistent hyperglycaemia and impaired postprandial glucose tolerance. **Drug interactions**: octreotide may reduce the requirements for the antidiabetic drugs insulin, metformin, repaglinide and the sulphonylureas. Octreotide increases plasma concentrations of administered bromocriptine.

Clinical scenario: Dr JB, a 57-year-old GP, tried to ignore pains in the joints of his hands, but when a colleague told him he looked acromegalic, he had himself referred to the local endocrine clinic, where biochemical investigations confirmed the initial diagnosis of acromegaly. His plasma GH level was elevated at 56 mU/l and failed to suppress when a glucose tolerance test was done. His plasma IGF-1 concentration was 6.5 times the upper limit of normal. An MRI scan of the pituitary revealed a pituitary macroadenoma arising from the pituitary fossa into the suprasellar space, which did not compress the optic chiasma. He responded well to pituitary surgery and subsequent radiotherapy, and many of the features of acromegaly resolved.

Clinical features associated with growth hormone deficiency (adults)

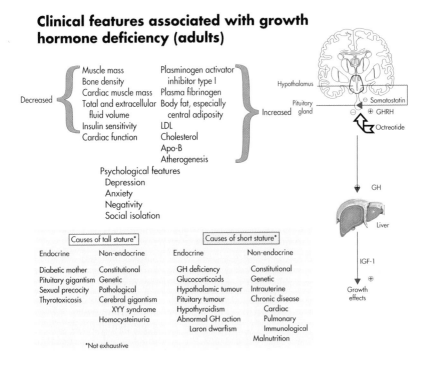

Decreased
Muscle mass
Bone density
Cardiac muscle mass
Total and extracellular
fluid volume
Insulin sensitivity
Cardiac function

Plasminogen activator
inhibitor type I
Plasma fibrinogen
Body fat, especially
central adiposity
LDL
Cholesterol
Apo-B
Atherogenesis

Increased

Hypothalamus
Pituitary gland
⊖ Somatostatin
⊕ GHRH
Octreotide
GH
Liver
IGF-1
Growth effects

Psychological features
Depression
Anxiety
Negativity
Social isolation

Causes of tall stature*		Causes of short stature*	
Endocrine	Non-endocrine	Endocrine	Non-endocrine
Diabetic mother	Constitutional	GH deficiency	Constitutional
Pituitary gigantism	Genetic	Glucocorticoids	Genetic
Sexual precocity	Pathological	Hypothalamic tumour	Intrauterine
Thyrotoxicosis	Cerebral gigantism	Pituitary tumour	Chronic disease
	XYY syndrome	Hypothyroidism	Cardiac
	Homocysteinuria	Abnormal GH action	Pulmonary
		Laron dwarfism	Immunological
			Malnutrition

*Not exhaustive

89 Treatment of thyroid disorders

The thyroid gland, situated anteriorly in the neck, secretes thyroxine (T_4) and **triiodothyronine** (T_3), which affect development, growth and metabolism. Their synthesis and secretion are controlled by the hypothalamic–pituitary axis. Hypothalamic TRH and a synthetic analogue **protirelin** cause release of TSH from the anterior pituitary. **Somatostatin** inhibits TRH release. TSH stimulates thyroid hormone production and release. Circulating T_3 and T_4 are largely bound to plasma proteins. The axis is regulated by levels of circulating thyroid hormones. Thyroid disorders are usually hypothyroidism or hyperthyroidism (thyrotoxicosis).

Hypothyroidism (called myxoedema in severe cases) is characterised by lethargy, sensitivity to cold, bradycardia, slow speech, and skin coarsening and thickening. Mental facilities are impaired and during development hypothyroidism can cause cretinism. An autoimmune disease, Hashimoto's thyroiditis (lymphadenoid goitre), causes hypothyroidism through development of autoantibodies to proteins involved in thyroid hormone production. Inadvertent use of excess radioiodine therapy may produce hypothyroidism. Iodine deficiency causes a non-toxic goitre, through an increase in pituitary thyrotrophin, which causes the gland to swell. Thyroid carcinoma is associated with hypothyroidism.

Hyperthyroidism (thyrotoxicosis) results in an excessively high metabolic rate, causing loss of weight with fatigue, increased appetite, excitability and nervousness. There is abnormally high sensitivity to heat, tachycardia, tremor, hyperthermia and sweating. The most common forms are Graves' disease (exophthalmic goitre or diffuse toxic goitre) and toxic nodular goitre. Toxic nodular goitre results from a benign neoplasm or adenoma. Amiodarone, an anti-dysrhythmic drug, contains iodine and may cause either hypo- or hyperthyroidism.

Treatment of hypothyroidism involves the administration of oral T_4 as **levothyroxine sodium** or T_3 as **liothyronine sodium**. ECG should be done initially to eliminate the possibility of ischaemia. With infants, treatment should be started immediately after diagnosis because of danger of permanent mental handicap. Levothyroxine sodium is the standard maintenance therapy. Doses in children and infants should be chosen after assessment of plasma T_4 and TSH levels, growth assessment and clinical response. Hypothyroid coma should be treated with intravenous liothyronine sodium. **Adverse effects** reflect over-dosage, which produce the symptoms of thyrotoxicosis.

Treatment of hyperthyroidism depends on the cause and may be surgical (usually when the thyroid obstructs respiration) or with drugs. **Radioactive iodine** (^{131}I) is taken orally and concentrated in the thyroid. It is useful for thyrotoxicosis in cardiac disease, if patients relapse after thyroidectomy or if other treatments are precluded. The **thiourylenes carbimazole**, which is metabolised to the active form, **methimazole**, and **propylthiouracil** are used orally. They may act by inhibiting the iodination of thyroglobulin. Carbimazole may suppress bone marrow and patients must be monitored for infections, particularly sore throat, and white cell counts taken. Treatment must be stopped immediately if neutropenia is detected. Iodine may be used during preparation for thyroidectomy, although its efficacy is disputed.

Propranolol counteracts some cardiovascular effects of hypothyroidism, e.g. agitation, dysrhythmias, tachycardia and tremor. It is useful in neonatal thyrotoxicosis but contraindicated in asthma.

Clinical scenario: A 33-year-old saleswoman was referred to the endocrinology clinic by her GP. Over 3 months she had lost 2 stone in weight, despite a normal diet. She had also developed sweating, palpitations and diarrhoea, and complained of feeling anxious most of the time. On examination she had a fine tremor in both hands. There was a regular tachycardia with a rate of 110 per minute. Her thyroid gland was palpable and there was a bruit heard. Eye movements were normal but lid lag and proptosis were noted. Blood tests revealed a depressed TSH and elevated T_3 and T_4, confirming thyrotoxicosis. Carbimazole and propranolol were prescribed and the patient was advised that if she developed any viral-type symptoms then she should have her white cell count checked immediately. After 6 months on treatment she was euthyroid and a course of ^{131}I was given.

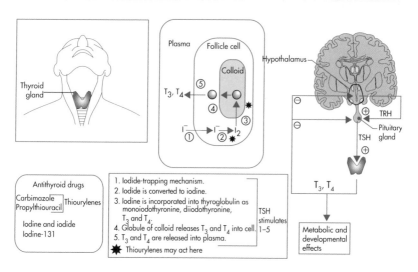

1. Iodide-trapping mechanism.
2. Iodide is converted to iodine.
3. Iodine is incorporated into thyroglobulin as monoiodothyronine, diiodothyronine, T_3 and T_4.
4. Globule of colloid releases T_3 and T_4 into cell.
5. T_3 and T_4 are released into plasma.
✳ Thiourylenes may act here

Antithyroid drugs
Carbimazole
Propylthiouracil │ Thiourylenes

Iodine and iodide
Iodine-131

TSH stimulates 1–5

Metabolic and developmental effects

90 Treatment of adrenal disorders

The adrenal glands are situated above each kidney (**A**) and consist of an inner medulla, which secretes the catecholamines epinephrine and norepinephrine, and an outer cortex, which consists of the outer zona glomerulosa, that produces aldosterone, and two inner zones, the thicker middle zone (the zona fasciculata) and a thinner zona reticularis, both of which produce cortisol and androgens. Cortisol's physiological actions (which should not be confused with the pharmacological actions of the synthetic glucocorticoids) are in intermediary metabolism, in which it stimulates hepatic gluconeogenesis, an anabolic action, whereas it is catabolic in muscle and adipose tissue, where it promotes tissue breakdown to mobilise glucose. Cortisol is involved in the maintenance of diurnal rhythms linked to light and dark and plays a permissive role in stress, where it allows greater utilisation of epinephrine by the tissues. Aldosterone is a mineralocorticoid promoting sodium re-uptake in the kidney.

Adrenal insufficiency is deficient secretion of cortisol and/or aldosterone and may be primary, through destruction of adrenocortical tissue, or secondary to tumours of the brain or pituitary gland. Primary adrenal insufficiency (Addison's disease) is autoimmune destruction of adrenocortical tissue. Aldosterone deficiency occurs in Addison's disease or through other causes. Patients may initially suffer an addisonian crisis with hypotensive collapse, fever and abdominal pain. High circulating ACTH and melanocyte-stimulating hormone (MSH) cause skin pigmentation and there is chronically low plasma Na^+ and high plasma K^+. Diagnosis is by injection of a biologically active fragment of ACTH, which with a non-responsive adrenal cortex does not result in an increase in plasma cortisol. Patients are given glucocorticoid and mineralocorticoid replacement, using prednisolone and fludrocortisone, respectively. Pituitary tumours may cause secondary adrenal insufficiency, when ACTH will cause cortisol release. Also, patients suffer the effects of cortisol lack, but not the pigmentation.

Adrenal hyperfunction causes **Cushing's syndrome**, a set of symptoms resulting from excess glucocorticoid secretion. **Cushing's disease** is a specific form of the syndrome caused by excess ACTH secretion by a pituitary tumour. The syndrome may be caused iatrogenically (drug induced) through the use of chronic, high-dose glucocorticoids.

Excess cortisol production may be accompanied by excess adrenal androgen secretion (see below). The features of Cushing's syndrome are shown in (**A**).

Treatment of Cushing's syndrome involves the surgical removal of the ACTH-secreting tumour if possible, or its destruction by irradiation. Microsurgical techniques have improved the precision of pituitary surgery, and drug treatments are ancillary to these. Drugs used include **ketoconazole**, a drug normally used to treat fungal infections, and **metapyrone**, which inhibits the enzyme 11β-hydroxylase in the adrenal cortex.

Virilism is excess production of adrenal androgens and in women results in, for example, hirsutism and alopecia (scalp hair loss). Congenital virilising adrenal hyperplasia results from a deficiency of enzymes involved in cortisol and aldosterone synthesis. This is usually treated with cortisol and mineralocorticoid replacement. Women may be treated with an anti-acne drug, **co-cyprindiol**, which is a mixture of an anti-androgen, **cyproterone acetate**, and the synthetic estrogen **ethinylestradiol**.

Clinical scenario: A19-year-old young woman was seen in A&E with dizziness. For the preceeding few months she had experienced dizziness when standing, loss of appetite and abdominal pains. On examination, her blood pressure was 110/60 supine and 80/40 when standing. There was pigmentation of her buccal mucosa and also along skin creases in both hands. Blood tests revealed hyponatraemia and hyperkalaemia. A short Synacthen test was performed which confirmed Addison's disease and she was commenced on hydrocortisone and fludrocortisone. Her symptoms improved and she was discharged from hospital a few days later. Subsequent investigations confirmed the presence of adrenal autoantibodies.

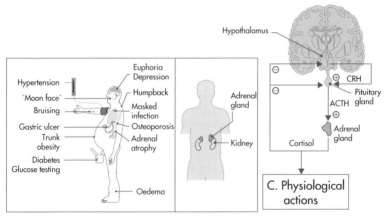

A. Features of Cushing's syndrome (excess glucocorticoids)

Reprinted from *Trounce's Clinical Pharmacology for Nurses* by Ben Greenstein (2004), page 207, with permission from Elsevier.

B. Anatomical location of the adrenal glands

C. Physiological actions

91 The sex hormones

The **female steroid hormones** important for reproduction are the **estrogens**, particularly **estradiol**, and the progestogenic hormone **progesterone**. Estradiol is synthesised by the developing ovarian follicle and progesterone by the corpus luteum after ovulation. Both are secreted into the circulation where they are largely bound to specific plasma proteins. Estradiol produces the typical female body shape. It promotes the proliferation of the uterine endometrium and prepares it for the action of progesterone by stimulating progesterone receptor synthesis. Progesterone renders the endometrium secretory to ready it for implantation of the fertilised ovum.

Both hormones regulate their biosynthesis through feedback mechanisms to the hypothalamus and anterior pituitary gland, by altering the release of the hypothalamic peptide **gonadotrophin-releasing hormone (GnRH)** and of the pituitary gonadotrophins **luteinising hormone** (**LH**) and **follicle-stimulating hormone** (**FSH**). In primates, GnRH is released into the portal circulation in a pulsatile manner, every 60–90 minutes, and the pulse interval may determine the ratio of LH/FSH secretion. During follicular development, the sex hormones exercise a negative feedback action on release of gonadotrophins from the pituitary gland but, when the egg is ready, estradiol exerts a positive feedback action on the brain and pituitary to cause a massive release of LH, which ruptures the ripe follicle and releases the ovum into the fimbria of the oviduct. After ovulation, if the egg is fertilised, the corpus luteum continues to produce progesterone until the placenta takes over production, otherwise the corpus luteum regresses, menstruation occurs and the cycle is repeated (**B**).

Estradiol under certain circumstances is considered to be carcinogenic, and can exacerbate and accelerate the progression of breast cancer, which is why women diagnosed with breast cancer before the discovery of **tamoxifen** routinely underwent bilateral oophorectomy and adrenalectomy to remove all sources of endogenous estradiol.

The discovery of the actions of estradiol and progesterone produced the oral contraceptives and HRT and modern fertility treatments. The discovery and characterisation of the estrogen and progesterone receptors led to the development of the estrogen receptor antagonist tamoxifen for the treatment of breast cancer, the selective estrogen receptor modulators (SERMs) and of the progesterone receptor antagonist **mifepristone** (RU486) as an abortifacient (**D**).

The discovery of the pulsatile release of GnRH from the hypothalamus produced a fertility treatment and the discovery that continuous exposure of the pituitary to GnRH causes sterility produced a treatment for prostate cancer.

The **male sex hormone testosterone** is synthesised by the testicular Leydig cells in response to LH. The germinal epithelium produces spermatozoa in response to FSH. Testosterone in turn exerts a negative feedback effect on both LH and FSH release. Testosterone is **androgenic**, i.e. it promotes the development and maintenance of the male sex organs, accessory sex organs and the secondary sexual characteristics, such as deep voice, beard and male body hair distribution. It is also anabolic, by promoting and maintaining muscle mass. Testosterone is a hormone but also a prohormone and is metabolised in target tissues to another active androgen, 5α-dihydrotestosterone (**C**). Testosterone and synthetic analogues are used to treat delayed puberty and to increase weight.

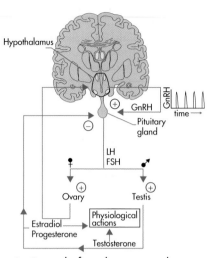

Hypothalamus

GnRH
Pituitary gland

LH
FSH

Ovary
Testis

Estradiol
Progesterone

Physiological actions

Testosterone

A. Control of sex hormone release

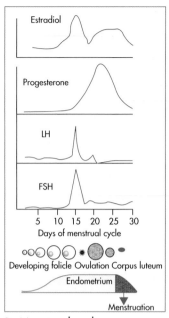

Estradiol

Progesterone

LH

FSH

5 10 15 20 25 30
Days of menstrual cycle

Developing follicle Ovulation Corpus luteum

Endometrium

Menstruation

B. Menstrual cycle

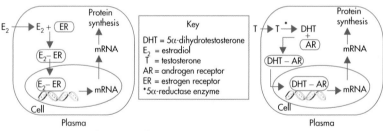

E_2 → E_2 + ER → Protein synthesis

mRNA

E_2– ER

E_2– ER → mRNA

Cell

Plasma

Key

DHT = 5α-dihydrotestosterone
E_2 = estradiol
T = testosterone
AR = androgen receptor
ER = estrogen receptor
*5α-reductase enzyme

T → T* → DHT + AR → Protein synthesis

mRNA

DHT – AR

DHT – AR → mRNA

Cell

Plasma

C. Mechanism of action of androgens and estrogens

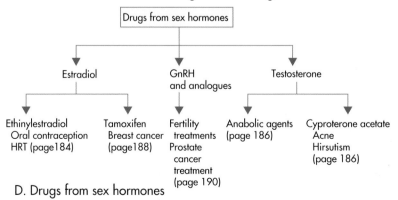

Drugs from sex hormones

Estradiol

GnRH and analogues

Testosterone

Ethinylestradiol
Oral contraception
HRT (page 184)

Tamoxifen
Breast cancer
(page 188)

Fertility
treatments
Prostate
cancer
treatment
(page 190)

Anabolic agents
(page 186)

Cyproterone acetate
Acne
Hirsutism
(page 186)

D. Drugs from sex hormones

92 Oral contraceptives

Oral contraceptives (OCs) are either combined, containing an estrogen (usually **ethinylestradiol**) and a **progestogen**, or **progestogen only**. Combined contraceptives may be **monophasic**, containing fixed amounts of the two steroids, or **biphasic** or **triphasic**, containing varying amounts of the steroids in sequential fashion to mimic the menstrual cycle (**A**). The bi- or triphasic OCs are generally prescribed for women who either do not have withdrawal bleeding or have breakthrough bleeding with monophasic OCs. OCs may be either low-strength estrogen or standard-strength estrogen. The progestogens used include **etynodiol**, **levonorgestrel** and **norethisterone** or the newer third-generation progestogens **desogestrel** and **gestodene**, which have fewer androgenic effects, cause fewer changes in lipoprotein metabolism and are more potent than the older progestogens, although they are associated with an increased incidence of venous thromboembolism. This form of contraception is now available also as a transdermal patch, containing **ethinylestradiol** and **norelgestromin**.

The combined OC is taken daily for 21 days followed by 7 pill-free days. It is taken daily, when its efficiency is 99%. **Mechanism of action**: ethinylestradiol inhibits FSH release, which prevents development of the ovarian follicle; the progestogen inhibits LH release, which prevents ovulation, and produces an endometrial mucus that reduces sperm motility (**B**). Withdrawal of the progestogen after 21 days precipitates menstruation. The **progestogen-only** pill is taken continuously and inhibits LH release, reduces sperm motility and may also block implantation of a fertilised ovum. This OC reduces the chances of pregnancy by about 90%. It is available also in parenteral form as: (i) a depot preparation of **medroxyprogesterone acetate** for intramuscular injection; (ii) an implant rod containing **etonogestrel**, which is implanted subdermally in the lower surface of the upper arm; and (iii) an intrauterine progestogen-releasing device containing **levonorgestrel**.

OC use and pregnancy risk: Missed pills increase the chance of pregnancy, especially at either the beginning or the end of a cycle of OC use, thus increasing the pill-free interval. The next should be taken as soon as the omission is discovered, but it should be realised that protection is lost for at least 7 days after missing the pill, even if the course is continued.

Combined OCs are associated with several health risks (**C**), including increased risk of **venous thromboembolism** (**VT**), particularly with higher doses of estrogen. The risk is greatest within the first year, although this risk is smaller than the risk of pregnancy. The risk is lowest with the third-generation OCs. For all combined OCs the risk does increase with age and women over 50 are usually advised not to continue. **Precautions** include a family history of VT, obesity, long-term immobilisation and varicose veins, and OCs are **contraindicated** in women with at least two of these conditions. **Arterial disease risk factors** include a family history of arterial disease, diabetes mellitus, hypertension, smoking, obesity, migraine and age (35 years or over). Women with two of these factors should avoid combined OCs. Other **contraindications** include pregnancy, liver disease, SLE, cardiovascular problems, e.g. heart disease associated with pulmonary embolism and TIAs without headaches. For these patients, and for heavy smokers, the progestogen-only pill may be a viable alternative. Breast cancer is a relatively low risk with the combined OC, and is generally confined to the breast.

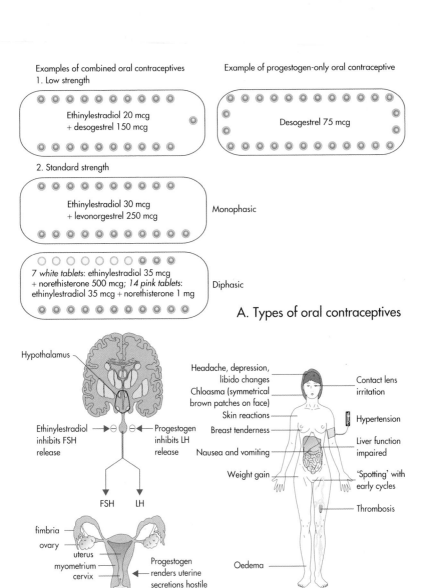

Examples of combined oral contraceptives
1. Low strength

Ethinylestradiol 20 mcg
+ desogestrel 150 mcg

Example of progestogen-only oral contraceptive

Desogestrel 75 mcg

2. Standard strength

Ethinylestradiol 30 mcg
+ levonorgestrel 250 mcg

Monophasic

7 *white tablets*: ethinylestradiol 35 mcg
+ norethisterone 500 mcg; *14 pink tablets*:
ethinylestradiol 35 mcg + norethisterone 1 mg

Diphasic

A. Types of oral contraceptives

Hypothalamus

Ethinylestradiol
inhibits FSH
release

Progestogen
inhibits LH
release

FSH   LH

fimbria
ovary
uterus
myometrium
cervix
vagina

Progestogen
renders uterine
secretions hostile
to sperm; may
also inhibit
implantation

Headache, depression,
libido changes
Chloasma (symmetrical
brown patches on face)
Skin reactions
Breast tenderness
Nausea and vomiting

Weight gain

Contact lens
irritation

Hypertension

Liver function
impaired

'Spotting' with
early cycles

Thrombosis

Oedema

B. Mechanism of action of OCs   C. Side-effects of combined OCs

93 Hormone replacement therapy

Hormone replacement therapy (HRT) is the clinical use of sex hormones or derivatives during and after menopause to prevent and ameliorate the unwanted effects following cessation of ovarian function. HRT includes androgen replacement in cases of, for example, delayed puberty or hypogonadism in the male.

HRT is now used by an estimated 20 million women worldwide.[26] Currently HRT is recommended for short-term use, but not for chronic use, when the risks may outweigh the benefits.[27]

Early clinical manifestations of menopause reflect declining estrogens and include vasomotor reactions ('hot flushes'), skin thinning and wrinkling, loss of pubic and axial hair, and emotional problems. **Later manifestations** include bone loss acceleration with danger of fractures, and lipid changes, including increased circulating cholesterol and a rise in LDL with a decline in LDL receptors (**A**).

Preparations for HRT include a combination of a low-potency estrogen such as oral estradiol, which is readily metabolised, and a progestogen, or estradiol alone (**B**). Ethinylestradiol is not used. Conjugated equine estrogens, or estradiol valerate together with a progestogen such as levonorgestrel or norethisterone, are prescribed orally or as patches, *which should be not placed anywhere near the breast.* Estradiol alone may be administered as a nasal spray, a gel or an implant, together with cyclical progestogen administration (**C**). **Estradiol, estriol** and **estrone** are prescribed orally as tablets, or estriol alone. The androgens **testosterone** or **tibolone** are sometimes prescribed for adjuvant therapy for menopausal symptoms.

Adverse effects and precautions with HRT: Adverse effects include nausea, vomiting and other GIT upsets, oedema, weight gain, breast tenderness, glucose intolerance, jaundice, blood lipid changes, libido and mood changes, headache, dizziness and hypersensitivity reactions (**D**). Reactions against contact lenses may occur. Uterine fibroids may become enlarged. It is currently felt that **the long-term risks** of, for example, VT, cardiovascular disease and gynaecological cancers, notably ovarian cancer and endometrial cancer in women with an intact uterus, outweigh the advantages.[27] **Precautions** include the presence of antiphospholipid antibodies due to risk of thrombosis, although SLE is not necessarily a contraindication.

HRT in the male: Androgens may be used to treat hypogonadism in men and delayed puberty in boys. Androgens are widely misused by both men and women in sport as anabolic agents to improve performance.

Preparations: Testosterone or its esters, e.g. **testosterone undecenoate, enantate** or **propionate**, are formulated as gels, transdermal patches, oily injections or mucoadhesive buccal tablets. **Adverse effects** include androgenic effects such as hirsutism, alopecia and accelerated epiphyseal closure in prepubertal boys. Testosterone and other androgens may initiate or aggravate prostate cancer. **Risks and precautions** include prostate cancer, hepatic, renal or cardiovascular impairment, diabetes and hypercalcaemia due to skeletal metastases. Prostate monitoring is advisable during treatment. Androgens are **contraindicated** in male breast cancer, hypercalcaemia, where there is a history of primary liver tumours, nephrotic syndrome, pregnancy and breastfeeding.

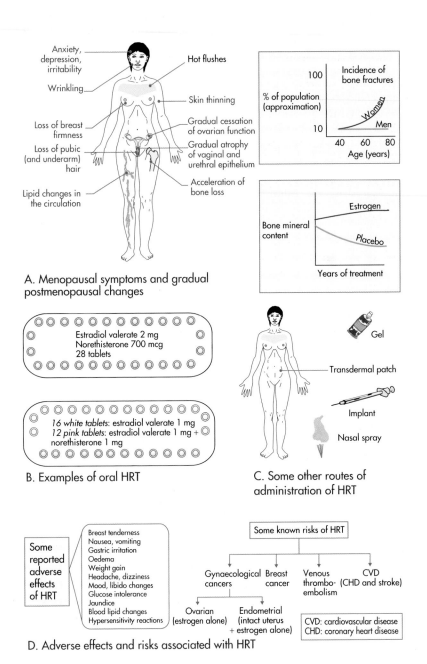

Anxiety, depression, irritability

Wrinkling

Loss of breast firmness

Loss of pubic (and underarm) hair

Lipid changes in the circulation

Hot flushes

Skin thinning

Gradual cessation of ovarian function

Gradual atrophy of vaginal and urethral epithelium

Acceleration of bone loss

Incidence of bone fractures

100

% of population (approximation)

10

Women

Men

40   60   80
Age (years)

Bone mineral content

Estrogen

Placebo

Years of treatment

A. Menopausal symptoms and gradual postmenopausal changes

Estradiol valerate 2 mg
Norethisterone 700 mcg
28 tablets

16 white tablets: estradiol valerate 1 mg
12 pink tablets: estradiol valerate 1 mg + norethisterone 1 mg

B. Examples of oral HRT

Gel

Transdermal patch

Implant

Nasal spray

C. Some other routes of administration of HRT

Some reported adverse effects of HRT

Breast tenderness
Nausea, vomiting
Gastric irritation
Oedema
Weight gain
Headache, dizziness
Mood, libido changes
Glucose intolerance
Jaundice
Blood lipid changes
Hypersensitivity reactions

Some known risks of HRT

Gynaecological cancers

Breast cancer

Venous thrombo-embolism

CVD (CHD and stroke)

Ovarian (estrogen alone)

Endometrial (intact uterus + estrogen alone)

CVD: cardiovascular disease
CHD: coronary heart disease

D. Adverse effects and risks associated with HRT

94 Drug treatment of breast cancer

Breast cancer: Treatment options for breast cancer are **local** and **systemic**. Local treatments are surgery and irradiation. In many cases both options are needed. Systemic treatments are **chemotherapy, hormonal therapy** and **biological** therapy. Treatment choices depend on: (i) properties of the cancer; (ii) stage; (iii) the patient's general health; and (iv) the patient's own choices. Surgery may be: breast saving (partial breast removal) or complete removal (mastectomy); radical mastectomy (removal of underarm lymph nodes) is now rarely done; and irradiation, usually localised to the breast, which limits adverse effects. Following surgical removal of the tumour, all women should be considered for adjuvant treatment because micrometastases may escape surgery. The treatment will depend on the estrogen receptor (ER) status of the primary tumour, the risk of recurrence and menopausal status.

ER-positive tumours contain estrogen receptors and physiological estrogens can exacerbate the cancer; thus, estrogen receptors are blocked using **tamoxifen**, an estrogen receptor antagonist (**B**). Estrogens are biosynthesised by aromatisation of the A-ring (see opposite), and **aromatase inhibitors** such as **exemestane** (a steroid), or **anastrozole and letrozole** (non-steroidal), which block aromatisation, are also options for ER+ tumours. Aromatase inhibitors are prescribed for postmenopausal women who cannot take tamoxifen. Cytotoxic drugs may be used as supplements.

ER-negative tumours require chemotherapy. It is indicated if the cancer is diagnosed as HER2[30]-positive, ER negative, with a high growth rate or with lymphatic and vascular invasion. Chemotherapy for first-line therapy for metastatic breast cancer, or for advanced cancer, may employ either **anthracycline antibiotics**, e.g. **mitoxantrone** (an anthracycline derivative), or **doxorubicin** may be used, or cyclophosphamide, or a combination of methotrexate and fluorouracil and cyclophosphamide. The choice will depend on whether the drugs have been previously used as adjuvant therapy, and on the distribution and rate of progression of the disease. The NICE has recommended that the **taxanes docetaxel** and **paclitaxel** be used for advanced breast cancer when other cytotoxic therapy has failed or is inappropriate.[31]

Biological therapy currently is the use of **trastuzumab**, a recombinant humanised monoclonal antibody directed against the HER2 protein. It is licensed for patients with metastatic breast cancer who over-express HER2 at level 3+ (see opposite) and who do not respond to other forms of therapy, or for whom anthracyclines and taxanes would be inappropriate. See NICE[31] for more details. Cost, as with the other biological treatments, is a significant consideration, because the cost of a 38-week combination course of trastuzumab and paclitaxel is approximately £9600 for paclitaxel and £15 500 for trastuzumab, although precedent suggests that prices may come down when patents expire.

The prognosis for breast cancer depends on several factors, including the **stage** of the cancer when first diagnosed. Mortality has fallen by at least 20%, due mainly to earlier detection and better treatment. The smaller the tumour, the less likely metastasis will have occurred. The second factor is the **grade** of the cancer – the more abnormal the tissue appears histologically, the higher the grade. Ductal carcinoma *in situ* (DCIS) is carcinoma of cells lining the milk ducts of the breast and is curable (grade 0). Historically, patients diagnosed with cancers less than 2 cm across with no lymph node involvement have a 70–78% chance of surviving at least 10 years after diagnosis. Every case is, however, unique, since cancers grow at different rates and treatment efficacy varies with the individual.

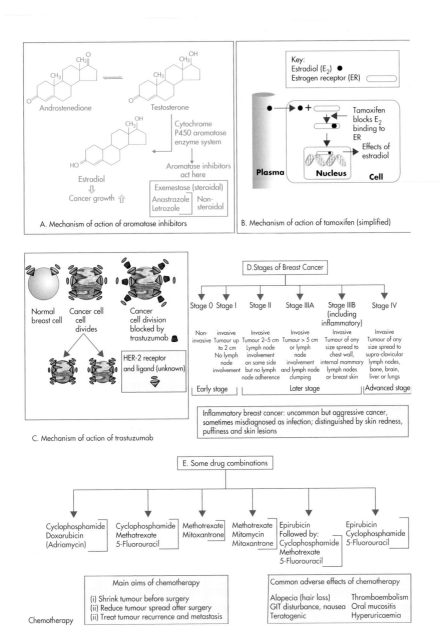

A. Mechanism of action of aromatase inhibitors

B. Mechanism of action of tamoxifen (simplified)

C. Mechanism of action of trastuzumab

D. Stages of Breast Cancer

Stage 0	Stage I	Stage II	Stage IIIA	Stage IIIB (including inflammatory)	Stage IV
Non-invasive	Invasive Tumour up to 2 cm No lymph node involvement	Invasive Tumour 2–5 cm Lymph node involvement on same side but no lymph node adherence	Invasive Tumour > 5 cm or lymph node involvement and lymph node clumping	Invasive Tumour of any size spread to chest wall, internal mammary lymph nodes or breast skin	Invasive Tumour of any size spread to supra-clavicular lymph nodes, bone, brain, liver or lungs

| Early stage | Later stage | Advanced stage |

Inflammatory breast cancer: uncommon but aggressive cancer, sometimes misdiagnosed as infection; distinguished by skin redness, puffiness and skin lesions

E. Some drug combinations

| Cyclophosphamide Doxorubicin (Adriamycin) | Cyclophosphamide Methotrexate 5-Fluorouracil | Methotrexate Mitoxantrone | Methotrexate Mitomycin Mitoxantrone | Epirubicin Followed by: Cyclophosphamide Methotrexate 5-Fluorouracil | Epirubicin Cyclophosphamide 5-Fluorouracil |

Chemotherapy

Main aims of chemotherapy

(i) Shrink tumour before surgery
(ii) Reduce tumour spread after surgery
(ii) Treat tumour recurrence and metastasis

Common adverse effects of chemotherapy

Alopecia (hair loss)	Thromboembolism
GIT disturbance, nausea	Oral mucositis
Teratogenic	Hyperuricaemia

95 Ovarian and prostate cancer

Ovarian cancer may start in epithelial or germ cells. Known risk factors include early menarche and childless adulthood. A familial history increases the risk. In about 80% of women it is associated with the presence of a cell surface marker (CA125) in serum, although CA125 may be present in the absence of ovarian cancer. Drug treatments to increase fertility may increase the risk. There are defined stages of ovarian cancer (**A**) and more than 75% of cases are diagnosed at an advanced stage.

Treatment: At diagnosis, malignancy has usually spread to surrounding tissues and complete hysterectomy may be needed. Radiotherapy is complicated by effects on surrounding organs. **Chemotherapy** is generally preferred initially, and first-line therapy is usually a platinum-based compound, e.g. **carboplatin** or **cisplatin**, either alone or in combination with **paclitaxel**. **Cisplatin**, like the alkylating agents, reacts with DNA to cause intrastrand DNA cross-linking, probably between adjacent guanine residues of the DNA. This reaction breaks the hydrogen bonds between guanine and cytosine residues, resulting in DNA denaturation. It is administered intravenously by slow injection or infusion. **Adverse effects** include severe nausea and vomiting, which can be treated with a $5\text{-}HT_3$ receptor antagonist, e.g. **ondansetron**. Cisplatin is nephrotoxic, and concomitant hydration and diuresis must be provided. It is also ototoxic, and may cause anaphylactic reactions and peripheral neuropathies. **Carboplatin**, a derivative of cisplatin, is less nephrotoxic, neurotoxic and ototoxic. It is, however, more myelotoxic. **Paclitaxel** is a taxane. It stabilises microtubules in a polymerised state, resulting in mitotic arrest. It is administered as an infusion. **Adverse effects** include hypersensitivity reactions and require routine premedication with antihistamines, including an H_2-receptor antagonist, and a corticosteroid. Bradycardia, asymptomatic hypotension, arrhythmias, myelotoxicity, peripheral neuropathy and alopecia are other adverse effects. Patients who fail to respond may be given pegylated liposomal doxorubicin HCl.[32]

Prostate cancer may be diagnosed with newer assays for free and total PSA (prostate-specific antigen) in plasma and for pre-PSA. It may be treated with surgery, radiotherapy and drugs, or left untreated, depending on patient age and the tumour stage (**B**). Surgery may be radical prostatectomy, orchidectomy (orchiectomy; removal of the testes) or transurethral resection. Radiotherapy is an option if the tumour is still localised.

Pharmacological approaches use hormone therapy to stop testosterone production by pituitary down-regulation and with anti-androgens to block testosterone and dihydrotestosterone at the androgen receptor. Pituitary down-regulation is achieved using stable gonadorelin analogues including **goserelin, leuprorelin** and **triptorelin**. When using analogues it is important to administer an anti-androgen such as **cyproterone acetate, flutamide** or **bicalutamide**. This precaution diminishes the initial flare of LH release from the pituitary, which can cause a dangerous surge of testosterone release before its later shutdown.

Chemotherapy utilises drugs including **mitoxantrone** (**mitozantrone**) and **epirubicin**, both chemically related to the antibiotic doxorubicin. Mitoxantrone has dose-related cardiotoxicity; epirubicin is less cardiotoxic. Both may cause bone marrow suppression. **Estramustine**, an example of a so-called 'magic bullet', is a combination of mustine, a nitrogen mustard and an estrogen. **Docetaxel**, a taxane, is used with prednisolone for hormone-refractory metastatic prostate cancer.

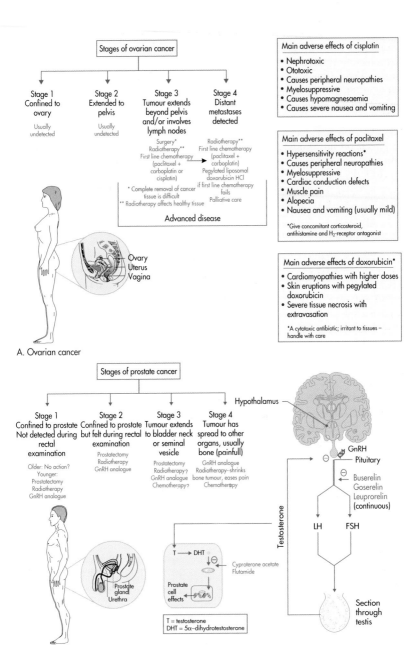

A. Ovarian cancer

Stages of ovarian cancer

Stage 1
Confined to ovary

Usually undetected

Stage 2
Extended to pelvis

Usually undetected

Stage 3
Tumour extends beyond pelvis and/or involves lymph nodes

Surgery*
Radiotherapy**
First line chemotherapy (paclitaxel + carboplatin or cisplatin)

* Complete removal of cancer tissue is difficult
** Radiotherapy affects healthy tissue

Stage 4
Distant metastases detected

Radiotherapy**
First line chemotherapy (paclitaxel + carboplatin)
Pegylated liposomal doxorubicin HCl if first line chemotherapy fails
Palliative care

Advanced disease

Ovary
Uterus
Vagina

Main adverse effects of cisplatin

- Nephrotoxic
- Ototoxic
- Causes peripheral neuropathies
- Myelosuppressive
- Causes hypomagnesaemia
- Causes severe nausea and vomiting

Main adverse effects of paclitaxel

- Hypersensitivity reactions*
- Causes peripheral neuropathies
- Myelosuppressive
- Cardiac conduction defects
- Muscle pain
- Alopecia
- Nausea and vomiting (usually mild)

*Give concomitant corticosteroid, antihistamine and H_2-receptor antagonist

Main adverse effects of doxorubicin*

- Cardiomyopathies with higher doses
- Skin eruptions with pegylated doxorubicin
- Severe tissue necrosis with extravasation

*A cytotoxic antibiotic; irritant to tissues – handle with care

B. Prostate cancer

Stages of prostate cancer

Stage 1
Confined to prostate Not detected during rectal examination

Older: No action?
Younger:
Prostatectomy
Radiotherapy
GnRH analogue

Stage 2
Confined to prostate but felt during rectal examination

Prostatectomy
Radiotherapy
GnRH analogue

Stage 3
Tumour extends to bladder neck or seminal vesicle

Prostatectomy
Radiotherapy?
GnRH analogue
Chemotherapy?

Stage 4
Tumour has spread to other organs, usually bone (painfull)

GnRH analogue
Radiotherapy–shrinks bone tumour, eases pain
Chemotherpy

Prostate gland
Urethra

Hypothalamus

GnRH
Pituitary

Buserelin
Goserelin
Leuprorelin
(continuous)

LH   FSH

Testosterone

T → DHT
Cyproterone acetate
Flutamide

Prostate cell effects

T = testosterone
DHT = 5α–dihydrotestosterone

Section through testis

96 Type 1 diabetes mellitus

Type 1 diabetes mellitus is an autoimmune disease of the pancreas, which destroys pancreatic islet β-cells. This results in a life-threatening deficiency of insulin. It commonly presents in young children and adults and is more prevalent in populations originating from northern Europe. There are both environmental and genetic contributory factors. There appears to be an association in type 1 diabetes with HLA haplotypes DR3 and DR4 of the major histocompatibility complex (MHC) on chromosome 6.

Insulin is normally released in response to a rise in blood glucose levels. After a meal, insulin removes glucose from the circulation and promotes its uptake into the tissues via glucose transporters and also promotes glucose conversion to glycogen and lipids. In addition insulin promotes the conversion of fatty acids to lipids, and the uptake of amino acids into liver and skeletal muscle, where they are incorporated into protein. Insulin is therefore an anabolic hormone.

Insulin lack results in a failure by the tissues to take up circulating glucose and the resulting hyperglycaemia deprives tissues of a major energy source; they respond with glycogenolysis, lipolysis and gluconeogenesis, all of which are catabolic. Excess glucose is excreted in the urine. The catabolic reactions generate ketone bodies and a dangerous ketosis, which if untreated leads to coma and death. Patients also face the ever-present problems of peripheral neuropathies, especially in the extremities, caused by the high circulating levels of glucose, which if not dealt with can cause retinal damage and blindness, and gangrene.

Treatment is with parenteral or inhaled human insulin and a carefully controlled diet. Human insulin is now prepared using recombinant DNA techniques, which eliminates problems of cross-species immune reactions. Preparations may be short, medium or long acting and come in several delivery forms (**A**). Treatment aims to maintain insulin levels within physiologically safe limits, i.e. about 4–9 mmol/l, which is achieved through regular and frequent patient-controlled monitoring of insulin blood levels, using glucose monitors (**B**). A typical treatment regimen might be to administer short-acting insulin 15–30 minutes before the three main meals and intermediate-acting insulin at night; alternatively, both short- and intermediate-acting insulins may be given before breakfast and supper. Insulin may be administered by injection using a syringe, a syringe pen or a pump, or orally by inhalation. Ongoing patient education and support by health professionals are essential.

Adverse effects of insulin are generally related to over-dosage, which causes hypoglycaemia, with dizziness, tremor, sweating and abnormal behaviour. Unless treated, convulsions, coma and death occur. It is relieved by giving sugar or glucose orally, or carefully by intravenous infusion if patients are unconscious. Glucagon or analogues may be given subcutaneously or intramuscularly. Other symptoms of insulin overdose include skin eruptions and pruritis at injection sites.

Transplantation of human islet β-cells into patients with type 1 diabetes is an interesting new avenue of research.

Clinical scenario: A 19-year-old boy with type 1 diabetes mellitus presented with vomiting, fever and breathlessness. His mother, who was with him, mentioned that he had had a cold for the last 3 days and, as he had not been eating, he had not taken his insulin injection that morning. He had been diagnosed with diabetes 5 years previously and usually took an injection of short-acting insulin 30 minutes before meals and an intermediate-acting preparation at night. On examination he was drowsy, dehydrated and hypotensive. His respiratory rate was 30 per minute and he smelt characteristically sweet. A peripheral capillary blood glucose measurement was 28 mmol/l and his arterial pH was 7.2. Urine dipstick testing was positive for ketones, glucose and protein. He was diagnosed with diabetic ketoacidosis and promptly started on treatment with rapid intravenous fluid replacement and intravenous insulin on a 'sliding scale', oxygen, and given antibiotics for a presumed chest infection. After 36 hours of treatment on this regimen his urine became free from ketones and he was transferred back on to his usual regimen of subcutaneous insulin without any complications.

A. Insulin injections

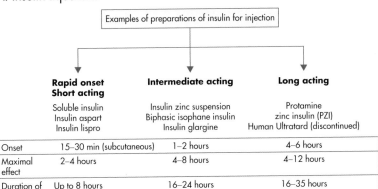

	Rapid onset Short acting	Intermediate acting	Long acting
	Soluble insulin Insulin aspart Insulin lispro	Insulin zinc suspension Biphasic isophane insulin Insulin glargine	Protamine zinc insulin (PZI) Human Ultratard (discontinued)
Onset	15–30 min (subcutaneous)	1–2 hours	4–6 hours
Maximal effect	2–4 hours	4–8 hours	4–12 hours
Duration of action	Up to 8 hours	16–24 hours	16–35 hours

Examples of preparations of insulin for injection

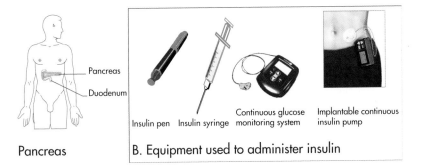

Pancreas
Duodenum

Insulin pen   Insulin syringe   Continuous glucose monitoring system   Implantable continuous insulin pump

Pancreas

B. Equipment used to administer insulin

97 Type 2 diabetes mellitus (NIDDM)

Type 2 diabetes occurs in approximately 85% of diabetic patients. Patients have the symptoms of insulin deficiency, and sometimes a reduced cellular responsiveness to insulin. Blood glucose is raised, with glycosuria, although ketoacidosis is less common in type 2 than in type 1 diabetes. Type 2 diabetes may be genetically linked. Patients with type 2 diabetes present with an apparent insulin resistance and may have a deficiency of insulin through an exhausted pancreas. Patients may be hyperinsulinaemic and may present with infection. Historically, type 2 diabetes has been a problem of the middle-aged and older patient, but younger patients are now presenting with it because of the increase in obesity. Type 2 diabetes may be distinguished from type 1 because patients with type 1 respond to a glucose infusion with a flat insulin response (A).

The primary aim of treatment is to control plasma glucose and lipids and to lower blood pressure, if raised. Patients are encouraged to give up smoking and lose weight (B). Patients face the risks of MI, neuropathy, retinopathy and renal failure. Most patients are overweight and, before drugs are prescribed, dietary control may be tried in order to reduce the fasting blood sugar below 9 mmol/l, and plasma cholesterol no higher than 6.5 mmol/1. ACE inhibitors may be prescribed to reduce blood pressure if diet fails. Blood pressure should be reduced, if possible, to about 145/85.

Drugs are prescribed after 6 months if dietary strategies fail. The principal orally active drugs available (C) are the biguanide **metformin**, if patients are overweight, and oral sulphonylureas such as **glibenclamide, glipizide** and **gliclazide**, if they are not, unless metformin is contraindicated. Oral sulphonylureas act by augmenting insulin release and are therefore active only if the pancreatic islets are healthy. Gliclazide is popular because the peak response is achieved after about 5 hours and the therapeutic effect may last up to 24 hours. Therefore it may be taken before breakfast and gives cover through lunch and supper. Also, it is rarely associated with hypoglycaemic episodes. **Adverse effects** of oral sulphonylureas include constipation, diarrhoea, nausea and vomiting, and hypersensitivity reactions. Relatively rarely, they may cause cholestatic jaundice. Sulphonylureas are contraindicated during pregnancy or when breastfeeding, and in ketoacidosis, hepatic or renal impairment, and porphyria.

The **thiazolidinediones pioglitazone** and **rosiglitazone** appear to reduce resistance to insulin, resulting in lower plasma glucose, and may be prescribed alone or with metformin or a sulphonylurea, although a thiazolidinedione–metformin combination is generally favoured. The prandial glucose regulators **nateglinide, repaglinide** and **acarbose** reduce postprandial plasma glucose. They are taken before eating and should not be taken if a meal is omitted. **Acarbose** inhibits α-glucosidase, which converts carbohydrate to glucose. If, however, the patient's islets fail to release insulin, the hormone will need to be prescribed. **Adverse effects** of acarbose include flatulence, diarrhoea and abdominal distension; hypoglycaemia and hypersensitivity reactions may occur with nateglinide and GIT disturbances with the thiazolidinediones. The thiazolidinediones, acarbose, nateglinide and repaglinide are all contraindicated during pregnancy and breastfeeding, and in patients with hepatic impairment, and acarbose is contraindicated in inflammatory bowel diseases such as Crohn's disease and ulcerative colitis. Liver function as well as plasma glucose and insulin should be monitored in patients prescribed the thiazolidinediones, nateglinide, acarbose and repaglinide.

Clinical scenario: A 53-year-old businessman was advised to make an appointment with his GP by the practice nurse. For the past 2 years he had been attempting to prevent the progression of type 2 diabetes mellitus by lifestyle modification. He was obese, smoked 20 cigarettes every day and drank 30 units of alcohol a week. His efforts at weight loss and smoking cessation were unsuccessful and his HbA_{1c} was steadily rising. On examination his blood pressure was elevated at 160/90 and there was reduced fine touch sensation in his left foot. Renal function was normal and there was no retinopathy. His cholesterol, however, was elevated at 5.6 mmol/l. He was commenced on metformin at 500 mg twice a day, simvastatin 20 mg at night for the cholesterol and ramipril, an ACE inhibitor, for the high blood pressure, at a dose of 1.25 mg, increasing to 2.5 mg daily after 2 weeks. He was also referred to a local smoking cessation coordinator. One year later his HbA_{1c} was still elevated and gliclazide 40 mg once a day was added to the metformin, which was also increased.

A. Insulin release during a constant glucose infusion   B. Treatment strategies for diabetes

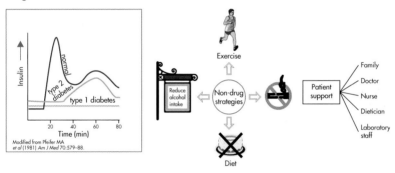

C. Anti-diabetic drugs

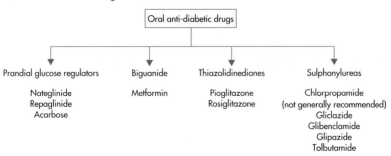

98 Osteoporosis

Osteoporosis is loss of bony tissue and is associated with morbidity and mortality. It is characterised by 'fragility fractures', defined as fractures after a fall, often involving the hip. Other common fractures include the spine and distal radius (Colles' fracture). Primary osteoporosis in women is caused by a combination of estrogen deficiency and age. In men the cause is less clear but probably includes age-related falls in circulating estrogen and androgen. Bone loss begins during the fifth decade of life. In both sexes peak bone mass is determined by nutrition, physical exercise, vitamin D, calcium, sex hormones and genetic status. The menopause accelerates the rate of bone loss. Other known risk factors include glucocorticoid drugs, ethnic origin, and history of thyroid disease, alcoholism and smoking. Osteoporosis is diagnosed using DEXA scans (dual-energy X-ray absorptiometry).

Prevention and treatment of osteoporosis: Patients should take calcium and vitamin D supplements regularly. **Bisphosphonates** prevent or slow the rate of bone loss at and after the menopause (**A**). Bisphosphonates currently used in the UK are **alendronic acid, disodium etidronate, disodium pamidronate, ibandronic acid, risendronate sodium, sodium clodronate, strontium ranelate, tiludronic acid** and **zoledronic arid**. They prevent bone loss in the hip and spine in healthy women at the menopause and in older patients with existing osteoporosis. Most are given as tablets taken once a week. Disodium pamidronate and zoledronic acid are formulated as intravenous infusions. Bisphosphonates are used also to treat the hypercalcaemia of malignancy and Paget's disease of bone (osteitis deformans). They are absorbed onto hydroxyapatite crystals in bone and reduce the rate of bone turnover by slowing the rates of bone growth and dissolution.

Clinical note: Patients are advised to swallow bisphosponates whole with plenty of water before breakfast, and while sitting or standing upright, and to take no food for at least 30 minutes after taking the tablets. This is because of the danger of oesophageal reflux, with possible oesophageal ulceration. Administration should be once weekly to reduce further the risk of GIT problems.[32]

Adverse effects with bisphosphonates include GIT upsets, such as oesophageal reactions, regurgitation, dyspepsia, gastric distension and diarrhoea. Because of their mechanism of action they can cause hypoglycaemia. They may cause other adverse effects, including hypersensitivity reactions, central effects, including hallucinations, renal problems, hyperphosphataemia and myalgia. They are generally contraindicated in pregnancy, breastfeeding and pre-existing oesophageal abnormalities or other conditions that delay gastric emptying, and should be used with caution in patients with renal or hepatic impairment, or with problems of calcium and phosphate metabolism.

Calcitonin is a hormone released by C cells in the thyroid gland that lowers blood levels of calcium and phosphate. It is used for patients who cannot tolerate bisphosphonates, to treat hypercalcaemia associated with malignancy and the pain of Paget's disease of bone. It may be administered as a nasal spray or an intramuscular or subcutaneous injection. **Teriparatide**, a recombinant fragment of parathyroid hormone, is also available (**B**).

HRT is used to prevent osteoporosis, but its prolonged use is now discouraged because of cardiovascular risks. **Raloxifene**, an SERM, is licensed to treat osteoporosis.

Clinical scenario: A 75 year-old woman with smoking-related chronic obstructive pulmonary disease (COPD) fell whilst shopping in the supermarket. She was unable to weight-bear and was admitted to hospital for treatment. There she was diagnosed with a fractured neck of her femur, which was repaired by the orthopaedic surgeons. During her post-operative recovery, it was noted that she had received several courses of steroids for infective exacerbations of her COPD during the past 4 years. A diagnosis of osteoporosis was made and she was started on a calcium/vitamin D combination and weekly alendronate. The calcium supplement resulted in constipation, which was treated with lactulose. The alendronate caused oesophagitis, which was controlled with lansoprazole.

A. Drug treatments for ostesporosis

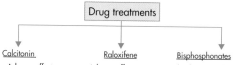

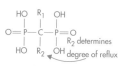

Bisphosphonic acid

Calcitonin

Adverse effects:
allergic reactions
in nose if inhaled,
or at site of injection;
diarrhoea, nausea,
vomiting

Raloxifene

Adverse effects:
thrombophlebitis,
venous thromboembolism,
peripheral oedema,
leg cramps, hot flushes,
hypertension,
breast discomfort

Bisphosphonates

Alendronic acid
Disodium etidronate
Disodium pamidronate
Ibandronic acid
Residronate sodium
Sodium clodronate
Strontium ranelate
Tiludronic acid
Zoledronic acid

Sodium alendronate

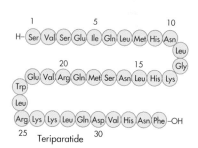

Teriparatide

Teriparatide is a recombinant fragment containing the biologically active region of human parathyroid hormone, marketed in the UK by Eli Lilly under the name Forsteo.®

B. Teriparatide

Preparation
Prefilled pen for subcutaneous injection, to treat post-menopausal osteoporosis
Action: Promotion of new bone formation
Adverse effects include nausea, vomiting, reflux and haemorrhoids; polyurea, muscle cramps, vertigo
Precautions include renal impairment
Contraindications: Paget's disease of bone, increased baseline risk of osteosarcoma, previous radiation therapy to bone, pre-existing hypercalcaemia, unexpained raised alkaline phosphatase, pregnancy, breastfeeding.

99 Gastro-oesophageal reflux disease

Gastro-oesophageal reflux disease (GERD) is inflammation of the oesophagus. The most common form is **reflux oesophagitis**, caused by frequent regurgitation of gastric juices as a result of abnormal relaxation of the lower oesophageal sphincter (**A**). It may be associated with a hiatus hernia. Other contributory causes include pregnancy, constipation and obesity. Symptoms are mainly regurgitation of bitter-tasting fluid, 'heartburn' and perhaps difficulty swallowing. Some patients may be hoarse and have breathing difficulties. Symptoms may be exacerbated by smoking, binge eating, or simply by bending over or lifting something. Complications may include stricture of the oesophageal canal, bleeding (which may lead to iron deficiency), ulceration and Barrett's oesophagus, when the normal squamous oesophageal epithelium is replaced by columnar epithelium, which is associated with a risk of malignancy.

The approach to treatment depends on the diagnosis and severity of symptoms. These may be severe, with the risk of erosion and malignancy, and require immediate investigation (see Clinical scenario 1 opposite), or mild, or non-erosive, when lifestyle changes and antacids, when necessary, may be the first choice (**B**). These are insoluble aluminium- or magnesium-based compounds that neutralise acid and provide symptomatic relief, e.g. **aluminium hydroxide** and **magnesium carbonate, hydroxide** or **trisilicate**. Aluminium hydroxide is available as chewable tablets, capsules or a suspension. Magnesium carbonate is available as an oral suspension, and magnesium trisilicate may be dispensed as an oral suspension. Compound formulations include **co-magaldrox**, a mixture of aluminium and magnesium hydroxides. **Adverse effects** of antacids are related to their adsorptive properties, their degree of solubility and their potential misuse. Aluminium salts constipate and magnesium salts are laxative. They interfere with drug action, e.g. aluminium salts adsorb drugs such as tetracyclines and inhibit their absorption from the GIT. Activated dimethicone (**simeticone**), an antifoaming agent, may be added to formulations to treat flatulence, and alginates may be included, which act as 'rafts' that float on the surface of the gastric contents, thus protecting the gastric mucosa and lessening the occurrence of reflux.

Histamine H_2-receptor antagonists such as **cimetidine, famotidine, nizatidine** and **ranitidine**, and **proton pump inhibitors**, e.g. **esomeprazole, lansoprazole, omeprazole, pantoprazole** and **rabeprazole**, are now regarded as treatments of choice for GERD, although proton pump inhibitors are more effective. **Adverse effects** of H_2-receptor antagonists include GIT disturbances and relatively rare hepatic impairment, which is a precaution or contraindication to their use. Impotence has been reported, especially with cimetidine. Proton pump inhibitors produce a similar pattern of adverse effects, and may mask the presence of gastric ulcers.

Motility stimulants are dopamine antagonists e.g. **domperidone** and **metoclopramide**. They (i) enhance the power of oesophageal sphincter contraction, (ii) stimulate gastric emptying and (iii) speed up the passage of small bowel contents. **Adverse effects** include acute dystonic reactions consisting of facial and ocular spasms, especially in children and young women. These may be treated with an injection of **procyclidine**, an antimuscarinic drug. In addition to drugs, **lifestyle changes** should be instituted, if necessary (see Clinical scenario 2 opposite).

Clinical scenario 1: Mr PO, a 62-year-old accountant who worked at home, presented to his GP with difficulty in swallowing and a feeling of acute discomfort when he tried to eat. He admitted to a drinking habit during the working day and he smoked two packets of cigarettes daily. He had lost about 6 kg of weight during the previous 2 months. The GP immediately sent him to hospital where a barium meal revealed a severe oesophageal stricture with an abnormal mucosal pattern. The appearance was typical of a stricture associated with a benign tumour, which was confirmed after taking biopsies. The tumour was removed and the patient advised to stop smoking and to moderate his alcohol intake.

Clinical scenario 2: Ms DR, a 52-year-old secretary, suffered from moderate hypertension for which she took nifedipine, was obese and had been taking antacids regularly for heartburn and burning reflux. She was partial to fish and chips, drank several cups of coffee and smoked a packet of cigarettes daily. She went to her GP complaining of a severe burning sensation in her chest, and was referred to a gastroenterologist who performed endoscopy and diagnosed GERD. Nifedipine, a calcium channel blocker that can lower oesopageal sphincter tone, was stopped and bendroflumethiazide, a thiazide diuretic, prescribed instead for the hypertension She was advised to lose weight, cut down or stop smoking, reduce her intake of fatty foods and coffee, and take antacids more sparingly.

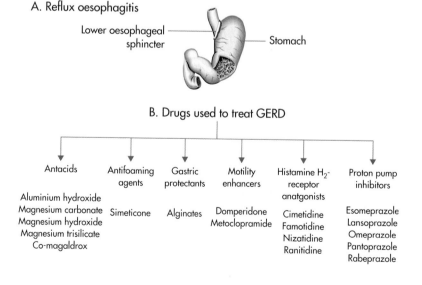

A. Reflux oesophagitis

Lower oesophageal sphincter

Stomach

B. Drugs used to treat GERD

Antacids	Antifoaming agents	Gastric protectants	Motility enhancers	Histamine H₂- receptor anatgonists	Proton pump inhibitors
Aluminium hydroxide Magnesium carbonate Magnesium hydroxide Magnesium trisilicate Co-magaldrox	Simeticone	Alginates	Domperidone Metoclopramide	Cimetidine Famotidine Nizatidine Ranitidine	Esomeprazole Lansoprazole Omeprazole Pantoprazole Rabeprazole

100 Gastric and duodenal ulceration and *H. pylori*

Gastric and duodenal ulcers are lesions of the mucous membrane (**A**). Many are caused by bacterial infection with **Helicobacter pylori**. Other potentially ulcerative factors, such as diet, lifestyle and stress, are now believed to be contributory but not necessarily causal. Drugs, e.g. NSAIDs, may cause ulcers. **Symptoms:** ulcers may be symptomless; the most common symptom is burning pain between the breastbone and navel. Other symptoms include nausea, vomiting, belching, weight and appetite loss, and fatigue. **Complications** include bleeding, obstruction, particularly at the junction between the antral part of the stomach and duodenum, and perforation, when gastric contents escape into the sterile environment of the peritoneum, causing peritonitis. **Diagnosis** may involve a barium meal, endoscopy, tissue biopsies, and blood and ^{13}C-labelled urea breath tests for infection.

Drug treatment involves (i) eradicating infection and (ii) ulcer-healing agents, including **proton pump inhibitors, H$_2$-receptor antagonists, chelating drugs, prostaglandin analogues** and **carbenoxolone**. *H. pylori*, if present, is usually effectively eradicated using triple therapy with a 1-week course of amoxicillin and either **clarithromycin** or **metronidazole** and a proton pump inhibitor. There is, however, a high relapse rate. **Ranitidine bismuth citrate** may be substituted for a proton pump inhibitor if the latter is contraindicated or not tolerated. Treatment for more than 1 week may produce more effective eradication but is generally not recommended because of adverse effects of the drugs and consequent poor compliance

Chelating agents form complexes with metal ions, thereby neutralising them. **Tripotassium dicitrobismuthate** is used together with two antibacterials and a proton pump inhibitor as part of a 2-week treatment for resistant cases of *H. pylori*. **Adverse effects** include nausea and vomiting, and both tongue and faeces may be darkened. It is **contraindicated** in pregnancy and with severe renal impairment. Bismuth is toxic, causing encephalopathy in higher doses, but at the time of writing no cases have been reported with the doses of tripotassium dicitrobismuthate used so far to treat ulcers. **Sucralfate** is a complex of sucrose and aluminium sulphate and may act by coating the mucosa, thus shielding it from acid and pepsin. **Adverse effects** include nausea, vomiting, diarrhoea, vertigo, dizziness and back pain. It should be used with caution when pregnant or breastfeeding, or in patients with severe renal impairment.

Misoprostol, a synthetic prostaglandin, has protective and secretion-inhibitory actions and promotes healing of both duodenal and gastric ulcers. It is administered in tablet form and is useful as a prophylactic treatment against the occurrence of NSAID-induced ulcers. **Adverse effects** include vaginal and intermenstrual bleeding, diarrhoea and abdominal pain. It is **contraindicated** in women of child-bearing age because of the danger of inadvertent abortion, and is used in these patients only if there is serious danger of ulceration with NSAIDs; these patients should be advised to take adequate contraception measures during treatment with misoprostol.

Carbenoxolone sodium is a synthetic derivative of glycerrhizinic acid, which is extracted from liquorice. It is formulated together with aluminium hydroxide, magnesium hydroxide and alginic acid as a chewable tablet. **Adverse effects** include hypokalaemia with consequent impairment of skeletal and cardiac muscle function, sodium retention and hypertension. Prolonged use may result in both kidney and muscle damage.

Clinical scenario: Mrs HP, a 30-year-old laboratory technician who often ate spicy curries and enjoyed an evening drink, started getting indigestion some hours after her evening meal and treated it with OTC antacids which helped at first, but the discomfort persisted. She was given ranitidine by a colleague and the symptoms subsided for a while but returned with severe pain above the navel. She went to her GP who sent her to the gastroenterology unit at the local hospital where after endoscopy and a ^{13}C-labelled urea breath test they diagnosed a duodenal ulcer. Triple therapy with a 1-week course of amoxicillin 1 g twice daily, clarithromycin 500 mg twice daily and esomeprazole 20 mg twice daily was prescribed. She was advised to lay off the spicy foods, cut down or stop alcoholic drinks until she was better, and not take medicines from colleagues or friends.

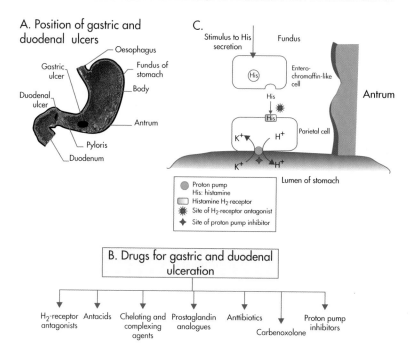

A. Position of gastric and duodenal ulcers

B. Drugs for gastric and duodenal ulceration

C.

Pancreatitis is inflammation of the pancreas and may be acute or chronic. Acute pancreatitis requires immediate hospitalisation. Around 50% of cases are caused by obstruction of the pancreatic duct by gallstones and alcoholism accounts for most of the others. Peptic ulcers, trauma, major abdominal or cardiac surgery, and some prescription drugs, e.g. oral contraceptives, may precipitate acute pancreatitis. Acute pancreatitis may be secondary to, for example, intrabiliary rupture of a hyatid cyst. Pancreatic inflammation is mediated by activation of enzyme systems within the pancreas, which 'autodigest' pancreatic tissue. Full recovery is possible, although relapses do occur. **Chronic pancreatitis**, however, is incurable because of irreversible tissue damage. Almost all cases in the West are a result of chronic alcohol excess whereas in tropical countries malnutrition related to tapioca (cassava) intake is a principal cause. Cystic fibrosis or haemochromatosis may be causative. Pancreatitis may be secondary to other conditions.

Symptoms include upper abdominal pain radiating through to the back, nausea, vomiting, abdominal distension because of fluid leakage, mild hyperpyrexia, and raised blood, urine and peritoneal fluid amylase. With chronic hyperpyrexia, eating causes pain and patients may fast and lose weight; insulin and glucagon lack may cause symptoms of diabetes mellitus, and lipase deficiency causes fat malabsorption with resultant steatorrhoea. **Diagnosis** includes ultrasound for gallstones and measurement of pancreatic amylase, and a CT scan of the abdomen may be done.

Treatment: Acute pancreatitis requires analgesia, usually an opiate, and fluids, both colloid and crystalloid. Patients will need referral to the intensive therapy unit if prognosis is poor. Initial aims are to stop further progression of local disease and to prevent remote organ failure. Patients may be hypoxic and require ventilation or increased inspired oxygen. Early visual examination of the pancreas and ducts may be needed using ultrasound. ERCP (endoscopic retrograde cholangiopancreatography), which achieves duct decompression, especially if the patient is jaundiced with severe pancreatitis and gallstone involvement is suspected. Broad-spectrum antibiotics are of proven prophylactic value for sepsis of necrosed pancreatic tissue. Mild acute pancreatitis may resolve within days. If there is any biliary aetiology, cholecystectomy (surgical removal of the gallbladder) should be done once acute symptoms have settled. After discharge patients must stop all alcohol. They should be gradually weaned off opiates to try to avoid the development of dependence. Patients who fail to put on weight or with persistent pain must be re-evaluated for development of chronic pancreatitis.

Chronic pancreatitis is treated with a variety of measures, mainly to try to stop organ damage and reduce the probability of future attacks. Strategies include: (i) stopping alcohol intake; (ii) prescribing a low-fat diet to reduce pancreatic load; and (iii) prescription of oral pancreatic enzymes, e.g. **pancreatin**, a porcine extract of pancreas. Patients are advised to take pancreatin with or shortly after meals to minimise GIT metabolism, and not to take pancreatin with hot food, because it is inactivated by heat. Dosage is titrated against stool consistency, size and frequency. It is irritant to buccal membranes and should be swallowed immediately.

Clinical scenario: A 50-year-old gentleman with a history of alcoholism was admitted with abdominal pain and vomiting. The pain had started gradually that afternoon and increased dramatically in severity. The pain was located in the upper epigastric region and radiated through to his back. On examination he was distressed, sweating, and tachycardic. He was breathless but oxygen saturations in air and chest, arterial blood gases and abdominal X-rays were normal. His abdomen was tender to palpation. Blood tests revealed markedly elevated amylase which confirmed acute pancreatitis. He was treated with IV opiates for analgesia and metoclopramide for nausea and vomiting and given oxygen via a face mask. He was started on a reducing regime of chlordiazepoxide. Subsequent ultrasound examination of his pancreas was unremarkable.

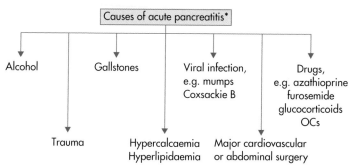

Causes of acute pancreatitis*

- Alcohol
- Gallstones
- Viral infection, e.g. mumps Coxsackie B
- Drugs, e.g. azathioprine furosemide glucocorticoids OCs
- Trauma
- Hypercalcaemia Hyperlipidaemia
- Major cardiovascular or abdominal surgery

Indicators of poor prognosis include:*

Age > 55 years
Glucose > 10 mmol/l
LDH > 600 iu/l
Calcium < 2 mmol/l
Urea > 16 mmol/l
Po_2 < 60 mmHg (< 8 kPa)
* Not comprehensive

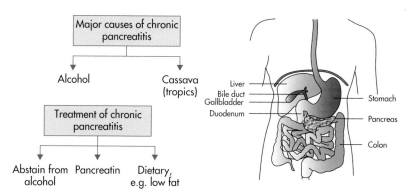

Major causes of chronic pancreatitis

- Alcohol
- Cassava (tropics)

Treatment of chronic pancreatitis

- Abstain from alcohol
- Pancreatin
- Dietary, e.g. low fat

Liver
Bile duct
Gallbladder
Duodenum
Stomach
Pancreas
Colon

Relationship of bile duct to gallbladder and liver

102 Small bowel disorders: Coeliac disease and carcinoids

The **small bowel** consists of the duodenum, jejunum and ileum. It is the major site of absorption of most food and drugs, and so any disorders of the small bowel will have a serious impact on nutrition and the efficacy of drug action. Small bowel disorders that impair absorption and thus nutrition include **coeliac disease, carcinoid tumours, diarrhoea** and **malabsorption**. GIT surgery may cause problems with small bowel absorption.

Coeliac disease is a type 4 hypersensitivity reaction to gluten, a blanket term for glutenin and acid-insoluble prolamines, including the gliadin found in cereals, notably wheat, rye, oats and barley (**A**). Consequences of the hypersensitivity reaction include cryptic hyperplasia and villous atrophy in the small bowel with resultant malabsorption. Patients present with growth retardation, unexplained anaemia, weight loss, diarrhoea and oral aphthous ulcers, which occur as small red and white spots in the mouth. It is **diagnosed** using antigliadin antibodies (**B**), anti-endomysial[34] antibodies and upper gastrointestinal endoscopy with a jejunal biopsy. Complications of coeliac disease include hyposplenism, increased risk of small bowel lymphoma, osteomalacia and dermatitis herpetiformis.[35] **Treatment** (**C**) includes: (i) strict adherence to a gluten-free diet; (ii) supplementation with calcium, folate and iron; and (iii) food supplements regarded as drugs by the Advisory Committee on Borderline Substances. Other causes of villous atrophy include hypogammaglobinaemia, lymphoma, tropical sprue and Whipple's disease.

Carcinoid tumours (**D**) arise from neuroendocrine, enterochromaffin cells in the lamina propria of the intestinal mucosa, most commonly in the ileum and appendix. **Symptoms** reflect the release of 5-HT from the tumour, and include: (i) intussusception (telescoping of bowel segments) or obstruction; (ii) right heart valvular stenosis (although a bronchial carcinoid or an atrial septal defect may affect the left heart); (iii) skin flushing; (iv) bronchospasm; (v) diarrhoea; and (vi) weight loss. Diagnosis (**E**) includes urine tests for 5-HIAA (5-hydroxyindoleacetic acid), ultrasound and X-rays, especially to chest, MRI, 123-MIBG scintigraphy and γ-octreotide scans to localise tumours.

Nomenclature note: Carcinoid syndrome refers to the occurrence of liver secondaries that release 5-HT into the systemic circulation. Normally, the liver will metabolise any hormone arising from non-metastatic GIT carcinoids.

Treatment (**F**) is dictated by the location of the primary and the presence of metastases. Surgical treatment includes bowel resection and embolisation of, for example, liver metastases. Drug treatments include the α-blocker **phenoxybenzamine** for flushing, and the diarrhoea may be treated with **methysergide** and **cyproheptadine**, although methysergide is associated with potentially serious adverse effects, especially retroperitoneal and mediastinal fibrosis. **Octreotide**, a long-acting somatostatin analogue, suppresses secretions from neuroendocrine cells, including carcinoids. Lymph or liver metastases of carcinoid tumours may be treated with interferon alfa, an immunomodulating drug, which is available also as a pegylated preparation to prolong its action, when it is prescribed as interferon alfa-2a or interferon alfa-2b. Carcinoid (and other neuroendocrine) tumours resistant to neuroendocrine treatment, or when relapse occurs, may require chemotherapy.

Clinical scenario: The presentation of a carcinoid tumour depends on its site of origin. Stomach carcinoids are usually discovered incidentally unless the patient presents with obstruction of the gastric outlet, bleeding or upper abdominal pain. Bronchial carcinoids usually arise in the proximal bronchus, are slow growing, and produce symptoms of haemoptysis (coughing up of blood) and bronchial obstruction. Appendiceal and small bowel tumours are mostly silent, and therefore advanced when identified. Presentation of acute appendicitis and presentation of appendiceal carcinoids are virtually indistinguishable. Small bowel tumours usually grow slowly and are often revealed through weight loss and abdominal pain. Malignant small bowel tumours cause mechanical obstruction because of fibrosis in the bowel mesentery. Carcinoids can occur rectally and are discovered during rectal examination or lower endoscopy.

A. Gluten and coeliac disease

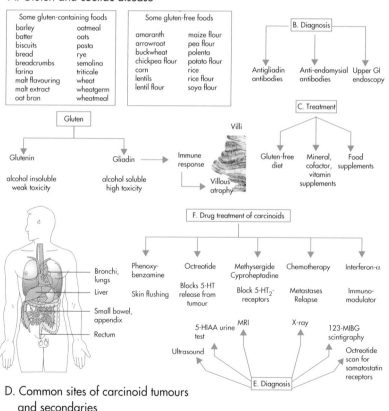

Some gluten-containing foods
- barley
- batter
- biscuits
- bread
- breadcrumbs
- farina
- malt flavouring
- malt extract
- oat bran
- oatmeal
- oats
- pasta
- rye
- semolina
- triticale
- wheat
- wheatgerm
- wheatmeal

Some gluten-free foods
- amaranth
- arrowroot
- buckwheat
- chickpea flour
- corn
- lentils
- lentil flour
- maize flour
- pea flour
- polenta
- potato flour
- rice
- rice flour
- soya flour

B. Diagnosis
- Antigliadin antibodies
- Anti-endomysial antibodies
- Upper GI endoscopy

C. Treatment
- Gluten-free diet
- Mineral, cofactor, vitamin supplements
- Food supplements

Gluten
- Glutenin — alcohol insoluble weak toxicity
- Gliadin — alcohol soluble high toxicity

Villi

Immune response → Villous atrophy

F. Drug treatment of carcinoids
- Phenoxybenzamine — Skin flushing
- Octreotide — Blocks 5-HT release from tumour
- Methysergide Cyproheptadine — Block 5-HT$_2$-receptors
- Chemotherapy — Metastases Relapse
- Interferon-α — Immunomodulator

Bronchi, lungs
Liver
Small bowel, appendix
Rectum

E. Diagnosis
- 5-HIAA urine test
- MRI
- X-ray
- 123-MIBG scintigraphy
- Ultrasound
- Octreotide scan for somatostatin receptors

D. Common sites of carcinoid tumours and secondaries

103 Diarrhoea and malabsorption

Diarrhoea is the passage of liquid stools with abnormal frequency, accompanied by an increase in stool weight above 200 g daily. Risk factors include poor sanitation, contaminated water supply, poor hygiene during food preparation and the season of the year. Causes of malabsorption are numerous (**A**), and include viral infection, laxatives, malabsorption, lactase deficiency, bacterial toxins, amoebiasis and shigellosis. Diarrhoea coupled with bloody stools may be a symptom of a serious underlying condition, e.g. colorectal cancer, Crohn's disease, ischaemic colitis, ulcerative colitis, pseudo-membranous colitis or schistomiasis. The prognosis of infective diarrhoea depends on geographical location. In less developed countries diarrhoea is the principal cause of death in children aged under 5 years. Diarrhoea is not a significant mortality factor in developed societies.

Investigation: Persistent unexpected diarrhoea requires taking a history and per rectum examination to exclude a rectal tumour. Stool culture and microscopic examination for cysts, parasites and ova may be necessary. Biochemistry for electrolyte disturbance, folate and iron assay, and small bowel radiology and gastroscopy with duodenal biopsy should be done if symptoms suggest small bowel involvement. Sigmoidoscopy (examination of the rectum and sigmoid colon) should be done if large bowel involvement is suspected.

The treatment of diarrhoea (**B**) depends on underlying cause and severity and on the nutritional status of the patient. Principal aims include: (i) maintenance of electrolyte and fluid balance; (ii) reduction in gut motility; and (iii) eradication of infective organism if detected.

Electrolyte and fluid balance should be a primary aim when treating diarrhoea, especially for infants and very young children. Glucose solutions are effective because glucose and sodium are co-transported back from the lumen into the epithelial cell in both the ileum and the kidney nephron. Preparations for oral rehydration therapy (ORT) are available as powders for reconstitution in water. They should have not only sodium and glucose (or another carbohydrate such as cooked rice starch) but also an alkalising agent to prevent acidosis. A typical dose might contain sodium chloride 470 mg, potassium chloride 300 mg, disodium hydrogen citrate 530 mg and glucose 3.6 g, to be dissolved in 200 ml of water.

Travellers' diarrhoea is often the result of unaccustomed cuisine or failure to heed local warnings regarding the condition of the tap water. Travellers should take ORT and antimotility drugs. Antibiotics are usually not needed because infections with organisms such as *Escherichia coli* are usually self-limiting.

Antimotility agents treat uncomplicated acute diarrhoea, but are not recommended in young children or infants, for whom fluid and electrolyte balance should be rapidly provided. **Opiates** used include **codeine phosphate**, and **diphenoxylate** and **loperamide**, both of which are pethidine congeners that do not significantly cross the blood–brain barrier. Codeine phosphate and loperamide are also anti-secretory. Neither codeine nor loperamide should be used with abdominal distension or in ulcerative colitis or antibiotic-associated colitis. **Co-phenotrope**, a mixture of diphenoxylate and atropine, is recommended for rehydration for adults and adolescents aged over 16.

Antibacterial therapy is not indicated in simple gastroenteritis because many infections are viral, and bacterial infections are generally self-limiting. In the UK, *Campylobacter* species is the commonest bacterial infective agent, and **erythromycin** or **ciproflaxin** may be prescribed.

Clinical scenario: Diarrhoea is symptomatic of several underlying conditions. It may result from problems that alter the motility of the gut, which may involve one of the following: (i) damage to the autonomic nervous system, or surgical intervention including vagotomy and diabetic autonomic neuropathy. Irritable bowel syndrome and thyrotoxicosis may alter GIT motility, resulting in diarrhoea. (ii) Osmotic changes in the GIT are a possible cause of diarrhoea, e.g. those caused by lactase deficiency, osmotic laxatives, magnesium sulphate or sucrose, which has been prescribed for infants to treat constipation. (iii) Secretory problems may be the cause of diarrhoea. Diarrhoea may be produced by bacterial infections, e.g. infections produced by *Vibrio cholerae* or *E. coli*. Malabsorption or increases in the deposition of bile salts into the lumen after cholecystectomy are other secretory causes of diarrhoea.

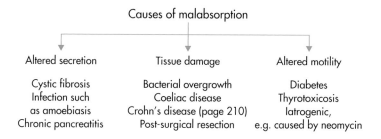

Causes of malabsorption

Altered secretion	Tissue damage	Altered motility
Cystic fibrosis	Bacterial overgrowth	Diabetes
Infection such	Coeliac disease	Thyrotoxicosis
as amoebiasis	Crohn's disease (page 210)	Iatrogenic,
Chronic pancreatitis	Post-surgical resection	e.g. caused by neomycin

A. Causes of malabsorption*

*For NHS-allowed food treatments see BNF, Appendix 7, Borderline Substances

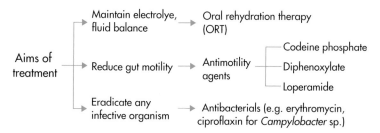

B. Diarrhoea aims of treatment

Ulcerative colitis (UC) is chronic inflammation and ulceration of the colon and rectum, with periods of remission and relapse. The distal terminal of the ileum may be affected, when it is termed **backwash ileitis**. Known associations include sclerosing cholangitis (inflammation of the bile ducts) and primary biliary cirrhosis. Curiously, smokers almost never get UC, and it sometimes develops after smoking is discontinued.[36] Causes and disease predictors are not known, although both UC and Crohn's disease appear to share similar susceptibility genes on chromosomes 2, 3, 7 and 12. HLA factors may also be important predictors of disease. Prolonged or chronic stress can exacerbate UC, although a causative role is not established. Drugs, e.g. NSAIDs, may precipitate an attack. **Symptoms** include diarrhoea, often with blood, pus and mucus, and hyperpyrexia. **Diagnosis** involves stool analysis to exclude bacterial infection, endoscopy with biopsy, barium enema and X-ray, and blood biochemistry. **Complications** include malnutrition, inflammation of the abdominal cavity, eyes, skin and joints, and increased risk of rectal and colon cancer within about 10 years of first presentation of UC. UC may be mild, moderate or fulminant (severe) – see (**B**).

Medical treatment of UC (**A**) aims to treat an attack and maintain the patient in remission. Supplementary measures are used during remission (**C**). Anti-inflammatory drugs aim to present 5-aminosalicylic aid (5-ASA) to the large bowel. These include: **balsalazide**, a pro-drug metabolised to 5-ASA; **mesalazine**, which is 5-ASA in a pH-dependent acrylic coat that disintegrates in the distal ileum and proximal colon; **olsalazine**, which consists of two molecules of 5-ASA linked by a diazo bond that is cleaved in the large bowel by colonic bacteria; and **sulfasalazine**, a combination of 5-ASA and the sulphonamide sulfapyridine. 5-ASA is released in the large bowel and sulfapyridine is absorbed, with resultant adverse actions of the sulphonamides. Drugs are **administered** orally as tablets or capsules, or as an enema or suppository, and their site of action is the large bowel. The active moiety is 5-ASA, which may act by inhibiting superoxide generation, neutrophil chemotaxis, and leukotriene and prostaglandin synthesis. 5-ASA may also scavenge free radicals. Aminosalicylates may be used to treat an acute attack but are generally more useful for maintaining the patient in remission. **Adverse effects** of aminosalicylates include: (i) blood dyscrasias (blood abnormalities) – patients must report symptoms such as bruising, purpura (skin rashes from bleeding into skin), or fever, sore throat or general malaise; (ii) hypersensitivity reactions; (iii) exacerbation of colitis symptoms; (iv) nausea, vomiting and abdominal pain; and (v) nephritis. **Caution** is needed in pregnant or breastfeeding patients and those with renal impairment.

Corticosteroids used include **budesonide, hydrocortisone** and **prednisolone**. These may be formulated as tablets, or foams for rectal administration suppositories, or for parenteral administration. They are not recommended for chronic use because of side-effects. **Immunosuppressants** used include **azathioprine, ciclosporin** and **mercaptopurine**. These are used in severe attacks of UC and to avoid extended use of corticosteroids. They inhibit cell division and suppress normal function in cells such as bone marrow and the GIT. **Antibiotics**, e.g. ciprofloxin, clarithromycin and metronidazole, are used when inflamed tissues become infected. **Heparin** has been found useful in attacks of UC, although its mechanism of action is unknown.

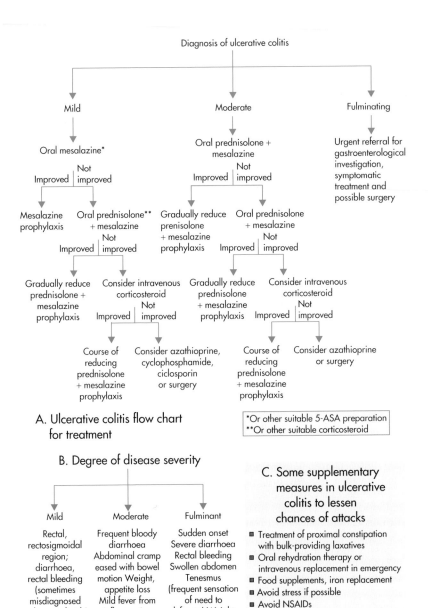

Diagnosis of ulcerative colitis

Mild

Oral mesalazine*

Improved | Not improved

- Mesalazine prophylaxis
- Oral prednisolone** + mesalazine
  - Improved | Not improved
    - Gradually reduce prednisolone + mesalazine prophylaxis
    - Consider intravenous corticosteroid
      - Improved | Not improved
        - Course of reducing prednisolone + mesalazine prophylaxis
        - Consider azathioprine, cyclophosphamide, ciclosporin or surgery

Moderate

Oral prednisolone + mesalazine

Improved | Not improved

- Gradually reduce prenisolone + mesalazine prophylaxis
- Oral prednisolone + mesalazine
  - Improved | Not improved
    - Gradually reduce prednisolone + mesalazine prophylaxis
    - Consider intravenous corticosteroid
      - Improved | Not improved
        - Course of reducing prednisolone + mesalazine prophylaxis
        - Consider azathioprine or surgery

Fulminating

Urgent referral for gastroenterological investigation, symptomatic treatment and possible surgery

*Or other suitable 5-ASA preparation
**Or other suitable corticosteroid

A. Ulcerative colitis flow chart for treatment

B. Degree of disease severity

Mild

Rectal, rectosigmoidal region; diarrhoea, rectal bleeding (sometimes misdiagnosed as haemorrhoids)

Moderate

Frequent bloody diarrhoea Abdominal cramp eased with bowel motion Weight, appetite loss Mild fever from inflammation Inflammation of eyes, skin, joints

Fulminant

Sudden onset Severe diarrhoea Rectal bleeding Swollen abdomen Tenesmus (frequent sensation of need to defecate) Weight, appetite loss Weakness, fatigue

C. Some supplementary measures in ulcerative colitis to lessen chances of attacks

- Treatment of proximal constipation with bulk-providing laxatives
- Oral rehydration therapy or intravenous replacement in emergency
- Food supplements, iron replacement
- Avoid stress if possible
- Avoid NSAIDs

105 Large bowel disorders II: Crohn's disease[37]

Crohn's disease is chronic inflammation of the GIT, which, unlike UC, is confined to the mucosa and transmural, i.e. extends through all the layers of the gut wall. Crohn's disease often presents as an overlap syndrome with UC. Sites commonly affected are the distal ileum, large bowel and often the anus, although the rectum is frequently unaffected. The **cause** is unknown; **predisposing factors** include heredity, diet, infection and absorbed toxins, which may produce symptoms, e.g. arthritis, skin lesions and uveitis. Mycobacterial infection may be a cause. Controversy exists over the MMR vaccine and the development of Crohn's disease. **Symptoms** depend to some extent on the site of the lesions, but generally include abdominal pain, fever, fatigue, aphthous ulcers, ankylosing spondylitis (a seronegative arthritis affecting the spine, and particularly the hip joint), arthritis, erythema nodosum (skin flushing and shin tenderness), uveitis, weight loss and failure to thrive in children. The list of investigations is shown in (**A**). Strictures may form in severe cases and surgery may be indicated.

Treatment of Crohn's disease is aimed at symptomatic control. At initial diagnosis, the patient may be prescribed **prednisolone**, which usually reduces symptoms within 4 weeks. **Budesonide**, another glucocorticoid, is effective in producing a remission, especially when treating acute inflammation of the ileum and ascending colon. An advantage of budesonide is its formulation as a controlled-release capsule, which reduces the amount of absorbed steroid. **Prednisolone** may also be applied topically, e.g. as a **foam** that is released from an applicator inserted into the rectum. It is safe to use in pregnancy to treat left-sided colitis and rectal inflammation, but is **contraindicated** with strictures, fistulae and bowel infections, and for patients with a history of adverse reactions to glucocorticoids.

Patients in whom corticosteroids are contraindicated may be prescribed a 5-ASA compound, e.g. **balsalazide**, **sulfasalazine**, **mesalazine** or **olsalazine**. Patients who fail to respond to steroids or 5-ASA therapy may be prescribed immunosuppressants, e.g. **methotrexate** or **azathioprine**, when regular blood checks must be done. Improvement may not be noticed for 4–6 weeks after initiating azathioprine therapy. For this reason, patients who can take glucocorticoids should be given a course of glucocorticoid therapy to cover them (unless contraindicated) until the immunosuppressant produces relief.

Infliximab, a 'biologic' drug that neutralises TNF-α, produces a remission in mild-to-moderate Crohn's disease, and is used in combination with drugs, e.g. azathioprine, when patients appear to have a reduced incidence of relapse than when on azathioprine alone. **Nataluzimab,** another biologic drug that inhibits α_4-integrins, blocks neutrophil invasion of tissues, and is potent in treating symptoms and producing remission in Crohn's disease resistant to infliximab.

Cholestyramine, a bile acid sequestrant, may control diarrhoea in patients who do not respond to treatment, and those in whom the terminal ileum has had to be removed. Patients on prolonged use of cholestyramine may require supplemental therapy with vitamins A, D, E and K.

Metronidazole, an antibiotic used to treat anaerobic bacterial infection, is used to treat infected fissures and fistulae (abnormal connections between two hollow organs, e.g. between a burst anal fistula and the skin). Drug interactions with metronidazole include lithium, oral anticoagulants and phenobarbital, and alcohol is contraindicated due to a disulfiram-like effect with the drug. Metronidazole may produce peripheral neuropathies.

Clinical scenario: A 57-year-old Slovakian woman, who came to visit her family in the UK, was referred to hospital suffering from diarrhoea, anorexia, fever and severe pain in the lower right abdominal quadrant. She had lost over 10 kg in weight over 5 months. There was no blood in her stools, which also tested negative for infective organisms. Blood biochemistry revealed nothing abnormal and she tested negative for *Entamoeba histolytica*, *Yersinia enterocolitica* and HIV. She was a non-drinker and smoked only after a meal. Chest X-rays showed up normal. Colonoscopy revealed a lesion in the ascending colon. Endoscopy suggested a malignant tumour and biopsies showed chronic inflammation and non-caseating granulomas. (Caseation is degeneration of diseased tissue into a cheese-like mass, often associated with tubercular lesions). Oesophagogastro-duodenoscopy revealed an erythematous gastric mucosa while the small bowel appeared healthy. Crohn's disease was diagnosed and she was prescribed budenoside 3 mg three times daily and balsalazide at a loading dose of 2.25 g three times daily. She did not respond to treatment and, if anything, became worse with persistent pain and fever. After consultation with colleagues a thoracic CT scan was done and showed up changes in the apical segments of the lung. More biopsies were taken from the tumour which this time were stained using the Ziehl – Neelsen stain, an acid-fast carbol fuchsin stain. The test was positive and the patient was put onto a course of combination therapy with Rifater® (*Hoechst Marion Roussel*), a combination of rifampicin, isoniazid, ethambutol and pyrinazidamide. Within 15 days the stools were normal and there was no diarrhoea. Temperature returned to normal and the patient was discharged with a letter to her doctor in Slovakia, recommending follow-up colonoscopy and that the patient be prescribed antitubercular medication.

A. Investigations for Crohn's disease

Abdominal X-ray
Barium enema
Barium meal + follow-up
Bone density scan
Colonoscopy
CT scan
Flexible sigmoidoscopy
Hydrogen breath test
Intestinal permeability test
Leukocyte scan
MRI
Schilling test (ability to absorb vitamin B_{12} from the bowel)
Sigmoidoscopy
Small bowel enema
Ultrasound

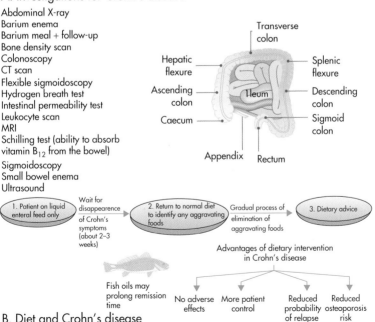

B. Diet and Crohn's disease

106 Constipation

Constipation is the infrequent passage of a dry, hard stool, sometimes accompanied by abdominal pain and a bloated abdomen. There are several known causes (**A**), and the main factor is insufficient fluid in the large bowel, because of either excessive resorption or inadequate fluid intake. Advice should be sought before using laxatives. Persistent constipation, particularly if accompanied by pain, may reflect an underlying complaint. Constipation is more common in children, the elderly and women, particularly when premenstrual or pregnant. Constipation that alternates with diarrhoea may be symptomatic of, for example, irritable bowel syndrome.

Laxatives should be used only if dietary measures are ineffective or if straining, e.g. in angina, is to be avoided. Ideally, laxatives should not be absorbed, should be non-toxic and non-irritant and should not interfere with nutrient, vitamin and drug absorption. Laxatives (**B**) may be bulk forming, faecal softeners, osmotic or stimulant. Bowel cleansing solutions, e.g. effervescent $MgCO_3$ solutions, are used to clear the bowel of faeces before operations, and are not laxatives.

Bulk-forming laxatives include ispaghula husk (psyllium seeds), sterculia, methylcellulose and bran. Adequate fluid intake is essential to avoid intestinal obstruction with these laxatives. Patients should, if possible, resort to high-fibre foods with fruit juices in the first instance. Bulk-forming laxatives are indicated when stools are hard and small (i.e. dehydrated), and when patients have anal fissures, chronic diarrhoea in diverticular disease, colostomy, haemorrhoids, ileosotomy, irritable bowel syndrome and UC. **A precautionary note**: preparations are usually supplied dry for reconstitution in water, and fatalities through asphyxiation have occurred, particularly in the elderly, who attempt to swallow dry granules. They are contraindicated in cases of colonic atony, faecal impaction and swallowing difficulties. Methylcellulose is also contraindicated in infective bowel disease.

Faecal softeners include **methylcellulose, liquid paraffin, arachis oil, glycerol** and **non-ionic surfactants**, e.g. **docusate sodium**. Bulk-forming laxatives also soften stools. They are useful when patients have haemorrhoids or anal fissure. Some may be taken orally or applied as enemas. Glycerol is administered as a suppository, and also stimulates rectal motility as a mild irritant. Liquid paraffin, the traditional remedy, causes lipoid pneumonia with regular use and reduces the absorption of fat-soluble vitamins from the gut. They are generally contraindicated in children under 3 years.

Osmotic laxatives draw water into the large bowel and include saline purgatives, e.g. magnesium sulphate (Epsom salts) and phosphate salts (for rectal administration). Lactulose is a semi-synthetic disaccharide converted by large bowel bacteria into osmotically active acids. Its use is associated with flatulence and distension (**C**), and action may be delayed by a few days. Macrogols are a group of polymers of ethylene glycol.

Stimulant laxatives increase gut motility and are taken on an empty stomach, preferably at bedtime, as they take 8–12 hours to act. They may cause cramps through their contractile effects. Many are anthraquinones, including **dantron** (potentially carcinogenic) and **senna**. These release the active principle emodin in the small bowel, where it is absorbed and increases motility of the large bowel. **Bisacodyl** directly stimulates nerve endings on the bowel wall. **Docusate sodium** (dioctyl sodium sulphosuccinate) is used as an adjunct to bowel radiology.

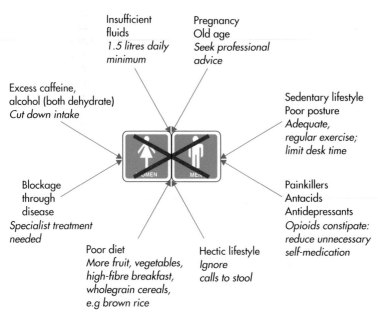

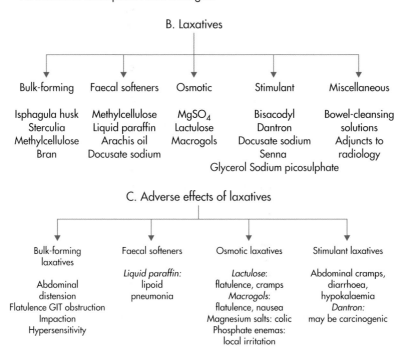

A. Causes of constipation and strategies

B. Laxatives

Bulk-forming	Faecal softeners	Osmotic	Stimulant	Miscellaneous
Isphagula husk	Methylcellulose	MgSO$_4$	Bisacodyl	Bowel-cleansing
Sterculia	Liquid paraffin	Lactulose	Dantron	solutions
Methylcellulose	Arachis oil	Macrogols	Docusate sodium	Adjuncts to
Bran	Docusate sodium		Senna	radiology

Glycerol Sodium picosulphate

C. Adverse effects of laxatives

Bulk-forming laxatives	Faecal softeners	Osmotic laxatives	Stimulant laxatives
	Liquid paraffin:	*Lactulose:*	Abdominal cramps,
Abdominal	lipoid	flatulence, cramps	diarrhoea,
distension	pneumonia	*Macrogols:*	hypokalaemia
Flatulence GIT obstruction		flatulence, nausea	*Dantron:*
Impaction		Magnesium salts: colic	may be carcinogenic
Hypersensitivity		Phosphate enemas:	
		local irritation	

107 Gastrointestinal infections I: Bacterial infections

Gastrointestinal infections may be bacterial, viral, parasitic or worm infections. Infection damage may be (i) localised to mucosal inflammation, e.g. amoebiasis or shigellosis, or (ii) invasive, to other tissues such as blood and liver, e.g. hepatitis A. Symptoms are grouped into: (i) diarrhoea; (ii) dysentery, which is severe diarrhoea with blood, mucus and pus; (iii) enterocolitis, which is inflammation of both small and large bowels; and (iv) gastroenteritis, which is inflammation of the stomach and intestine. Diarrhoea without blood and pus usually indicates enterotoxin activity, while the presence of blood and pus in faeces indicates mucosal destruction and invasion by the infection.

Bacterial infection: Clinically important bacterial pathogens of the GIT include *Bacillus cereus, Campylobacter, Clostridium perfringens, E. coli, Salmonella, Shigella, Vibrio parahaemolyticus* and *Yersinia enterocolitica*. Antibiotics can themselves cause diarrhoea. Clindamycin, as well as some broad-spectrum antibiotics, allows the proliferation of *Clostridium difficile*, which produces enterotoxins and consequent diarrhoea.

Treatment choice requires prior identification of the causative organism, investigation of its resistance to antibiotics and investigation of the patient with regard to: (i) known hypersensitivities; (ii) state of immunocompetence; (iii) ethnic origin or travel history; (iv) hepatic and renal health; (v) disease severity; (vi) ability to tolerate drugs by mouth; (vii) existing medication; and (viii) whether the patient is on OCs, pregnant or breastfeeding. Urgent treatment may require prescribing before the infection is diagnosed and intravenous administration. The choice of drug should, however, be reconsidered in the light of further knowledge. Patients should also be made aware of the reasons for the need to complete a course of antibiotic treatment, unless adverse effects intervene.

Specific examples: (i) Biliary tract infections require either a cephalosporin or gentamicin. (ii) Erythromycin or ciproflaxin is suitable for *Campylobacter* sp. (iii) Ciproflaxin or trimethoprim is suitable for severe **shigellosis** and **invasive salmonellosis**, when ciproflaxin should be used in trimethoprim-resistant cases. Mild shigellosis may not require antibiotics. (iv) **Peritonitis** may be treated with a combination of a cephalosporin or gentamicin with metronidazole or clindamycin. (v) **Typhoid fever** (*Salmonella typhi*) may be treated with cefotaxime, ciproflaxin or chloramphenicol, which is, however, associated with potentially dangerous adverse effects. (vi) Antibiotic-associated colitis may be treated with oral metronidazole or vancomycin, which is, however, associated with vancomycin-resistant enterococci, and should be used only if necessary. (vii) **Peritoneal dialysis-associated peritonitis** may be treated by adding ceftazidime or vancomycin (but see above) to the dialysis fluid.

Prevention of infection during procedures in the GIT utilises administration of antibiotics, e.g. when operating on the stomach or oesophagus, resection of colon or rectum or ERCP, when, for example, a single dose of intravenous gentamicin, ciprofloxacin or metronidazole may be administered, after testing for resistance.

Gastrointestinal tuberculosis is very uncommon in the UK, but prevalent in developing countries. Treatment is as for pulmonary tuberculosis.

Superinfection is caused by another organism resistant to an antibiotic being used to treat an identified infection. The resistant organism may be one that normally is benign and inhabits the body. It may become pathogenic only when other benign bacteria are destroyed by the antibiotic. It may, on the other hand, be a resistant strain of the primary infective organism, e.g. meticillin-resistant *Staphylococcus aureus* (MRSA).

Clinical scenario: Primary spontaneous bacterial peritonitis is diagnosed when there are pathogenic bacteria in peritoneal fluid without evidence of any intra-abdominal infection source. Secondary bacterial peritonitis is a peritoneal infection secondary to an abdominal source of infection, e.g. perforation of the viscera through colonoscopy, necrotising enterocolitis or volvulus (twisting of the bowel). Other causes include appendicitis, liver failure and peritoneal dialysis. Infective bacteria commonly responsible include *Staph. aureus*, *Streptococcus pneumoniae* and Gram-negative enteric bacilli. Less common infections include *Haemophilus influenzae and Neisseria meningitidis*. About 10% of patients may be asymptomatic, while symptoms may include diarrhoea, hypotension, rebound tenderness, abdominal pain, hyperpyrexia, weakness and decreased bowel sounds. Paracentesis generally reveals bile, blood and free air if the gut is perforated, and white blood cells are often grossly raised. In secondary bacterial peritonitis glucose is usually less than 60 mg/dL, lactate is greater than 30 mg/dl and total protein may be well above 1 g/l. Antibiotic treatment initially might be with the cephalosporin cefotaxime or ceftriaxone plus an aminoglycoside, e.g. gentamicin, in the case of of secondary bacterial peritonitis.

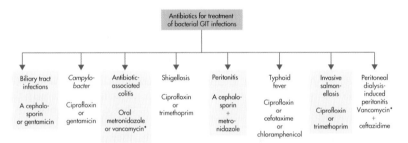

Causes of infection and treatment strategies
*But see text

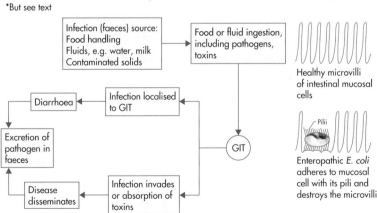

108 Gastrointestinal infections II: Protozoan infections

Protozoa are single-celled organisms and the smallest members of the animal kingdom. There are three clinically important species:

1. *Cryptosporidium parvum* has a high rate of occurrence in AIDS-prevalent countries, is usually transmitted to humans via farm animals in milk or water and invades the small intestinal mucosa, and its released toxin causes severe diarrhoea and cramps.

2. *Entamoeba histolytica* is a tropical species, transmitted as cysts in human faeces, and is passed on by carrier food handlers or in contaminated water. It invades the mucosa and may form localised ulcers or spread over the whole colonic mucosa, causing amoebic dysentery with blood and pus in the stools. The parasite may migrate to the liver, where it causes an abscess.

3. *Giardia lamblia* attaches itself to the brush border of the upper small intestine and may be asymptomatic, but may cause diarrhoea, abdominal cramp and steatorrhoea. The disease may be mild and run a 7- to 10-day course, but in immunocompromised patients it may become chronic. Stools of infected individuals are malodorous, loose and fatty (steatorrhoea).

Treatment: Cryptosporidiosis, when diagnosed, is usually left untreated unless it occurs in children or the elderly, or in patients who are immunocompromised. In the USA and India, where cryptosporidiosis is prevalent, it is treated with the macrolide antibiotic **azithromycin** together with paromomycin. Immuno-compromised patients or children are often given another antibiotic, **nitazoxamide**, which is effective in treating protozoan infections.

Entamoeba histolytica is treated with **metronidazole** or **tinidazole**. Metronidazole is a synthetic nitroimidazole with an action that targets the genomic activity of the organism, and is the drug of choice for amoebiasis (**A**). It is also effective in treating *Trichomonas vaginalis*, a sexually transmitted flagellate protozoan, and *Giardia lamblia*. Both drugs are potent against anaerobic bacteria and protozoa, and are effective for acute invasive amoebic dysentery. They are useful also if the amoeba has reached the liver. **Administration** of metronidazole is either orally as tablets or intravenously (**B**). **Adverse effects** of metronidazole and tinidazole include nausea, headache, upper abdominal pain, a metallic taste and, more rarely, skin rashes, urticaria, vaginal candidiasis, haemolysis and pancreatitis. A disulfiram-like effect with alcohol may occur. After long use, peripheral neuropathies may occur. **Contraindications** include pregnancy, breastfeeding and porphyria. **Drug interactions**: metronidazole enhances the activity of oral anticoagulants. Tinidazole has a similar profile.

Patients who pass *E. histolytica* cysts in their stools but are asymptomatic are treated with **diloxanide furoate**, which is relatively innocuous for adverse effects and kills the amoeba in the bowel lumen but not in the tissues.

Giardia lamblia is treated with metronidazole, tinidazole or, more rarely, **mepacrine hydrochloride** (quinacrine), which is a specific inhibitor of the parasite's glutathione reductase system, while sparing that of the host. The drug is unlicensed for use in the UK. **Adverse effects** of mepacrine include skin yellowing and discoloration of the palate; plus nausea, vomiting and CNS disturbances. It is sometimes used to treat discoid SLE. **Contraindications** include psoriasis; it should be used with **caution** in patients with a history of psychosis or hepatic impairment.

Clinical scenario: Miss AL, a 19-year-old gap student who had returned from a year's stay in Calcutta was referred to hospital complaining of diarrhoea with abdominal pain. She explained that she had suffered similar symptoms some months previously but they had resolved without treatment. *Entamoeba histolytica* cysts were identified in her stools and she was prescribed metronidazole at a dose of 800 mg every 8 hours for 5 days. The symptoms cleared but returned about a year later with increased severity. A colonoscopy was done and it showed severe inflammation of the terminal ileum and the caecal pole. The distal rectum showed some loss of vascularity. Biopsies were taken and histology showed up many trophozoites, several of which contained red blood cells. Fluorescein antibody tests and cellulose acetate precipitant (CAP) tests were positive. She was prescribed metronidazole 800 mg three times a day for 5 days followed by diloxanide furoate 500 mg three times a day for 10 days.

CH_2CH_2OH

O_2N ... N ... CH_3

N

Metronidazole is
a nitroimidazole

Actions: Antibacterial
        Amoebicidal
        Trichomonicidal
        Anti-inflammatory
        Immunosuppressive

Mechanism of action:
metronidazole is reduced intracellularly
by the organism, and then disrupts
DNA helical structure.

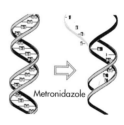
Metronidazole

A. Metronidazole: structure and action

Routes of administration of metronidazole:

Oral (availability ~ 90%)
Intravenous
Intravaginal
Topical

Liver first-pass metabolism of metronidazole:

35–65% by glucuronide conjugation,
hydroxylation and oxidation

Tissue distribution of absorbed metronidazole:

Most tissues, including bile, bone, CSF,
peritoneal fluid, pleural fluid, saliva,
seminal fluid, vaginal fluids
Crosses placenta, enters breast milk

Plasma protein binding of metronidazole:

Weakly protein bound (~8–12%)

B. Pharmacokinetics of metronidazole

109 Gastrointestinal infections III: Worm infections

Worm infestations are treated with **anthelmintics**, drugs that are directed against helminths, i.e. any of the parasitic worms. These include the **nematodes** (roundworms, e.g. *Ascaris lumbricoides*; hookworms, e.g. *Ancylostoma duodenale*; threadworms [pinworms], e.g. *Enterobius vermicularis*) and tapeworms. The commonest tapeworm in humans is *Taenia saginata*, which is transmitted to them in undercooked or raw beef (**A**). Most inhabit the small bowel, although *Trichuris trichiura*, a whipworm, inhabits the large bowel.

Worm infestation produces relatively mild abdominal discomfort, although some, e.g. *Ascaris*, can cause GIT obstruction when present in large numbers. Their larvae may migrate through the lungs and cause pneumonitis (acute respiratory distress), often with eosinophilia. In poorer countries, worm infections cause malnutrition in children. Trichuris infections may cause chronic diarrhoea and strongyloides infections may be fatal in immunocompromised patients in disseminated strongyloidiasis, when many thousands of their larvae invade other tissues. Hookworm larvae penetrate the skin and lungs and can cause pneuomonitis and dermatitis. In the GIT these worms feed on blood cells and can cause anaemia when diet is poor. Tapeworm infections are usually asymptomatic.

Diagnosis is generally through the identification of eggs or larvae in fresh stools. Perianal application of clear Sellotape may reveal threadworm eggs, which are laid in this area of the GIT. Tapeworms release body segments called proglottides, which are packed with eggs, and these are excreted with the faeces (**B**). Patients may experience nausea due to the sensation of passing these large segments.

Threadworms, roundworms and **hookworms** are treated with anthelmintics, and in the case of threadworms with strict hygiene to prevent autoinfection (**C**). Enterobius infection in one family member usually means that the whole family is infected and must be treated. The drug of choice for threadworms is **mebendazole**, and proprietary preparations are sold OTC. Mebendazole is also used to treat hookworm, roundworm and *Trichuris trichiura* (whipworm) infections. To treat threadworms, it is taken orally as a chewable 100 mg single-dose tablet for anyone aged over 2 years, and the dose repeated after 2 weeks if re-infection occurs. Adverse effects include diarrhoea and hypersensitivity reactions. When treating *Trichuris* or *Ascaris* spp. (roundworms), the dose is taken twice daily for 3 days.

Piperazine is supplied as a powder for reconstitution in water or milk for oral administration at night for adults and in the morning for children, with a follow-up dose after 14 days. Children and infants receive lower doses. For roundworm, piperazine is repeated at monthly intervals for up to 3 months. **Adverse effects** include nausea, diarrhoea and hypersensitivity reactions, including urticaria and bronchospasm. Rarely, it may cause hyperexia, Stevens–Johnson syndrome (a hypersensitivity reaction usually expressed as erythema multiforme). **Contraindications** include epilepsy, pregnancy, particularly in the first trimester, and liver and kidney disease.

Tapeworms are treated with **niclosamide** (the most used) and **praziquantel**. In the UK niclosamide is prescribed on a named-patient basis. It is believed to irreversibly damage the head of the worm so that it cannot attach itself to the mucosal wall. Proglottides nevertheless continue to release eggs, so a laxative is usually given with niclosamide. It is administered orally. **Adverse effects** include nausea, vomiting, pruritis and abdominal pain. **Contraindications** include alcohol. Niclosamide should be used with caution in pregnancy and when breastfeeding.

Clinical scenario: Tapeworm infections that are relatively uncommon in the UK include those caused by *Diphyllobothrium latum*, or broadfish tapeworm, more usually found in Baltic countries. Infection is through eating uncooked infected fish. Symptoms include nausea, diarrhoea and vitamin B_{12} deficiency, especially since very large numbers of worms may accumulate through autoinfection within the gut. The tapeworm is treated with mepacrine. *Hymenolepis nana* (dwarf tapeworm) is carried on dogs and is about 40 mm long. Fleas may be important vectors. It infects children predominantly. *H. diminuta* is carried by rats, which can infect stored cereals. These species are treated with anthelmintics. *Trichinella spiralis* is a genus of minute nematode worm occurring mainly in temperate climates. They are ingested with uncooked or imperfectly cooked meat and infect the small intestine. The females produce larvae that bore through the intestinal wall and cause trichiniasis (trichinosis). The larvae can reach all parts of the body, and may colonise muscle where they encyst and cause myalgia and weakness. Other symptoms include periorbital and conjunctival oedema, and sometimes splinter haemorrhages and skin rashes. Diagnosis includes total blood count and muscle biopsy. Infection can be fatal. Treatment is symptomatic, using drugs such as thiabendazole and albendazole.

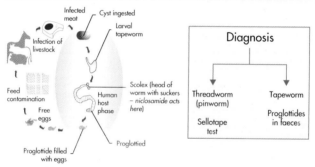

A. Tapeworm life cycle

B. Diagnosis

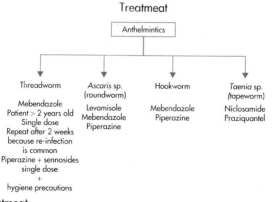

C. Treatmeat

110 Drugs and the liver: Hepatitis

A healthy liver is essential for the proper functioning of drugs, with respect to both drug efficacy and drug safety. After absorption from the GIT, drugs pass via the hepatic portal system into the liver, where they may be activated or inactivated. Many drugs, including the ciclosporin, antibiotics and amoxicillin, can damage the liver cell. Liver disease can render drugs toxic at therapeutic doses. In liver cirrhosis drugs may bypass the liver altogether, accumulate and become toxic. Drugs that can damage the liver include paracetamol, halothane, rifampicin, methotrexate, isoniazid and phenothiazines. Hepatitis is liver inflammation caused by several different viruses (**A**) and, less commonly, by bacteria, fungi and parasites. **Jaundice**, a common symptom of liver damage, is yellowing of the skin and the whites of the eyes, caused by excess blood levels of bilirubin, which the damaged liver cannot utilise for synthesis of bile. Jaundice may also be caused by, for example, gallstones or structural abnormalities of the biliary tree (**B**).

Infectious viral hepatitis can be due to a number of organisms (**A**). Risk factors include blood transfusion, body piercing and tattooing (HIV, hepatitis B and C), contaminated water, which may cause hepatitis A or B or parasitic infection, intravenous drug use with used needles, poor hygiene, maternofetal blood transmission (HIV, hepatitis B and C), and sexual intercourse. **Damage** to hepatocytes may be due to infection of the tissue either by the invading organism or, more usually, by immune-mediated reactions. **Presentation** with hepatitis includes abdominal pain, anorexia, diarrhoea, darkened urine, jaundice, hepatomegaly, which is often painful, fatigue, fever, pruritis, splenomegaly if viral, scleral icterus and skin rashes with, for example, hepatitis B, Lyme disease or syphilis. **Complications** of parasitic infestation, e.g. ascariasis, fascioliasis or schistosomiasis, include abscesses and biliary obstruction. Chronic hepatitis B and C may cause hepatocellular carcinoma, cirrhosis and portal hypertension. Hepatitis B and D co-infection may cause a fulminant hepatitis. Echinococcosis is associated with hydatid cyst formation and anaphylaxis and cyst rupture.

Treatment and vaccines: There is no treatment for hepatitis A, but a formaldehyde-inactivated vaccine is available, and is recommended for liver disease, haemophiliacs treated with factors VIII and IX, workers with the virus, patients infected with hepatitis B or C, travellers to high-risk areas and individuals whose sexual activities put them at high risk. **Hepatitis B** is generally more severe than hepatitis A, and about 10% of infected individuals become carriers. Treatment with large doses of interferon-α/β may be effective. The antiviral **lamivudine** is used for initial treatment and **adefovir** for chronic hepatitis B. A genetically biosynthesised, inactivated hepatitis B virus surface antigen (**HBsAg**) is available. Hepatitis C (HCV), the commonest cause of transfusion-associated hepatitis, has no vaccine and spreads through the same routes as hepatitis B. Blood donors should be routinely screened for HCV Patients are **treated with pegylated interferon-α** in combination with ribavirin for chronic hepatitis C. Hepatitis D virus (HDV) multiplies only in cells already infected with HBV There is no vaccine, but HBV vaccination protects against HIV. Bacterial, fungal and parasitic infections are treated as described (**C**).

A. Organisms causing infectious hepatitis*

Virus	Bacterium	Fungus	Parasite
Hepatitis A, B, C, D, E, G	*Salmonella typhi* (typhoid fever)	*Aspergillus* spp.	*Ascaris lumbricoides* (nematode)
Coxsackie	*Brucella melitensis* (brucellosis)	*Candida* spp.	*Clonorchis sinensis* (liver fluke)
Cytomegalo-virus	*Rickettsia rickettsii*	*Cryptococcus neoformans*	*Entamoeba histolytica* (amoebiasis)
Adenovirus	*Borrelia burgdorferi* (Lyme disease)	*Histoplasma capsulatum*	*Fasciola hepatica* (liver fluke)
HIV	*Treponema pallidum* (syphilis)	*Penicillium mameffei*	*Leishmania donovani* (leishmaniasis)
Epstein–Barr	*Coxiella burnetii* (Q fever)	*Trichosporon cutaneum* (Piedra)	*Plasmodium* spp. (malaria)
Herpes simplex			*Schistosoma* spp. (bilharzia)
Echovirus			*Toxocara canis* (toxocariasis)

Not exhaustive*

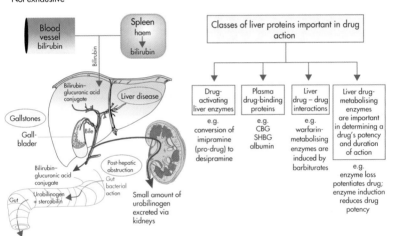

Classes of liver proteins important in drug action

Drug-activating liver enzymes
e.g. conversion of imipramine (pro-drug) to desipramine

Plasma drug-binding proteins
e.g. CBG SHBG albumin

Liver drug–drug interactions
e.g. warfarin-metabolising enzymes are induced by barbiturates

Liver drug-metabolising enzymes are important in determining a drug's potency and duration of action
e.g. enzyme loss potentiates drug; enzyme induction reduces drug potency

B. Biliary tree

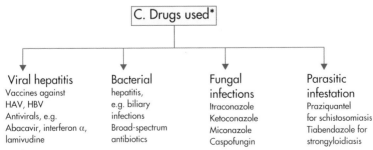

C. Drugs used*

Viral hepatitis
Vaccines against HAV, HBV
Antivirals, e.g. Abacavir, interferon α, lamivudine

Bacterial
hepatitis, e.g. biliary infections
Broad-spectrum antibiotics

Fungal infections
Itraconazole
Ketoconazole
Miconazole
Caspofungin

Parasitic infestation
Praziquantel for schistosomiasis
Tiabendazole for strongyloidiasis

Not exhaustive*

111 Alcoholism and the liver

In the UK, alcoholism and hepatitis are the two main causes of cirrhosis of the liver. Cirrhosis is the extensive development of liver scarring or fibrosis, when the liver can no longer regenerate normal liver tissue. Other causes include non-alcoholic fatty liver disease (NASH), Budd–Chiari syndrome, a blood vessel disease, autoimmune chronic active hepatitis and primary biliary cirrhosis. Alcoholism is a form of drug addiction that may be both genetically and socially influenced (A). At least 80% of alcoholic patients in the UK have co-existing medical problems, e.g. liver disease, pancreatitis, peripheral neuritis, hypertension and cardiomyopathy. Common psychiatric problems include serious cognitive impairment through cortical atrophy, depression, personality disorders and phobic states. Although symptoms may resolve with abstinence, the possibility of an underlying psychiatric problem that caused the addiction should be investigated.

Treatment involves: (i) abstinence; (ii) detoxification with long-acting benzodiazepines such as diazepam; (iii) alcohol avoidance with disulfiram and acamprosate; and (iv) intensive cognitive–behavioural therapy.

Treatment with drugs (B) includes the use of benzodiazepines, e.g. chlordiazepoxide and diazepam, which are prescribed to reduce the severity of alcohol withdrawal, but have to be used under close supervision because of the danger of dependence development.

Chlormethiazole (chlomethiazole) is a hypnotic–sedative structurally related to thiamine. It increases brain GABA activity and also inhibits alcohol dehydrogenase, thus lessening the severity of alcohol withdrawal. It is used only on an in-patient basis and is administered orally in capsule form. **Adverse effects** include drowsiness, tolerance and dependence, and enhancement of alcohol effects. **Precautions** include liver, kidney and lung disease, and elderly and drug-dependent patients. **Contraindications** include ongoing alcohol use, pregnancy and breastfeeding. Chlormethiazole passes into breast milk.

Disulfiram is an alcohol dehydrogenase inhibitor, which after alcohol ingestion rapidly causes an increase in acetaldehyde concentrations in blood, and the effects may last several hours. Reactions include vomiting, nausea, violent flushing, headache, tachycardia, breathlessness, headache and, in severe cases, hypotension and collapse. Patients on disulfiram may be advised to carry a warning card of the dangers of alcohol use while taking disulfiram. **Administration** is orally in tablet form with reducing dosage and not for more than 6 months. **Adverse effects** include initial drowsiness, vomiting, nausea, halitosis and loss of libido. More rarely, central effects including depression and mania may occur. **Precautions** include alcohol abstinence for at least 24 hours before use, liver, renal and respiratory diseases, epilepsy and diabetes. **Contraindications** include coronary artery disease, heart failure, hypertension, history of stroke and CNS disorders including depression, and history of suicide attempts and severe personality disorder, pregnancy and breastfeeding.

Acamprosate is prescribed to maintain alcohol abstinence. It binds to brain NMDA receptors, and modulates up-regulation of NMDA receptors, thereby inhibiting drug-seeking behaviour. It is prescribed orally as an enteric-coated tablet after abstinence has been achieved, used for 1 year, and continued after relapse, although effectiveness wanes if alcohol abuse after relapse becomes chronic. **Adverse effects** include skin rashes, abdominal pain and diarrhoea. **Precautions** include alcohol use; **contraindications** include pregnancy, breastfeeding, and severe renal or hepatic impairment.

Other interventions for severe liver cirrhosis include liver transplantation.

Clinical scenario: Mr PT, a 54-year-old bricklayer, was admitted to his local hospital after vomiting blood. His abdomen was distended and despite initial truculence he grudgingly admitted to a drinking habit, which sounded as though he exceeded 60 units of alcohol per week. Examination of his hands showed palmar erythema, leukonychia (pale nail cuticles), and Dupuytren's contracture of the ring and little fingers (forward curvature caused by contracture of the fascia in the fingers and palm). Abdominal examination suggested the presence of ascites fluid and hepatosplenomegaly. Prothrombin time was prolonged and the patient was given fresh plasma and an infusion of vitamin K. Somatostatin was infused to reduce blood flow into the splanchnic circulation. Liver function tests were consistent with hepatocellular jaundice. The haematamesis (vomiting of blood) was investigated by endoscopy, which revealed oesophageal varices, probably the result of portal hypertension. This was treated with sclerotherapy. The ascites was treated with a diuretic. The patient was deemed to be sufficiently psychologically stable to be treated as an out-patient, and was discharged and referred to local services for support. The patient agreed to a course of disulfiram and was warned of the consequences of taking alcohol while on the drug.

A. Development of alcoholism

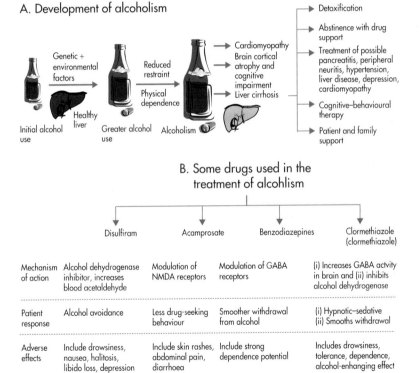

B. Some drugs used in the treatment of alcohlism

	Disulfiram	Acamprosate	Benzodiazepines	Clormethiazole (clormethiazole)
Mechanism of action	Alcohol dehydrogenase inhibitor, increases blood acetaldehyde	Modulation of NMDA receptors	Modulation of GABA receptors	(i) Increases GABA actvity in brain and (ii) inhibits alcohol dehydrogenase
Patient response	Alcohol avoidance	Less drug-seeking behaviour	Smoother withdrawal from alcohol	(i) Hypnotic–sedative (ii) Smooths withdrawal
Adverse effects	Include drowsiness, nausea, halitosis, libido loss, depression	Include skin rashes, abdominal pain, diarrhoea	Include strong dependence potential	Includes drowsiness, tolerance, dependence, alcohol-enhancing effect
Precautions	Alcohol abstinence 24 h before disulfiram; liver, renal disease, epilepsy, diabetes	Risk of treatment failure if alcohol taken during treatment	Tapering dosage necessary, over not more than 14 days; liver or renal impairment, pregnancy, porphyria	Kidney, liver, lung diseases, elderly patients, drug-dependent patients
Contra-indications	Cardiovascular disease, depression, history of suicide attempts, pregnancy, breastfeeding	Pregnancy, breast-feeding, severe liver or renal impairment	Sleep apnoea syndrome, respiratory depression, chronic psychosis, anxiety with depression	Ongoing alcohol use, pregnancy, breastfeeding

112 Asthma I: Introduction

Asthma, also called bronchial asthma, is chronic inflammation of the bronchial airways that causes bronchoconstriction and difficulty in breathing. The cause is unknown, although several attack precipitants have been identified: emotion, infections, allergens, chemicals, e.g. air pollution, drugs, e.g. antibiotics, aspirin, β-blockers and physical exertion. Important domestic allergens include pets, perfumes, cleaning sprays, house dust mites, grass and pollen, and certain foods, e.g. nuts. Atopy (a constitutional or hereditary hypersensitivity to allergens) is particularly strongly associated with asthma. In asthma, breathing difficulty is caused by broncho-constriction resulting from local release of inflammatory and constrictor chemicals including histamine, leukotrienes, inflammatory cytokines and bradykinin (C). Normally, bronchial patency is ensured by the sympathetic nervous system through the action of the neurotransmitter norepinephrine and circulating epinephrine on bronchial smooth muscle β$_2$-adrenoceptors. These when stimulated cause bronchodilatation. Asthmatics have a narrower safety margin as their bronchioles are chronically constricted, and an attack reduces patency even further (see opposite).

Clinical and safety note: The use of a non-selective β-antagonist is strictly contra-indicated in asthmatic patients, since this reduces the margin of safety even further.

Occurrence and symptoms: Disease onset occurs at any time of life, from early childhood to old age, and in the UK about 3.5 million people, of whom about half are children, suffer from asthma. At least 1000 fatal asthma attacks occur annually in the UK. Symptoms of an attack are predominantly difficulty in breathing, wheezing usually during expiration, and coughing up clear or yellowish-green sputum (presence of eosinophils). Other physical symptoms include atopic eczema, nasal polyps and hyperinflation of the chest. Status asthmaticus is a medical emergency that may occur after an inadequately controlled asthmatic attack. Patients need immediate ventilation with oxygen, bronchodilators and admission to the intensive care unit. Pregnancy requires very great patient care due to the dangers of maternal and fetal hypoxia.

Treatment of asthma is symptomatic and is aimed at: (i) preventing acute attacks and (ii) restoring normal breathing during an attack. The main pharmacological approaches are to prevent and treat attacks using (i) **sodium cromoglicate**, which blocks histamine release from mast cells (C), which is probably the least used of the asthma drugs; (ii) anti-inflammatory corticosteroids, which are taken either orally, e.g. **prednisolone**, or by inhalation, e.g. **beclometasone, fluticasone and budesonide**; (iii) both long- and short-acting β$_2$-receptor agonists, e.g. **salbutamol** and **terbutaline (short acting) and salmeterol (long acting)**; (iv) **theophylline**, which block phosphodiesterase and therefore maintains elevated intracellular levels of cyclic AMP; (v) short-acting antimuscarinic agents, e.g. **ipatropium**, which block broncho-constricting muscarinic ACh receptors; and (vi) leukotriene receptor antagonists **montelukast** and **zafirlucast**, which block the actions of the inflammatory leukotrienes at their receptors on bronchial smooth muscle fibres.

Clinical notes: 1. Sodium cromoglicate is ineffective in countering actions of already released histamine.
2. Historically, isoprenaline, a non-selective β-receptor agonist, was the first to be used as an inhaled drug, but caused fatalities due to stimulation of cardiac β$_1$-receptors.

Administration routes are an important feature of asthma treatment with drugs and inhalational administration is widely used, especially for inhaled steroids, anti-muscarinics, β$_2$-receptor agonists and cromoglicate (B). Doses are reduced because first-pass metabolism is side-stepped, so adverse effects are, theoretically, less of a problem. Dosage is controlled through the used of pressurised metered dose inhaler (A). The BNF provides detailed recommendation of asthma management.

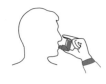

1. Remove mouthpiece cover and shake nebuliser vigorously

2. Hold nebuliser as shown and exhale gently, then..........

3. With mouthpiece in mouth start breathing in and press down to release medication and continue breathing in

4. Hold breath for about 10 seconds and then exhale slowly

A. Using a nebuliser

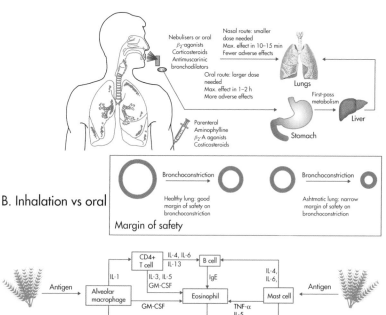

Nebulisers or oral β_2-agonists
Corticosteroids
Antimuscarinic bronchodilators

Nasal route: smaller dose needed
Max. effect in 10–15 min
Fewer adverse effects

Oral route: larger dose needed
Max. effect in 1–2 h
More adverse effects

Lungs

First-pass metabolism

Liver

Parenteral
Aminophylline
β_2-A agonists
Costicosteroids

Stomach

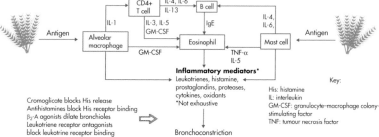

Bronchoconstriction

Bronchoconstriction

Healthy lung: good margin of safety on bronchoconstriction

Asthmatic lung: narrow margin of safety on bronchoconstriction

B. Inhalation vs oral

Margin of safety

Antigen

Alveolar macrophage

IL-1

CD4+ T cell

IL-4, IL-6 IL-13

B cell

IL-3, IL-5 GM-CSF

IgE

IL-4, IL-6,

GM-CSF

Eosinophil

Mast cell

Antigen

TNF-α IL-5

Inflammatory mediators*
Leukotrienes, histamine, prostaglandins, proteases, cytokines, oxidants
*Not exhaustive

Key:

His: histamine
IL: interleukin
GM-CSF: granulocyte–macrophage colony-stimulating factor
TNF: tumour necrosis factor

Cromoglicate blocks His release
Antihistamines block His receptor binding
β_2-A agonists dilate bronchioles
Leukotriene receptor antagonists block leukotrine receptor binding

Bronchoconstriction

C. Mechanisms of inflammation and of drug action

113 Asthma II: Anti-asthmatic drugs

Selective β₂-agonists: Salbutamol and **terbutaline** are synthetic, short-acting derivatives of epinephrine. They are formulated for inhalation or oral use in asthma, premature labour and other conditions of reversible airway obstruction. They are administered also by intravenous infusion in severe attacks of asthma, and they may be self-administered subcutaneously as a temporary measure before admission to hospital. **Salmeterol** and **formoterol** are longer-acting β₂-agonists. **Adverse effects** of β₂-agonists include fine tremor, palpitations (cardiac action) and hypokalaemia, especially with higher doses, headaches, nervous tension and paradoxical bronchospasm. **Precautions:** patients taking theophylline, corticosteroids and diuretics are particularly at risk of hypokalaemia. Other precautions include cardiovascular problems, especially arrhythmias, susceptibility to QT interval elongation and hypertension. Formoterol fumarate and salmeterol are indicated for chronic asthma, reversible airway obstruction, prevention of exercise-induced bronchospasm and chronic obstructive pulmonary disease (COPD).

Corticosteroids are effective prophylactic anti-inflammatory drugs in asthma but they become effective only 3–7 days after first administration. Their effectiveness lies in their anti-inflammatory action in reducing airway inflammation and mucus production. **Beclometasone (beclomethasone) dipropionate, budenoside** and **fluticasone propionate** are all taken by inhalation and appear to be equally effective. They are used by inhalation to treat mild-to-moderate acute attacks on a once-daily basis. If more cover is needed, a stepped approach, as described by the BNF, is recommended, where the patient takes regular prophylactic therapy using salbutamol or terbutaline, together with an inhaled corticosteroid such as beclometasone, stepping up if necessary to both short- and long-acting inhaled β₂-agonists salmeterol and formoterol. **Oral prednisolone** as a short course may be prescribed after an acute attack, and longer courses of lower-dose prednisolone together with inhaled corticosteroid may be necessary. **Adverse effects** are those associated with glucocorticoid use. Throat problems such as hoarseness and candiasis, which may be avoided by using spacers and can be treated with fungicidal throat lozenges, may occur with higher doses. In an emergency, or in acute attacks, **hydrocortisone** may be administered intravenously.

Sodium cromoglicate's prophylactic use in asthma is debatable. It is useful for protection against histamine release. In clinical trials, the leukotriene receptor antagonists **montelukast** and **zafirlukast** have reduced eosinophil counts in bronchoalveolar lavage fluid, induced sputum and peripheral blood. In some patients they may be at least as or more effective than inhaled corticosteroids, with which they also seem to have an additive effect. Both are available in tablet form. **Adverse effects** include headache, GIT upsets, hypersensitivity reactions, liver reactions and thrombocytopenia. They should be used with **caution** in the elderly, during pregnancy, and are contraindicated during breastfeeding and in patients with liver disease.

Ipratropium, an antimuscarinic agent, may be used by inhalation together with other agents in life-threatening attacks. It is also effective in COPD. **Tiotropium,** another antimuscarinic, is a long-acting bronchodilator licensed for COPD. **Contraindications** or **extreme precautions** are necessary in patients with glaucoma and prostatic hyperplasia. **Theophylline,** a xanthine, is rarely used in asthma except in emergencies, notably status asthmaticus. Current guidelines for treatment of acute asthma include IV magnesium sulphate and not intravenous theophylline. This is because the methylxanthines are very arrhythmogenic and may worsen a tachycardia, which often occurs in an acute asthma attack.

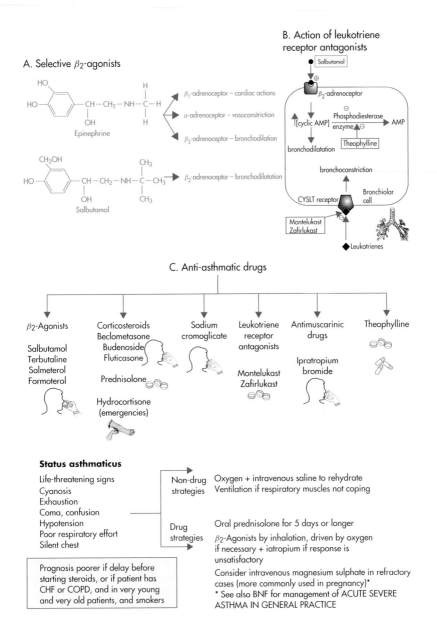

A. Selective β_2-agonists

HO—〔benzene ring〕—CH—CH$_2$—NH—C—H
β_1-adrenoceptor – cardiac actions
α-adrenoceptor – vasoconstriction
β_2-adrenoceptor – bronchodilation
Epinephrine

HO—〔benzene ring〕—CH—CH$_2$—NH—C—CH$_3$
β_2-adrenoceptor – bronchodilatation
Salbutamol

B. Action of leukotriene receptor antagonists

Salbutamol

β_2-adrenoceptor

[cyclic AMP] — Phosphodiesterase enzyme — AMP

Theophylline

bronchodilatation

bronchoconstriction

CYSLT receptor — Bronchiolar cell

Montelukast
Zafirlukast

Leukotrienes

C. Anti-asthmatic drugs

β_2-Agonists

Salbutamol
Terbutaline
Salmeterol
Formoterol

Corticosteroids

Beclometasone
Budenoside
Fluticasone

Prednisolone

Hydrocortisone
(emergencies)

Sodium cromoglicate

Leukotriene receptor antagonists

Montelukast
Zafirlukast

Antimuscarinic drugs

Ipratropium
bromide

Theophylline

Status asthmaticus

Life-threatening signs
Cyanosis
Exhaustion
Coma, confusion
Hypotension
Poor respiratory effort
Silent chest

Non-drug strategies
Oxygen + intravenous saline to rehydrate
Ventilation if respiratory muscles not coping

Drug strategies
Oral prednisolone for 5 days or longer
β_2-Agonists by inhalation, driven by oxygen if necessary + iatropium if response is unsatisfactory
Consider intravenous magnesium sulphate in refractory cases (more commonly used in pregnancy)*
* See also BNF for management of ACUTE SEVERE ASTHMA IN GENERAL PRACTICE

Prognosis poorer if delay before starting steroids, or if patient has CHF or COPD, and in very young and very old patients, and smokers

Chronic obstructive pulmonary disease (COPD) is an umbrella term for a number of respiratory problems including chronic bronchitis and emphysema, and smoking is the major cause. Emphysema is enlargement of and damage to the lung alveoli, resulting in reduced surface area for gas exchange. Chronic bronchitis is defined as a cough with expectoration of sputum for at least 3 months during 2 consecutive years, without symptoms of any other condition associated with sputum production. Other causes of COPD include occupational dust exposure, air pollution and α_1-antitrypsin deficiency. This group of enzymes inhibits protease activity, which if not inhibited results in tissue destruction. Cirrhosis of the liver is also a consequence of a phenotype of α_1-antitrypsin designated the ZZ phenotype. Smoking must be stopped immediately, whether or not enzyme deficiency is diagnosed. COPD is a chronic, slowly progressive condition of airflow obstruction and causes about 30 000 deaths per year in the UK. The symptoms of COPD include weight loss, wheezing, cor pulmonale (right ventricle enlargement caused by lung or pulmonary artery disease), central cyanosis, pursed lip breathing, flapping tremor and hyperinflation. COPD is distinguished from asthma by the use of spirometry (measurement of air volume inhaled and exhaled), patient history and clinical symptoms.

Treatment: Guidelines for treatment have been published by the NICE[38] and by the Global Initiative in Obstructive Lung Disease (GOLD)[39] (**A, B**). Treatments currently available are: (i) immediate abstinence from smoking; (ii) long-term oxygen therapy (LTOT); (iii) bronchodilators; (iv) lung volume reduction surgery for patients with emphysema; and (iv) lung transplantation for selected patients (extremely rare).

Drug treatment involves the use of short- and long-acting β_2-agonists and anticholinergic therapy (**C**). In the early stages of the disease these are administered via an inhaler. Short-acting β_2-agonists and anticholinergics can also be given via a nebuliser machine. This is used generally for acute exacerbations requiring hospitalisation, but patients with severe disease often have home nebulisers. Inhaled corticosteroids such as **beclometasone** are not as useful as in asthma, although they do reduce the incidence of infective exacerbations. Symptoms in moderate-to-severe cases of COPD may respond to combined therapy with an anticholinergic drug such as tiotropium and a long-acting β_2-agonist. **Antibiotics** and short courses of oral steroids may be needed if the patient presents with increased breathlessness and abnormally (for the patient) high volumes of purulent sputum.

Doxapram, a respiratory stimulant, is rarely used nowadays. It has been almost completely superseded by non-invasive ventilation via a tight-fitting mask. This has been shown to be effective in patients with acute exacerbations of COPD in the presence of acidosis caused by carbon dioxide retention.

LTOT may be prescribed in concentrations not exceeding 24–28% (controlled oxygen therapy) and initial treatment given in hospital in order to monitor blood gases before setting the dose for use at home. LTOT is given to patients for between 16 and 18 hours a day, and given in this fashion has been shown to extend life by up to 18 months. Oxygen can also be prescribed as an intermittent treatment for breathlessness of short duration and used as required by the patient.

Clinical scenario: Diagnosis of COPD and distinction from asthma rely on three routes of investigations, namely patient history, clinical symptoms and the use of spirometry. Confusion may arise when middle-aged patients who are smokers present with, for example, mild exertional dyspnoea. Also, not all patients who present with symptoms of COPD are smokers, although it is recognised that smoking does contribute 80–90% of the risk of COPD in the western hemisphere. Wheezing and coughing are usually indicative of COPD, but must be considered together with the patient's history. If there is a family history of atopy, then this is suggestive of asthma rather than COPD. Some practitioners consider that respiratory symptoms that respond to administration of an inhaled β_2-agonist exclude COPD. A productive cough may be a predictor of COPD, although any tentative diagnosis should take into account spirometric data, which are important in determining whether there is airway obstruction and COPD. Age is an important consideration in the differential diagnosis of asthma and COPD, since the mean age at presentation with asthma has been found in some studies to be significantly lower than that when presenting initially with COPD; however, diagnosis must depend also on other symptoms, and on the results of spirometry ($FEV_1/FVC < 70\%$).

A. GOLD recommendations of treatment of COPD

- Long-acting rather than short-acting bronchodilators are more effective for treating moderate-to-severe COPD
- Inhaled glucocorticoids are suitable only for patients with severe COPD
- Exacerbation of COPD in patients without acidotic respiratory failure is most effectively managed by nurse-administered homecare
- Rehabilitation programmes should be at least 2 months in duration

---

B. Joint recommendations of American and European Thoracic Societies for diagnosis and treatment of COPD (abridged)

- A diagnosis of COPD should be considered in patients with symptoms of cough, sputum production or dyspnoea, or a history of risk factors for COPD. Patients with airflow obstruction at a relatively early age, and especially with a family history of COPD, should be tested for α_1-antitrypsin deficiency
- All patients should have BMI, height, weight and respiratory rate measured
- Treatment aimed at ending tobacco dependence and use should be a high priority
- Pharmacological intervention should be initiated and patient-specific drug evaluation carried out
- Patients with COPD-related restricted activities, exercise intolerance, dyspnoea or other respiratory symptoms should be considered for pulmonary rehabilitation
- Lung volume reduction surgery or lung transplantation may improve spirometry results, exercise capacity, dyspnoea, lung volume, general life quality and prognosis for survival
- Nocturnal hypoxaemia of COPD disturbs sleep and measures should be taken to limit cough and dyspnoea

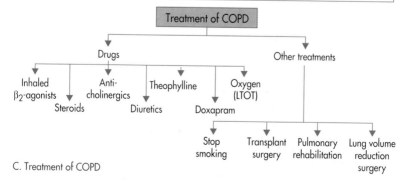

C. Treatment of COPD

115 Tuberculosis I: Principles of treatment

Tuberculosis (TB) is an infectious bacterial disease, usually of the lungs, caused by *Mycobacterium tuberculosis*. The disease is now re-emerging as a serious health problem, mainly in developing countries, because of HIV, poverty and malnutrition. TB can be caught by inhalation of aerosols caused by coughing and sneezing and from contaminated hands, but is more commonly spread through prolonged close proximity to an infected individual. Those most at risk (**A**) include AIDS (acquired immune deficiency syndrome) patients, drug abusers, alcoholics, health carers in contact with patients (unless immunised), and patients immunocompromised through diseases such as diabetes or after major surgery (**A**). **Testing** for TB includes the **tuberculin (Mantoux) test**, when a small quantity of the tuberculin protein, which is extracted from bacterial culture, is injected intradermally. A strong red flare 48–72 hours later is positive, and confirmed by sputum testing. A mild flare is common, but is not necessarily positive.

Common symptoms include swollen lymph glands, particularly in the neck, appetite and weight loss, exhaustion, pleurisy, non-productive cough, nocturnal sweating and, in advanced cases, haemoptysis.

An **intradermal vaccine** against TB is available. This is the BCG (Bacillus Calmette–Guérin) vaccine, a live, attenuated strain derived from *Mycobacterium bovis*. Vaccination is recommended for certain groups (**C**). **Contraindications and precautions** (as for all live vaccines) include acute illness, pregnancy, immunodeficiency, e.g. AIDS (absolute contraindication), patients undergoing chemo- or radiotherapy for malignancy, and patients on corticosteroids until adequately withdrawn from these.

Treatment of TB aims to prevent the emergence of resistant organisms, and to eradicate the infection completely. To achieve these aims, treatment is usually in two phases: (i) an **initial phase**, using a combination of at least three drugs, and (ii) a **continuation phase** using two drugs (**C**). The choice of drugs is determined by the sensitivity of the bacillus, the properties of the drug and the particular needs of the patient. For example, drugs vary in their ability to penetrate tissues and to sterilise tubercular lesions: **pyrazinamide** and **isoniazid** easily penetrate the CSF and are therefore useful in meningeal TB. Patient supervision is critical in eradicating the infection, and is not always possible, especially in developing countries, with patients of no fixed abode, or who do not have sufficient rest, nursing and nutrition. Monitoring, if possible, should include regular urine examination, e.g. with rifampicin, and tablet counts.

Special needs patients: Immunocompromised patients, especially HIV-positive patients, may have multi-resistant strains of *M. tuberculosis,* and drug sensitivity should be tested for. Young children taking **isoniazid**, which may cause optic neuritis, are not easily tested for optical disturbances and need special care. **Ethambutol** is actually contraindicated in optic neuritis. Many of the drugs are metabolised by the liver and hepatic impairment requires liver function tests and regular blood counts. Isoniazid, which is associated with peripheral neuropathies and commonly prescribed, should be used with caution or not at all in patients who are HIV positive, diabetic or alcohol dependent, or have renal impairment, or poor nutritional status.

Social and economic factors also determine the efficacy or otherwise of anti-tubercular drugs, e.g. the under-regulated use of antibiotics in livestock has contributed to bacterial resistance.

116 Tuberculosis II: Drugs

Isoniazid is structurally similar to pyridoxine (**A**). It penetrates phagocytic cells, and is effective against both intracellular and extracellular micro-organisms. **Mechanism of action**: isoniazid inhibits synthesis of the bacterial cell wall. It is bacteriostatic and also possibly bactericidal to *M. tuberculosis*. **Pharmacokinetics**: it is soluble in aqueous media and rapidly absorbed from the GIT. It penetrates into the CSF, and is acetylated in the liver and excreted via the kidneys. Peak plasma concentrations are achieved within 1–2 hours. Some patients are fast acetylators of isoniazid, and with poor checks on compliance these patients may receive inadequate cover. **Adverse effects** include peripheral neuritis at high doses, or those seen in patients at risk of neuropathies. Concurrent use of **pyridoxine** reduces the risk. Other effects include central disturbances, optic neuritis, hypersensitivity reactions and blood dyscrasias. **Precautions** include pregnancy and breastfeeding, HIV, slow acetylators, hepatic and renal impairment, alcoholism, epilepsy and history of psychosis. Isoniazid is **contraindicated** in drug-induced liver disease.

Rifampicin: Used mainly for TB, it is also used to treat Legionnaire's disease and prophylactically in individuals with known close contact with meningococcal meningitis or *H. influenzae* (type b). **Mechanism of action:** rifampicin inhibits RNA synthesis. Resistance develops through mutations at the binding site, so it should be prescribed with other antibiotics to reduce resistance development. **Pharmacokinetics:** it is well absorbed orally,[40] taken once daily and readily penetrates phagocytes, lung cavities and abscesses. It is excreted mainly via the bile. **Adverse effects** include harmless orange dis-coloration of sweat, tears and urine, GIT disturbances, renal failure, thrombo-cytopenia, collapse and shock, urticaria and jaundice, and microsomal enzyme induction. **Precautions** include hepatic and renal impairment, pregnancy, breastfeeding and concurrent use of OCs. **Contraindication:** jaundice.

Ethambutol dihydrochloride is a synthetic, water-soluble compound, mainly used when there is a possibility of resistance to other drugs. **Mechanism of action**: it inhibits synthesis of arabinogalactan, a vital part of the bacterial cell wall. It potentiates the action of lipophilic drugs, e.g. rifampicin. **Pharmacokinetics:** it is administered orally and readily absorbed, and peak levels are achieved within 2–4 hours. It penetrates into the CSF only when the meninges are inflamed. It is excreted mainly unchanged via the kidneys and also to some extent via the bile. **Adverse reactions** are rare, the most common being dose-related retrobulbar (behind the eyeball) neuritis, which may cause red–green colour blindness and loss of visual acuity. This is more likely after prolonged therapy at higher doses (~25 mg/kg per day over several months). Doses of less than 15 mg/kg per day are considered less likely to produce this adverse reaction. Other reactions include (rarely) pruritis and urticaria. **Precautions** include dose reduction with renal impairment and regular visual testing (difficult in children). **Contraindications:** optic neuritis and poor vision.

Pyrazinamide is related to nicotinamide (**A**). **Mechanism of action:** at pH 5.5 it is bacteriostatic to mycobacteria in macrophages. **Pharmacokinetics:** pyrazinamide is slightly water-soluble, well absorbed from the GIT and penetrates the meninges. A long half-life (12–24 hours) allows once-daily doses. Excretion is mainly renal. **Adverse effects** include gout exacerbation, photosensitivity and hepatotoxicity. **Precautions** include liver disease, pregnancy and gout.[41] **Contraindications** include porphyria and liver damage. Several other antibacterial drugs are also used to treat TB (**B**).

Clinical scenario: A 34-year-old woman, who had been admitted to the UK 3 months previously from the Sudan to visit a relative, was referred by her GP, who suspected TB, to the respiratory unit of her local hospital. She complained of constant fatigue, breathlessness and a feeling of generalised malaise. She had a non-productive cough and had lost about 5 kg in weight over the previous 4 months. She had experienced neither night sweats nor haemoptysis. Tests revealed a mild hyperpyrexia (37.9°C) but she was not anaemic, nor was there any clubbing (thickening of the tissues at the base of the toenails and fingers). Crepitations (fine crackling sounds in the lungs heard using the stethoscope) were clearly audible. Her chest X-rays showed shadowing in the upper and middle lobes, and slight hilar enlargement. Her white cell count and haemoglobin were within the normal range and CRP was 243 mg/l. A Mantoux test yielded a positive result and sputum tested positive for acid-fast bacilli. Cultures produced *M. tuberculosis* and the GP's tentative diagnosis of pulmonary TB was confirmed. The patient was treated as an in-patient and a course of isoniazid, rifampicin and pyrazinamide was prescribed for 2 months, followed for a further 4 months with isoniazid and rifampicin. After 6 months the patient was discharged with no signs of infection in the sputum and a much healthier chest X-ray. The patient returned to the Sudan.

A. Structures of some antitubercular drugs

B. Some other antibacterial drugs used to treat TB

Drug	Indications	Adverse effects	Precautions	Contraindications
Capreomycin Peptide antibiotic from *Streptomyces capreolus*	Adjunct antibiotic if patient is resistant to first-line drugs	Nephrotoxic; ototoxic; blood dyscrasias; electrolyte disturbances; pain and induration (tissue hardening); sterile abscesses at injection site; hepatotoxic; vertigo	Hepatic, renal disease; monitor auditory, renal, hepatic, vestibular function; pregnancy (teratogenic in animal tests)	
Cycloserine Antibiotic; structural analogue of D-alanine produced by *Streptomyces orchidaceus*	Adjunct antibiotic if patient is resistant to first-line drugs	Potentially serious CNS toxicity that is dose related; keep oral doses below 0.75 g/day to reduce chance of CNS toxicity; allergic dermatitis, when drug should be stopped	Pregnancy and breastfeeding; monitor liver and kidney function; reduce dose if renal impairment	CNS problems, e.g. epilepsy, depression, psychosis, severe anxiety; alcohol dependence; porphyria
Rifabutin Derived from rifamycin; structurally related to rifampicin	Some use with rifampicin-resistant strains; prophylactic in *M. avium* and advanced mycobacterial infections in patients with advanced AIDS	GIT disturbances; jaundice; occasionally hepatitis; anaemia; uveitis with high doses; arthralgia; bronchospasm; discoloration of sweat, saliva, urine; fever; urticaria; corneal opacity (asymptomatic) with long usage	As for rifampicin; hepatic and renal impairment; pregnancy and breastfeeding	

117 Pneumonia

Pneumonia is infection of the lung parenchyma. Symptoms are those of infection, with fever and malaise, with respiratory symptoms of cough and chest pain. Signs on examination are bronchial breathing and dullness to percussion, and findings include consolidation on chest X-rays. Pneumonia may be classified: (i) by environmental circumstances as **community-acquired (CAP)**, **hospital-acquired** or pneumonia in **immunocompromised patients**, e.g. AIDS; (ii) after chest X-ray, as **lobar pneumonia**, which affects entire lobes, and is often caused by *Streptococcus pneumoniae*, lobular pneumonia, with multiple patchy shadows in a localised area, or bronchopneumonia, when multiple patchy areas are widespread; or (iii) by the infecting micro-organism, the most likely being *S. pneumoniae*. Several others, e.g. *Haemophilus influenzae*, *Legionella pueumophila*, *Mycoplasma pneumoniae* or *Staphylococcus aureus*, may be responsible. Bronchopneumonia may (rarely) be caused by *Staph. aureus* which, after influenza or another viral infection, may cause a secondary bronchopneumonia. This is treated with intravenous **fusidic acid** and **flucloxacillin**. In hospital-acquired pneumonia, patients in intensive care who need assisted ventilation are particularly susceptible to so-called 'coliforms', which are micro-organisms related to *E. coli* and *Pseudomonas aeruginosa* that may precipitate bronchopneumonia. Immunosuppressed patients and alcoholics may contract primary bronchopneumonia through infection with *Klebsiella pneumoniae*.

Guidelines have been published by the British Thoracic Society for management of community-acquired pneumonia,[42] which include recommendations for procedures to assess the need for hospitalisation and severity, pathogen identification and disease treatment. Severity assessment includes the 'CURB' prognostic assessment of **c**onfusion (abbreviated mental test score of 8 or less), **u**rea (raised > 7 mmol/l), **r**espiratory rate raised > 30/min and **b**lood pressure (low blood pressure: systolic pressure < 90 mmHg and/or diastolic blood pressure < 60 mmHg).

Treatment depends on: (i) severity of the pneumonia; (ii) identity of the infecting organism; (iii) resistance of the infecting organism to treatment and (iv) the patient's reactions, e.g. penicillin sensitivity. Blood and sputum cultures (if available) are recommended to identify the organism and its resistance profile. Severe cases need Gram stains, and rapid legionella screening is advisable, especially in severe cases or if there is an outbreak. Treatment should be started immediately if the clinical presentation fits pneumonia. The BNF recommends **amoxicillin** or ampicillin, or **erythromycin, clarithromycin** or **azithromycin** if patients are penicillin sensitive, for uncomplicated CAP. If staphylococci are suspected, then **flucloxacillin** should be added. **Cefotaxime** or **cefuroxime** is recommended for severe CAP of unknown aetiology and flucloxacillin added if Gram-negative enteric bacilli, *Legionella* sp. or staphylococci are suspected. Hospital-acquired pneumonia requires a broad-spectrum **cephalosporin**, e.g. **cefotaxime**, or **ceftazidime**, or an antipseudomonal β-lactam or penicillin. Very severe cases may need, in addition, the use of an **aminoglycoside**. Atypical pathogens, e.g. *Legionella* spp., require **erythromycin** and possibly the addition of **rifampicin**.

Other measures for patients with CAP who are not admitted to hospital include support and information re adequate rest, fluids and nutrition, help to stop smoking and treatment of pleuritic pain with simple analgesics, e.g. paracetamol. Health workers should be familiar with pulse oximetry, a non-invasive method for measurement of haemoglobin saturated with oxygen.

Clinical scenario: Pneumonia is an acute inflammation caused by infection and profound infiltration of neutrophils into and around terminal bronchioles and alveoli. Oedema and inflammation cause consolidation of the affected bronchopulmonary segment. Predisposing factors include influenza with the complication of *S. pneumoniae* infection, smoking, COPD, asthma, bronchiectasis, malignancy, cystic fibrosis, immunosuppression, drug abuse and hospitalisation, which is associated with Gram-negative infection. Patients with conditions including diabetes, cardiovascular disease, Parkinson's disease, neurological disorders and oesophogeal obstruction are at risk of aspiration pneumonia, which is caused by anaerobic micro-organisms originating in the oropharynx. Aspiration pneumonia is often confined to the right lung. Development of pneumonia is associated with cough and sputum production, which may include haemoptysis. Patients suffer pleuritic chest pain, dyspnoea, sometimes myalgia, general malaise, weakness, and, in severe cases, respiratory distress, cyanosis and, in older patients, mental confusion. Symptoms may be dependent on age, when younger patients present with more severe initial symptoms such as a sudden rigor (shivering, fever, sensation of cold and rapid rise in body temperature). Auscultation may reveal, depending on the consolidation, pleural friction murmur, crackles and bronchial breathing. Patients who are hypotensive, clammy and cold to the touch may have septicaemia.

SARS is severe acute respiratory syndrome, an atypical pneumonia that apparently originated in the Far East and which is now feared to be a potential health hazard in other areas of the world, and at least one case was reported in Canada. SARS is caused by a virus of the paramyxoviridae family, which includes the viruses responsible for mumps and measles. Symptoms include fever, myalgia, headache and respiratory symptoms such as shortness of breath, cough, sore throat and difficulty breathing. It is thought to be infectious. At the time of writing there are no recommended treatments for SARS, except the use of barrier techniques to contain it with admitted patients, while milder cases may be managed at home, provided that patients limit their contacts.

Avian flu is caused by an influenza virus that first appeared in poultry in Asia and that has apparently jumped to humans, who develop pneumonia. Autopsy tissue samples and nasopharyngeal throat swabs from victims have tested positive for the avian influenza flu virus H5N1, which is transmitted through direct person-to-person contact. Experience of the virus suggests that it has not yet mutated sufficiently to spread rapidly from human to human, although there are fears that mutation is a matter of time, which could result in an influenza pandemic. This fear is exacerbated by a recent outbreak of avian flu in migratory geese in China, which was reported to have killed 1500 birds.

Antibiotics for treatment of pneumonia

Bactericidal*	Bacteriostatic
Aminoglycosides	Chloramphenicol
Bacitracin	Clindamycin
β-Lactams	Ethambutol
Isoniazid	Macrolides
Metronidazole	Sulphonamides
Polymyxins	Tetracyclines
Pyrazinamide	Trimethoprim
Quinolones	
Rifampicin	
Vancomycin	

*Intended as a guide only; may depend on dose

Legionnaires' disease is caused by *Legionella pneumophila*, so called because it was identified after it caused pneumonia among conference members of the American Legion in 1976. This species has several serogroups, the commonest cause of disease being serogroup 1, which results in acute pneumonia. Symptoms include malaise, dry cough, headache, myalgia and fever (~40°C). Initially, it may be misdiagnosed as septicaemia, but respiratory infection soon asserts itself as the main illness. Complications including renal failure, thrombocytopenia and generalised GIT disturbances may occur. There is a serious possibility of mortality (UK: ~12% in 1996). Treatment is with antibiotics, either orally or intravenously, and erythromycin is often used, with added rifampicin in severe cases, and mechanical ventilation if necessary. The disease is not usually transmitted from human to human, and infection appears to originate from water storage appliances such as humidifiers and air-conditioning systems, where stagnation encourages bacterial proliferation. Pontiac fever, a mild form of Legionnaires' disease, which was first identified in Pontiac in the USA, produces flu-like symptoms, and is geaerally treated with antipyretics and anti-inflammatory drugs.

118 Cystic fibrosis

Cystic fibrosis (CF) is a hereditary disease, confined mainly to white populations. The incidence of CF in the UK is approximately 1:2500 babies, and is caused by a mutation of a gene on chromosome 7, which codes for a protein called cystic fibrosis transmembrane conductance regulator (CFTR), a chloride channel that enables chloride transfer out of the cell and also regulates sodium import into the cell. CF is an autosomal-recessive disease (**A**).

The overall consequence of a lack of CFTR is the prevention of normal sodium chloride concentrations within exocrine cells, resulting in high salt-containing and therefore viscous secretions. Abnormally high lung mucus viscosity traps bacteria in the bronchioles with resultant infection. The lungs and pancreas are the two organs most affected, although other organs may also be affected. Symptoms, which may present soon after birth, include coughing with copious sputum, breathing difficulty, wheezing and recurrent chest infections, including pneumonia and consequent impairment of lung function (**B**). In CF, pancreatic secretions into the bile duct are seriously impeded and dietary fats and fat-soluble vitamins A, D, E and K are not absorbed. This results in malnutrition, failure to thrive and in many cases the production of malodorous steatorrhoea, as well as other problems (**C**). Symptoms of variable severity often develop within the first postnatal year, although they do sometimes appear later in childhood. Approximately 10% of cases present shortly after birth, with meconium ileus, when the prenatal gut contents, the meconium, fail to be expelled and form an obstruction that may need urgent surgery to be removed.

Diagnosis is by a genetic test that probes for the gene, which can be done prenatally by chorionic villous sampling if there is a family history of CF. Postnatally, blood samples routinely taken 6 days after birth to screen for phenylketonuria or hypothyroidism may be tested for CF. The sweat test measures salt in skin sweat and, in older children or adults, cells are scraped from inside the cheeks and probed for the CF gene. The **prognosis** historically was poor, and babies might survive for a few months only or a few years at most. Today, with improved care, children with CF may live fairly normal lives into their 30s or 40s.

Treatment requires a wide, multifactorial input (**E**) involving paediatricians, dieticians, trained nurses and physiotherapists. Regular checks for growth rate and general health have to be made. Lung health requires regular **chest physiotherapy** to maintain the airways clear of thickened mucus. Regular, long-term **antibiotic therapy** is virtually essential in many cases. Acute bacterial attacks may require intravenous antibiotics. Antibiotics directed against *Pseudomonas aeruginosa* may be taken by inhalation, as well as β_2-**agonists** to dilate the bronchioles. **Dornase alfa**, which is glycosylated recombinant human deoxyribonuclease 1, may be administered by nebuliser as an inhalation to digest mucus and thin it. **Pancreatin** is used to enhance fat absorption and digestion, and both **steroidal** and **non-steroidal** anti-inflammatory drugs may be used when necessary. Constipation and CF-related diabetes may also need to be treated. In severe cases, oxygen may need to be given and lung or heart and lung transplantation may have to be done to save the patient. Regarding nutrition, the Advisory Committee on Borderline Substances (ACBS) does recommend that certain food products may be regarded as drugs for the purposes of treating some conditions that cause impaired nutrition, and CF is one of these.

Gene therapy for CF is currently being researched, but although preliminary work *in vitro* is promising it is not, at time of writing, clinically possible.

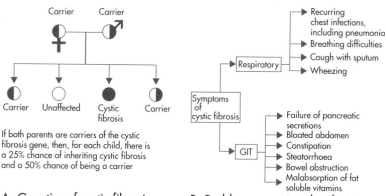

If both parents are carriers of the cystic fibrosis gene, then, for each child, there is a 25% chance of inheriting cystic fibrosis and a 50% chance of being a carrier

A. Genetics of cystic fibrosis

Symptoms of cystic fibrosis

Respiratory
- Recurring chest infections, including pneumonia
- Breathing difficulties
- Cough with sputum
- Wheezing

GIT
- Failure of pancreatic secretions
- Bloated abdomen
- Constipation
- Steatorrhoea
- Bowel obstruction
- Malabsorption of fat soluble vitamins

B. Problems associated with CF

C. Other problems associated with cystic fibrosis

- Hepatosplenomegaly
- Clubbing of fingers and toes
- Nasal polyps
- Male infertility due to failure of vas deferens development
- Female infertility due to uterine mucus thickness
- Diabetes

		Deleted in CF		
Nucleotide	– – – ATC ATC	TTT	GGT GTT – – –	
Amino acid	– – – Ile Ile	Phe	Gly Val – – –	
Amino acid number	506	508	510	

The deletion of three base-pairs in the CFTR gene results in the deletion of phenylalanine at position 508 of the CFTR protein, which is incorrectly folded. This is detected by the endoplasmic reticulum during post-translational processing and the protein is degraded. This deletion is responsible for about 75% of all cases of cystic fibrosis.

D. Δ F508 deletion in CFTR gene in cystic fibrosis

E. Treatment of cystic fibrosis

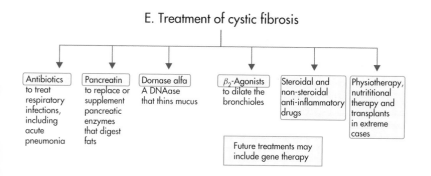

| Antibiotics to treat respiratory infections, including acute pneumonia | Pancreatin to replace or supplement pancreatic enzymes that digest fats | Dornase alfa A DNAase that thins mucus | β_2-Agonists to dilate the bronchioles | Steroidal and non-steroidal anti-inflammatory drugs | Physiotherapy, nutrititional therapy and transplants in extreme cases |

Future treatments may include gene therapy

119 Genitourinary systems I: Introduction

The genital and urinary (GU) systems are concerned with sexual reproduction and excretion of urine, respectively. In production and excretion of urine the kidneys are responsible for maintaining homoeostasis. The urethra is the final common pathway for expulsion of urine and spermatic fluid. Functionally, and in pathological terms, the urinary and genital tracts impinge on each other in that, for example, sexual intercourse can transmit urinary tract infections (UTIs). Benign prostatic hyperplasia (BPH), which is the most common GU problem in men, is associated with difficulties in micturition through compression of the urethra (A). In women, UTIs are the most common GU problem, partly because of the proximity of the anus to the relatively short urethra, through which faecal bacteria can migrate to the bladder (B). This is the most common route for infection, although in 20–30% of cases in women the skin micro-organisms *Staph. saprophyticus* and *Staph. epidermidis* are the infective agents. Urethral catheterisation and sexual intercourse may· facilitate UTIs. UTIs may occur in newborn males with congenital obstruction and in older men with acquired prostatic obstruction.

Generally, symptoms of renal disease (C) include altered frequency of micturition, urinary retention, haematuria, polyuria or oliguria (production of abnormally small volumes of urine) and dysuria (painful or difficult micturition). Patients may experience pain at any point along the renal tract, and in chronic cases patients may report anorexia and pruritis (itching), which is a common feature of chronic renal failure.

Sexually transmitted infections (STIs) are an ever-expanding medical problem (D). Common presenting symptoms include genital ulcers, urethral discharge and vaginal discharge, which may be a symptom of infection with one of a number of infecting organisms, including *Candida albicans*, *Chlamydia trachomatis*, *Neisseria gonorrhoeae* (gonococcus), *Treponema pallidum* (syphilis) and *Trichomonas vaginalis*. Vaginal discharge may accompany cervical polyps, herpes simplex (a sexually transmitted and contagious virus that may cause cold sores and genital herpes), neoplasia, chemical irritants or retained tampons. HIV, which causes AIDS, is transmitted through sexual intercourse, organ donation and contaminated blood products, across the placenta, during delivery and in breast milk. Another source is the use of shared needles and needle-stick injuries.

Neoplastic disease targets the GU systems. BPH is a feature of male ageing. Testicular tumours target predominantly younger men and are associated with metastases. Risk factors include cryptorchidism (undescended testes), ethnicity, because it is more prevalent in affluent white populations, a family history of testicular cancer and AIDS. Women may develop uterine or cervical cancer, the incidence of the latter now being greatly reduced through routine NHS screening services. Risk factors for cervical cancer include smoking, human papillomavirus (also responsible for warts), sexual promiscuity and HIV. Risk factors for uterine cancer, which is less common than cervical or ovarian cancer, include childlessness. In addition, late menopause, HRT, obesity and ovarian cysts, all of which increase exposure to endogenous estrogen, increase the risk of uterine cancer.

Drugs are used to treat GU infections and problems with micturition. They are used to increase urine flow, not only for local GU problems but for more widespread diseases, e.g. the use of diuretics in hypertension and heart failure.

A. The GU system in men

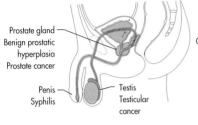

Prostate gland
Benign prostatic hyperplasia
Prostate cancer

Penis
Syphilis

Testis
Testicular cancer

B. The GU system in women

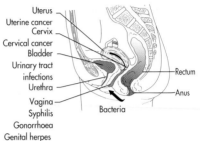

Uterus
Uterine cancer
Cervix
Cervical cancer
Bladder
Urinary tract infections
Urethra
Vagina
Syphilis
Gonorrhoea
Genital herpes

Rectum

Anus

Bacteria

C. Common presentations in renal disease

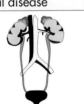

- Proteinuria – abnormally high protein in urine
- Haematuria – blood in urine
- Uraemia – nitrogenous waste products in blood, e.g. urea, creatinine
- Renal calculi (kidney stones)
- Hyperuricaemia – uric acid excess in blood
- Hypo- or hypernatraemia, hyper- or hypokalaemia
- Renal failure
- Oligouria, polyuria, dysuria
- Urinary incontinence – involuntary micturition (more common in women)
- Urinary tract infection
- Urethral, vaginal discharge

D. Symptoms and management of STIs

Common presenting symptoms STIs

Genital ulcers
Urethral discharge
Vaginal discharge

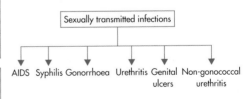

Sexually transmitted infections

AIDS Syphilis Gonorrhoea Urethritis Genital ulcers Non-gonococcal urethritis

Management of STIs

Correct diagnosis
Effective treatment
Tracing patient's sexual contacts
Patient follow-up
Patient education

120 Genitourinary systems II: Summary of tubule transport systems and sites of diuretic action

In order to understand the action of diuretics and their adverse effects, it is necessary to consider the normal function of the nephron and to know the sites of action of the diuretics, especially in terms of potassium loss. Any intervention that alters body water and osmolality has potential dangers, especially in the elderly and the very young.

The **proximal tubule**: After glomerular filtration has occurred, almost all of the filtered organic solutes, such as drugs, including diuretics, amino acids and glucose, and about 60% of water, 40% of NaCl and about 80% of HCO_3^- ions are reabsorbed here. The solutes are reabsorbed by specific transport systems in the tubule. The carbonic anhydrase (CA) inhibitor acetazolamide acts in the early part of the tubule. Normally, CO_2 diffuses from the luminal fluid into the tubule cell, where CA catalyses its conversion to $NaHCO_3$, which ionises and the HCO_3^- ion is transported back into the interstitial fluid. By inhibiting CA, acetazolamide prevents the reabsorption of HCO_3^-. NaCl is reabsorbed further along the tubule by a mechanism against which no diuretic is known to act. Osmotic diuretics such as mannitol act both here and in the collecting ducts, which can be rendered permeable to water (see below).

Loop of Henle: This consists of the thin descending limb, the thin ascending limb and the thick ascending limb (see opposite). Tubular fluid entering the thin descending limb is hypotonic relative to the interstitium, and so water is reabsorbed here. Therefore osmotic diuretics will be active in this limb.

The thick ascending limb is virtually impermeable to water, but has an energy (ATP)-requiring $Na^+/K^+/2Cl^-$ transporter in both the medullary and cortical regions that actively pumps NaCl back into the tubular cell. Approximately 35% of filtered NaCl is reabsorbed in the thick ascending limb. This results in hypotonic urine, and the thick ascending limb is thus also known as the 'diluting segment'. Some of the reabsorbed K^+ diffuses back into the lumen and this process powers the reabsorption of Ca^{2+} and Mg^{2+}. Normally, the urine that reaches the distal tubule is hypotonic. The so-called 'loop diuretics', which are very effective, and sometimes referred to as 'high ceiling' diuretics, inhibit the $Na^+/K^+/2Cl^-$ transporter in the ascending limb. In this case, the urine presented to the distal tubules is isotonic because it contains unreabsorbed NaCl and also Ca^{2+} and Mg^{2+}.

The **distal convoluted tubule**, like the thick ascending limb, is relatively impermeable to water. A NaCl transporter that is distinct from the $Na^+/K^+/2Cl^-$ transporter in the ascending limb reabsorbs approximately 10–15% of filtered NaCl here. The distal tubule NaCl transporter is blocked by the thiazide diuretics. Ca^{2+} ions are actively reabsorbed in the distal convoluted tubule via an apical calcium channel and a Na^+/Ca^{2+} exchanger in a process regulated by parathyroid hormone.

The **collecting tubule** reabsorbs less than 5% of the NaCl reabsorbed by the kidney but is nevertheless very important for diuretic action as it and the distal collecting duct are the site of action of the mineralocorticoids and therefore of the aldosterone antagonist diuretics. It is where most K^+ secretion occurs, although K^+ secretion here is not linked to Na^+ reabsorption. It is also unique in the nephron as the only site where water permeability can be changed by a hormone, namely antidiuretic hormone.

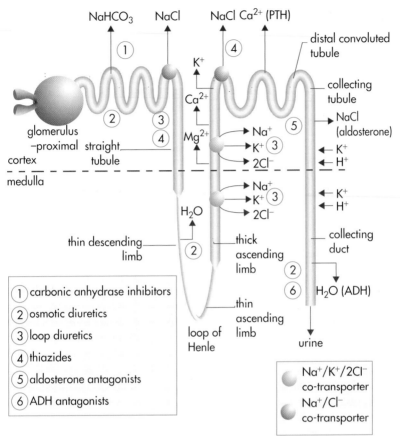

1 carbonic anhydrase inhibitors
2 osmotic diuretics
3 loop diuretics
4 thiazides
5 aldosterone antagonists
6 ADH antagonists

Na⁺/K⁺/2Cl⁻ co-transporter
Na⁺/Cl⁻ co-transporter

Tubular ion exchange and sites of action of diuretics

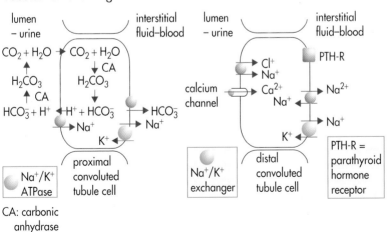

CA: carbonic anhydrase

121 Genitourinary systems III: Clinical uses of diuretics

Diuretics increase urine flow. Uses include hypertension, pulmonary and peripheral oedema, oliguria due to renal failure, ascites caused by liver failure and heart failure.

Loop diuretics are the most powerful, and act by inhibiting Na^+ reabsorption by 15–20% in the thick ascending limb of the loop of Henle. These include, principally, **furosemide, bumetanide** and **torasemide**, which are administered orally in tablet form.[43] **Therapeutic uses** include treating nephrotic syndrome, acute renal failure, hypertension resistant to thiazides, oedema, pulmonary congestion, and for reducing end-diastolic ventricular filling pressure and acute hypercalcaemia. **Adverse effects** include hypokalaemia, hyponatraemia, hypomagnesaemia, alkalosis, hyperuricaemia (which may precipitate a gout attack), ototoxicity, especially when injected, myalgia and hyperglycaemia. **Precautions:** treat hypovolaemia before use; pregnancy, porphyria, prostatic hyperplasia. **Contraindications** include renal failure with anuria and liver cirrhosis with pre-comatose states.

Thiazides include **bendroflumethiazide** (bendrofluazide), **chlortalidone, indapamide, metolazone, cyclopenthiazide** and **xipamide**. Diuresis is achieved through inhibition of Na^+ reabsorption in the early part of the distal tubule, and they are therefore not as potent as the loop diuretics. **Uses** include diabetic nephrogenic diabetes insipidus, oedema due to nephrotic syndrome, management of mild-to-moderate hypertension by reduction of peripheral vascular resistance and ascites caused by cirrhosis.[44] **Adverse effects** include postural hypotension, hyperglycaemia, hyperuricaemia, hyponatraemia, hypokalaemia, hypochloraemic alkalosis, hypercalcaemia, gout attacks and altered plasma lipid levels. **Precautions** include porphyria, pregnancy and breastfeeding, older patients, and patients with SLE and liver or renal impairment. **Contraindications** include Addison's disease, symptomatic hyperuricaemia, hyponatraemia, hypokalaemia and hypercalcaemia.

Potassium-sparing diuretics inhibit Na^+ reabsorption in the distal tubule (**amiloride** and **triamterene**) or the collecting ducts (**spironolactone** and **eplerenone**), and K^+ excretion is reduced. **Uses** include: (i) oedema; (ii) conditions causing excess mineralocorticoid production, e.g. in Conn's syndrome and ectopic ACTH production; (iii) secondary aldosteronism with water and salt retention, e.g. in congestive cardiac failure, hypovolaemia, nephrotic syndrome and hepatic disease; and (iv) with loop or thiazide diuretics to limit K^+ loss. **Adverse effects** include hyperkalaemia, gynaecomastia with spironolactone, and blue urine fluorescence with amiloride. **Precautions** include diabetes, pregnancy and breastfeeding, and elderly patients. Contraindications include patients on K^+ supplements, or who have hyperkalaemia or renal failure and, with spironolactone, Addison's disease and hyponatraemia.

Carbonic anhydrase inhibitors, principally **acetazolamide**, are weak diuretics used to treat acute and chronic glaucoma.

Diuretics and the elderly: Elderly patients often develop gravitational oedema with swollen legs and ankles, and should not be treated on a long-term basis with diuretics. They should be encouraged to use support stockings and should sit with their legs raised if possible. Elderly patients are prone to adverse effects of diuretics due to reduced renal function, and doses should be adjusted accordingly.

Diuretics and hypokalaemia: Patients on cardiac glycosides, notably digoxin, may be hypokalaemic. Caution is needed, especially with thiazides and loop diuretics. Caution should also be exercised with severe coronary artery disease, when hypokalaemia is dangerous.

Clinical scenario: An 83-year-old woman was referred to the elderly medicine admissions unit by her GP. He had seen her that day at the request of the patient's grand-daughter. The patient had been complaining of feeling out of sorts and tired for some weeks, and when the GP arrived at her flat he found her to be confused, drowsy and dehydrated. Although generally of good health, there was a past medical history of hypertension, which was treated with bendroflumethiazide and atenolol. The family had also noted that over the past 2 years there had been a deterioration in her short-term memory. On examination at the admissions unit the patient had impaired conciousness with a Glasgow Coma Score of 12 out of 15. She was dehydrated and bradycardic, and her blood pressure was 105/50. Neurological examination demonstrated generalised reduction in tone although reflexes were essentially normal. Investigations revealed a profound hyponatraemia, elevated white cell count and inflammatory markers, and leukocytes, protein and nitrites on a urine dipstick. The patient was diagnosed with a thiazide-induced hyponatraemia and dehydration complicated by a urinary tract infection. Both antihypertensives were stopped and the patient was resuscitated with intravenous crystalloid solutions and amoxicillin. Plasma sodium levels were monitored carefully. As the patient became euvolaemic her consciousness returned to normal. She was started on a normal diet and made a good recovery. It became apparent on the ward that her day-to-day blood pressure was actually normal and she was discharged on no regular medication.

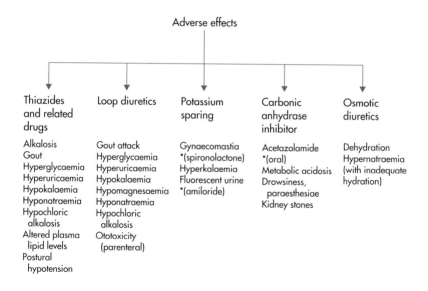

Adverse effects

Thiazides and related drugs
Alkalosis
Gout
Hyperglycaemia
Hyperuricaemia
Hypokalaemia
Hyponatraemia
Hypochloric
 alkalosis
Altered plasma
 lipid levels
Postural
 hypotension

Loop diuretics
Gout attack
Hyperglycaemia
Hyperuricaemia
Hypokalaemia
Hypomagnesaemia
Hyponatraemia
Hypochloric
 alkalosis
Ototoxicity
 (parenteral)

Potassium sparing
Gynaecomastia
*(spironolactone)
Hyperkalaemia
Fluorescent urine
*(amiloride)

Carbonic anhydrase inhibitor
Acetazolamide
*(oral)
Metabolic acidosis
Drowsiness,
 paraesthesiae
Kidney stones

Osmotic diuretics
Dehydration
Hypernatraemia
(with inadequate
 hydration)

The pharmacology of renal medicine can be broadly divided into two sections: the treatment of acute renal failure and the treatment of chronic kidney disease.

The functions of the kidneys are not confined to the production of urine, but also include acid–base balance, calcium metabolism, salt and water regulation, and regulation of haemoglobin levels, to name a few. Treatment of renal diseases is aimed at restoring these functions and maintaining homoeostasis.

Acute renal failure (ARF) is divided into three categories (**A**) according to the site of the pathology responsible for the renal insult: **pre-renal ARF**, **intrinsic renal ARF** and **post-renal ARF**.

Pre-renal ARF is generally caused by a reduction in blood flow to the kidney. This can be caused by shock syndromes such as cardiogenic shock following an MI or septic shock developing from meningitis, pneumonia or a UTI. Hypotension and subsequent renal failure are also common in surgical patients. Treatment is aimed at restoring blood flow to the kidneys. So, for example, in septic shock there would be aggressive fluid resuscitation, intravenous antibiotics and inotropic support if necessary.

Intrinsic renal ARF is less common than pre- or post-renal ARF and is caused by a direct insult to renal tissue. Examples include glomerulonephritis secondary to microscopic polyangiitis or Wegener's granulomatosis, or tubulointerstitial nephritis caused by NSAIDs. Treatment of the autoimmune disorders includes high-dose steroids and cytotoxic agents (methotrexate and cyclophosphamide). Renal replacement therapy is often required in the acute situation.

Post-renal ARF is caused by an obstruction to urinary drainage from the kidneys. The culprit lesion may be in the ureters, the bladder or the urethra. A very common cause of post-renal ARF is prostatic enlargement impinging on the urethra. Treatment is aimed at relieving the obstruction.

It is the complications of ARF that are responsible for the associated high mortality. These complications include acidosis, hyperkalaemia, uraemia and oedema (**B**).

Hyperkalaemia is caused by impaired potassium excretion and redistribution of intracellular cations. Cardiac toxicity occurs above 6.5 mmol/l, but treatment is often commenced before this. Infusions of insulin and dextrose are given over 30 minutes. Insulin stimulates cellular uptake of potassium and hydrogen ions and dextrose prevents subsequent hypoglycaemia. Salbutamol nebulisers are also used to stimulate cellular potassium uptake. These measures are effective only in reducing the concentration of plasma potassium by 0.6 mmol/l each. Calcium gluconate solution is also given in the acute situation to stabilise the myocardium.

Acidosis will often respond to treatment of the underlying condition, but can be partially reversed by infusions of varying strengths of sodium bicarbonate solution. These need to be used with caution, as their high sodium content can cause further fluid retention.

Renal function can deteriorate in addition to other pathologies such as acute or subacute heart failure. In such scenarios diuretics are used to relieve pulmonary oedema, optimising cardiac funtion and so improving renal perfusion. There is, however, little place for diuretics in the management of ARF and rather the emphasis lies in achieving euvolaemia.

Once all reversible pathologies have been treated, a decision is made whether to proceed to renal replacement therapy, i.e. plasma exchange, dialysis, etc.

A. Categories of acute renal failure

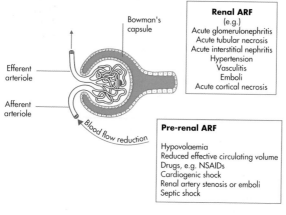

Bowman's capsule

Efferent arteriole

Afferent arteriole

Blood flow reduction

Renal ARF
(e.g.)
Acute glomerulonephritis
Acute tubular necrosis
Acute interstitial nephritis
Hypertension
Vasculitis
Emboli
Acute cortical necrosis

Pre-renal ARF

Hypovolaemia
Reduced effective circulating volume
Drugs, e.g. NSAIDs
Cardiogenic shock
Renal artery stenosis or emboli
Septic shock

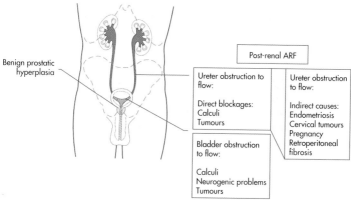

Benign prostatic hyperplasia

Post-renal ARF

Ureter obstruction to flow:

Direct blockages:
Calculi
Tumours

Ureter obstruction to flow:

Indirect causes:
Endometriosis
Cervical tumours
Pregnancy
Retroperitoneal fibrosis

Bladder obstruction to flow:

Calculi
Neurogenic problems
Tumours

B. Indications for acute dialysis

- Resistant hyperkalaemia
- Resistant acidosis
- Symptomatic uraemia
- Resistant pulmonary oedema
- Pericarditis

C. Complications of acute renal failure

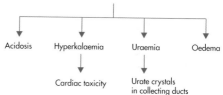

Acidosis   Hyperkalaemia   Uraemia   Oedema

Cardiac toxicity

Urate crystals
in collecting ducts

The management of **chronic renal disease (CRD)** is based on the principle of maximising and maintaining any remaining renal function and minimising the potential complications resulting from renal disease. The stages of renal disease are determined by the glomerular filtration rate (GFR) (**A**). The complications of renal disease can be broadly classified as: (i) anaemia; (ii) proteinuria and cardiovascular disease; (iii) acidosis; (iv) calcium metabolism; (v) nutrition; and (vi) maintaining euvolaemia/salt and water balance. One of the main manifestations of renal disease is **impaired salt excretion in urine**, causing water retention and oedema. This is assessed by examination of the patient's peripheries, skin turgor and jugular venous pressure, and auscultation of the lung fields. **Diuresis** is maintained using large doses of loop diuretics such as furosemide or bumetanide, which can be augmented with thiazide diuretics. Diuretics are also used to control hypertension, paramount in the management of patients with CRD. **Angiotensin-converting enzyme (ACE)** inhibitors are used in conjunction with diuretics for blood pressure control. These agents have also been shown to reduce proteinuria and so retard disease progression. **Cardiovascular risk** is further treated by lipid-lowering strategies and antithrombotic agents. Hyperkalaemia is a common problem in CRD as well as acute renal disease. ACE inhibitors are well-known hyperkalaemic agents and this adverse effect needs to be considered when prescribing. Some causes are given in (**B**).

Patients with CRD become anaemic through impaired secretion of erythropoietin from the juxtaglomerular apparatus in the kidneys, and also because uraemia affects the ability of the bone marrow to incorporate iron into red blood cells. Consequently, it is not only necessary to monitor haemoglobin levels, but also ferritin and transferrin saturation levels. Patients often require large doses of iron, which can be given intravenously. Erythropoietin is given as an injection three times weekly in chronic renal failure.[45] Diagnosis is given in (**B**).

CRD effects on bone: CRD has diverse effects on the skeleton, causing abnormal bone remodelling and mineralisation. In health, the kidney hydroxylates 25-hydroxycholecalciferol (25-hydroxyvitamin D) to 1,25-dihydroxycholecalciferol. In CRD, the failure of this mechanism results in low serum calcium levels and subsequent secondary hyperparathyroidism. This is also compounded by reduced secretion of phosphate. This is treated with calcium salts and **1α-calcidol**. Patients must, however, be monitored for development of hypercalcaemia, which heralds tertiary hyperparathyroidism. Other treatments to prevent these developments include phosphate binders and dietary phosphate restriction.

Also, acidosis and immobility adversely affect the skeleton. Autoimmune diseases and renal transplantation are often treated with **steroids** and immunosuppressants, both of which can result in osteoporosis. This is treated with **bisphosphonates**, although distinction between osteoporosis and hyperparathyroidism is important. Correcting acidosis is important in maintaining homoeostasis and optimising cardiac function. Oral **sodium bicarbonate** is used for this purpose. Review by a renal nutritionist is also important in regulating salt, protein and phosphate intake.

Stage	Description	GFR (ml/min per 1.73 m^2)	Prevalence (%)
1	Kidney disease with normal GFR	> 90	3.3
2	Kidney damage with mild GFR reduction	60–89	3
3	Kidney damage with moderate GFR reduction	30–59	4.3
4	Kidney damage with severe GFR reduction	15–29	0.2
5	Kidney failure	< 15	0.2

A. The stages of renal disease are determined by the GFR

Renal

Alport's syndrome
Amyloid
Bladder, urethral
  obstruction
Myeloma
Interstitial nephritis
Polycystic kidneys
Chronic pyelonephritis
Renal vascular
  disease

Drugs*

Ciclosporin
GOLD
NSAIDs
Penicillamine

*Not exhaustive

Extra-renal

Diabetes mellitus
Gout
Hypercalcaemia
Malignant hypertension
Renovascular disease
Vasculitis

B. Some causes of chronic renal disease

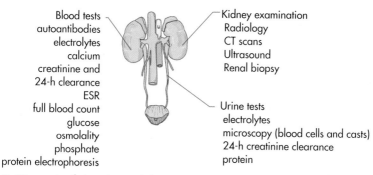

Blood tests
autoantibodies
electrolytes
calcium
creatinine and
24-h clearance
ESR
full blood count
glucose
osmolality
phosphate
protein electrophoresis

Kidney examination
Radiology
CT scans
Ultrasound
Renal biopsy

Urine tests
electrolytes
microscopy (blood cells and casts)
24-h creatinine clearance
protein

C. Diagnosis of chronic renal disease

124 Genitourinary systems VI: Urinary tract infections

Urinary tract infections are more common in women. A major factor is the shorter length of the female urethra and its proximity to the anus, because pathogenesis usually involves ascending urethral bacteria. The patient's bowel flora, including *E. coli*, *Klebsiella* sp. and enterococci, may cause infection, although the skin micro-organisms *Staph. saprophyticus* and *Staph. epidermis* also cause a significant number of UTIs in women (**A**). Bladder infection is more likely with pre-existing conditions, e.g. bladder stones, impaired emptying of the bladder, urinary stasis or obstruction or previous bladder epithelial damage. Pyelonephritis is bacterial infection of the kidneys, resulting from ascending infections in patients with faulty vesicoureteric valves, or as a complication of septicaemia. It may be acute or chronic.

Presenting symptoms of UTIs include malodorous urine, dysuria, haematuria and pain, and tenderness in the suprapubic area. Cystitis is a common condition (**B**). Acute pyelonephritis presents with pain in the loins, hyperpyrexia and systemic disturbances. In some patients, especially the elderly, symptoms could well be atypical, when patients complain of non-specific loss of well-being, nocturia and incontinence.

Diagnosis of UTIs involves: (i) the use of dipsticks, which detect elastase enzyme from eosinophils and urinary nitrites, produced by bacterial reduction of nitrates in urine, positive elastase and nitrites usually indicating the presence of a UTI; (ii) urine culture to identify the infection and microscopy; if, in a clean-catch midstream urine specimen, more than 100 000 of the same micro-organism are counted, then this provides confirmation of infection; and (iii) excretion urography, which will show anatomical abnormalities of the urinary tract.

Treatment of UTIs is with 3 to 5-day courses of antibiotics, e.g. **amoxicillin**, **nitrofurantoin** or **trimethoprim**, the choice of antibiotic dependent on antibiotic sensitivity tests and the response of the infection to initial treatment. Patients should take plenty of fluids both during and for several weeks after treatment. Some patients may relapse, and these should be prescribed low-dose prophylactic antibiotic treatment for 6–12 months. Acute pyelonephritis may make patients very ill, and they may need parenteral antibiotics, e.g. **ciprofloxacin**, **cefuroxime** or an **aminoglycoside** such as **gentamicin**. Patients with diabetes mellitus or other problems that involve the kidneys, or with abnormal urinary tracts, are more likely to fail initial treatment, and may develop complications such as renal papillary necrosis or perinephric abscesses with the accompanying risk of Gram-negative septicaemia. Abscesses require antibiotic therapy and may require surgical drainage.

During pregnancy, about 5–7% of women have significant bacteriuria, which, if untreated, may cause acute pyelonephritis. This poses a potentially serious risk to both mother and fetus from septic shock. Birth may be premature and infant weight low.

Non-pregnant, healthy women who develop acute cystitis (**B**) have little risk of complications, but if patients have pre-existing disease affecting the kidneys, e.g. diabetes mellitus, they are at risk of complications such as renal or perinephric abscesses.

Clinical scenario: Mrs BR, a 60-year-old widow, was admitted to hospital after persistent vomiting. She had a history of type 1 diabetes mellitus and ischaemic heart disease, pulmonary hypertension and pulmonary embolism, and had previously undergone percutaneous transluminal coronary angioplasty. She was listless and complained of abdominal pain. On examination, her abdomen was distended, although not tender. Her bowel sounds were sluggish and pneumaturia (bubbles of gas in urine, suggestive of bacterial action in the urinary tract) was noted. An abdominal radiograph revealed gas in the bladder and pneumoperitoneum (gas in the peritoneal cavity) showed up on chest X-ray. Exploratory laparotomy was done and revealed an emphysematous bladder. A course of cefpirone was prescribed and the presence of infection was confirmed by urine culture, which tested positive for *E. coli*. She recovered well and was discharged.

A. Micro-organisms responsible for UTIs

Micro-organism	Relative UTI incidence*	
	Hospital	Community
E. coli	45–55	80–90
P. vulgaris	10–12	5–10
Klebsiella	15–20	1–2
Enterobacter	2–5	–
Psudomonas	10–15	–
Enterococcus	10–12	< 1

*Data source: *Renal and Urinary Systems*, 2nd edn. S. Datta, N. Mirpuri, P. Patel, Mosby, Edinburgh, p. 76.

Tuberculosis
Tubulo-interstitial nephritis
Glomerulonephritis
Carcinoma
Ureteric neoplasm or stone
Haematological disorder

Infarcts
Papillary necrosis
Kidney stone

Parasites

Stones

Urethral tumour or infection

Prostate cancer
Benign prostatic hyperplasia

Some causes of haematouria

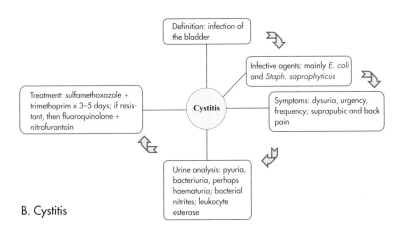

Definition: infection of the bladder

Infective agents: mainly *E. coli* and *Staph. saprophyticus*

Treatment: sulfamethoxazole + trimethoprim x 3–5 days; if resistant, then fluoroquinolone + nitrofurantoin

Cystitis

Symptoms: dysuria, urgency, frequency; suprapubic and back pain

Urine analysis: pyuria, bacteriuria, perhaps haematuria; bacterial nitrites; leukocyte esterase

B. Cystitis

125 Genitourinary systems VII: Urinary incontinence

Urinary incontinence is involuntary urination. Normally, continence is possible through (i) the sphincters at the bladder neck, and the urethral muscles, and (ii) detrusor muscle stability; this bladder muscle does not contract involuntarily. Also, the bladder wall can stretch to accommodate increasing volumes of urine. The mechanism of urine voiding involves decreased sympathetic drive, which relaxes the sphincters, and increased parasympathetic drive, which contracts the detrusor muscle. Continence is also under voluntary control through the activity of higher brain centres. Urinary incontinence is more common in women, and is distressing. Urinary incontinence is classified as stress incontinence, urge incontinence (detrusor instability incontinence), or overflow incontinence.

Stress incontinence, also called sphincter insufficiency, is involuntary loss of urine that may result through pelvic floor laxity after birth in mothers, in older multiparous and, more usually, obese women who have bladder neck sphincter impairment, and in men after prostatectomy, which may cause damage to the external sphincter. Urine is voided by an increase in intra-abdominal pressure, e.g. during or after coughing, laughing or standing up. **Treatment** involves pelvic floor exercises, which increase the muscle strength around the bladder outlet, and bladder training. **Drugs used** include **duloxetine**, a dual norepinephrine and serotonin (5-HT) re-uptake inhibitor which is now licensed for moderate-to-severe stress incontinence in women; it appears to be more effective when used together with pelvic floor exercises. Its **mechanism of action** is thought to be centrally by increasing urethral sphincter tone and contractility. **Administration** is oral. **Adverse effects**, which reflect non-selective potentiation of catecholaminergic and serotoninergic drives, include GIT upsets such as diarrhoea and constipation, nausea and vomiting, central effects such as increased libido and anxiety, and autonomic effects such as sweating, blurred vision and sexual dysfunction. **Precautions** include narrow angle glaucoma, depression, epilepsy, history of mania and concomitant use of anticoagulants. The drug should be withdrawn gradually. **Contraindications** include pregnancy, breastfeeding and liver disease. It is now also used as an antidepressant.

Urge incontinence occurs mostly in women, and is the involuntary voiding of urine together with a strong urge to urinate (C). The most common cause is detrusor instability. **Treatment:** mild cases sometimes respond to bladder retraining,[46] and severe cases are treated with antimuscarinic drugs. Those licensed are **flavoxate, oxybutynin, propiverine, solifenacin, tolterodine** and **trospium**. All are available for oral administration. **Adverse effects** reflect parasympathetic blockade. **Precautions** include elderly patients and those with any autonomic neuropathy. Antimuscarinic drugs may exacerbate congestive heart failure, coronary artery disease, hyperthyroidism, arrhythmias and prostate hypertrophy, and should be used with caution in liver disease and hiatus hernia with reflux oesophagitis. **Contraindications** include GIT obstruction or atony, myasthenia gravis, severe ulcerative colitis, urinary retention and severe bladder outflow obstruction.

Overflow incontinence is involuntary urination when the bladder is full. It occurs mainly in men with BPH with bladder outflow obstruction. There is danger of renal damage if the obstruction is not relieved with suprapubic or urethral catheterisation. Drug treatment is mainly with selective α-blocking drugs **alfuzocin, doxazocin, indoramin, prazocin, tamsulosin** or **terazocin**. They relax smooth muscle, thus increasing urine flow rate. **Adverse effects, precautions and contraindications** reflect generalised α_1-blockade.

Mechanism of action of duloxetine

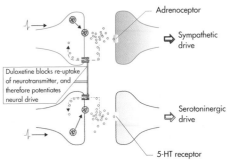

Duloxetine blocks re-uptake of neurotransmitter, and therefore potentiates neural drive

Adrenoceptor

Sympathetic drive

Serotoninergic drive

5-HT receptor

Pelvic floor exercise

Put pressure on the pelvic floor muscles by sitting on a hard seat or across a tightly rolled carpet or towel. When the bladder contracts and an urgent call to void urine happens, force five rapid squeezes of the pelvic floor muscles. This manoeuvre relaxes the bladder.

Some causes of detrusor instability 'urge incontinence'

- Alzheimer's disease
- Bladder hyperreflexia
- Benign prostatic hyperplasia
- Brain tumour
- Bladder stone
- Cough, sneeze, laughter
- Herniated spinal disc
- Loop diuretics
- Lower UTI or inflammation
- Natural ageing
- Parkinson's disease
- Stroke

Nocturnal enuresis

Most children are dry by 3 years, but bedwetting may persist, due to infection or, more usually for behavioural reasons. Non-pharmaceutical strategies are available, and drugs are usually inappropriate under age 7. Desmopressin as is sometimes prescribed short-term therapy, and care should be taken about fluid overload.

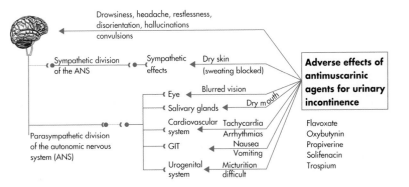

Drowsiness, headache, restlessness, disorientation, hallucinations convulsions

Sympathetic division of the ANS

Sympathetic effects

Dry skin (sweating blocked)

Eye — Blurred vision

Salivary glands — Dry mouth

Cardiovascular system — Tachycardia, Arrhythmias

GIT — Nausea, Vomiting

Parasympathetic division of the autonomic nervous system (ANS)

Urogenital system — Micturition difficult

Adverse effects of antimuscarinic agents for urinary incontinence

Flavoxate
Oxybutynin
Propiverine
Solifenacin
Trospium

Gonorrhoea is an STI transmitted by *Neisseria gonorrhoeae*, a Gram-negative intracellular diplococcus that infects epithelial cells, especially those of the GU tract, rectum, eye (conjunctiva) and pharynx. Transmission occurs during anal, oral or vaginal sex, and may affect the cervix, throat, anus and penis. Untreated gonorrhoea potentiates HIV infection because it renders an HIV-positive person more infective by increasing the numbers of HIV-infected cells in the mucosa of the mouth, throat and genitalia. Gonorrhoea is transmitted *in utero*, during parturition and may cause eye infections (ophthalmia neonatorum) in the baby if left untreated.

Symptoms: The incubation period may range from 2 to 15 days, approximately. In women it may be symptomless or include dysuria, vaginal discharge, which may be bloody, and sore throat. Complications include Bartholin's abscess[47] and salpingitis, which here refers to inflammation of the fallopian tubes. Men may develop epididymitis and prostatitis, and complain of a purulent urethral discharge, and homosexual men may complain of proctitis. Diagnosis is by Gram staining and cultures from swabs taken from the penis or urethra in men and from the endocervix in women. If gonorrhoea is disseminated, synovial fluid should be sampled for microscopy and blood culturing done.

Treatment for uncomplicated gonorrhoea is a single oral dose of 500 mg **ciprofloxacin**, a quinolone, whereas pharangeal infection requires treatment with **ceftriaxone**, a cephalosporin. Unfortunately, at least 10% of gonorrhoea cases in the UK are resistant to ciprofloxacin, and spectinomycin or ceftriaxone may have to be used instead. Complicated infections may need longer courses of treatment, and in all cases culture test should be carried out at least 72 hours after completing treatment.

Non-gonococcal urethritis (NGU) is, usually, infection with *Chlamydia trachomatis*, which may present with symptoms similar to those of gonorrhoea. NGU is diagnosed using PCR tests for chlamydial nucleic acids. Treatment is with **oxytetracycline** or **erythromycin** in pregnancy.

Syphilis is infection with *Treponema pallidum*. It is relatively uncommon in the UK. Transmission depends on the anatomical site of the syphilitic ulcer, and is through direct contact during anal, oral or vaginal sex. The organism is transmitted through minute skin abrasions during sexual activity. *T. pallidum* may also cross the placenta. The **symptoms**, if left untreated, have been classified as primary, secondary and tertiary stages (see opposite). Initially, after an incubation period ranging from about 10 to 100 days, a papule, less than 5 mm in diameter, develops on the skin at the site where infection occurred. The papule ulcerates, when it is called a chancre, which spontaneously heals within around 2–4 weeks. There may be more than one chancre or there may be no lesion. In babies with congenital syphilis, symptoms may appear between weeks 2 and 6 after parturition. Symptoms include failure to thrive, nasal discharge, and mucosal and skin lesions.

Diagnosis is done using the *T. pallidum* enzyme assay (EIA), which is confirmed using the *T. pallidum* haemagglutination assay (TPHA) and the Venereal Disease Reference Laboratory (VDRL) test. The VDRL test may be negative in untreated patients during the tertiary stage, or in patients who have been treated. In addition, the micro-organism can be seen in fluid taken from the lesion using dark-ground microscopy.

Treatment for primary and secondary syphilis is with intramuscular **procaine penicillin**, **erythromycin** or **doxycycline** for 10–14 days, and for 4 weeks in tertiary syphilis. Asymptomatic contact patients should be treated with doxycycline for 14 days.

Historical note: Guy de Maupassant, the 19th century French novelist who wrote *The Necklace*, arguably one of the finest short stories written, was infected with syphilis in his 20s. The only treatment available was mercury, administered either orally or directly to the syphilitic lesion. He passed through the primary, secondary and tertiary stages of syphilis, and during this period wrote his major works. Eventually, in the tertiary stages of syphilis, he lost his reason and suffered hallucinations and attempted to cut his throat. He was subsequently sectioned and died in a well-known asylum for the insane in Passy in 1893. It is not known whether his dementia was due to syphilis or the central toxic effects of mercury; both cause severe behavioural and motor changes. Conceivably, both the disease and the treatment contributed to his creative output and to his death.

Stages of syphilis if untreated

Primary: 10–90 days incubation, then papule develops at infection site and ulcerates. Lesion heals spontaneously within 2–4 weeks

Secondary: 3–10 weeks after appearance of primary lesion, possible symptoms include: skin rashes, except on face; wart-like perianal lesions (condylomata lata); malaise, fever, arthalgia, inflammation; symptoms disappear within 1 year in most patients, followed by a latent (hidden) period

Tertiary: after 2 years or more, symptoms of ongoing tissue damage appear. Granulomatous lesions (gummae) may appear on testes, skin, bone and liver. Cardiovascular symptoms include aortic regurgitation (reflux of blood into the left ventricle during diastole) and (uncommonly) thoracic aortic aneurysms. Neurosyphilitic conditions (rarely seen in the UK due to timely treatment) are progressive dementia, tremor, brisk reflexes and extensor plantar reflexes. Intracranial gummae may cause raised intracranial pressure

HIV is the human immunodeficiency virus, which causes AIDS, the acquired immune deficiency syndrome. **Transmission** is mainly through: hetero- and homosexual intercourse; contaminated needles; from mother to child during pregnancy, childbirth and in breast milk; dental accidents; contaminated blood products; and organ transplantation. However, in developed countries blood products have been screened since 1985. HIV is a retrovirus, with RNA that is transcribed into DNA, which is then incorporated into the host cell's genome. **Viral resistance** is due to high viral turnover and the rapid mutability of its reverse transcriptase. **Infection of host cells** occurs through binding of the HIV surface glycoprotein gp720 (**A**) mainly to CD4 receptors on host lymphocytes and, together with host chemokine co-receptors CXCR4 and CCRS, HIV penetrates into the host cell, in which it releases viral RNA. The host cell multiplies the virus. The progressive loss of CD4 helper cells results in immunodeficiency and renders the individual susceptible to opportunistic infections, some of which normally would not be considered pathogenic (**B**). Antibody abnormalities open the way for infections with encapsulated bacteria, e.g. *Haemophilus influenzae* and *Streptococcus pneumoniae*. During the latency period, the viral load and consequent immunodeficiency status grow despite lack of symptoms (**C**).

The different stages of HIV: Category A is primary AIDS infection when symptoms are relatively mild, e.g. those of glandular fever. Patients may develop mild lymphadenopathy or be without symptoms of AIDS other than being HIV positive. Category B patients develop mild infections, e.g. idiopathic thrombocytopenic purpura, herpes zoster that involves more than one dermatome or persistent vaginal candiasis. Category C patients develop symptoms of severe immunodeficiency affecting virtually all systems.

Treatment of AIDS: The approach is antiretroviral to reduce the plasma viral load as far as possible and keep it low. Combination therapy is used with at least three drugs to reduce resistance development (HAART).[48] Antiretroviral drugs fall into one of four groups: (i) **nucleoside/nucleotide reverse transcriptase inhibitors (NRTIs)**; (ii) **non-nucleoside reverse transcriptase inhibitors (NNRTIs)**, e.g. efavirenz; (iii) **protease inhibitors**; and (iv) **entry** or **fusion inhibitors**.

Nucleoside/nucleotide reverse transcriptase inhibitors are nucleoside analogues (**D**). **Zidovudine**, representative of this group, is structurally similar to thymidine and is incorporated into the growing viral RNA strand; this stops chain elongation by reverse transcriptase because, instead of an –OH group attached to the 3′ carbon chain, zidovudine has an $-N_3$ (azido) group, and bond formation with a phosphate group cannot occur. **Administration** may be oral or by intravenous infusion. Zidovudine is rapidly absorbed orally with a plasma half-life of 1 hour, and the intracellular half-life of the active triphosphate is about 3 hours. Unusually for nucleosides, which require active uptake into cells, zidovudine enters the cell by passive diffusion. **Adverse effects** include anaemia and neutropenia, lactic acidosis, GIT disturbances, anorexia, liver damage, pancreatitis, lipid-altering effects, arthralgia, myopathy and flu-like symptoms. **Precautions** include anaemia, chronic hepatitis B or C and renal impairment (**E**). **Contraindications** include abnormally low neutrophil counts and breastfeeding. **Resistance** develops because of rapid viral mutation and resistant strains of the virus are transmitted to other individuals. Also, with prolonged use, less of the drug is converted to the active triphosphate.

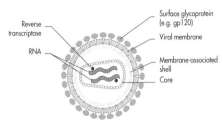

Reverse transcriptase
RNA

Surface glycoprotein (e.g. gp120)
Viral membrane
Membrane-associated shell
Core

A. Diagrammatic section through the human immuno deficiency virus (HIV)

C. Viral and gp120 antibody titres in AIDS

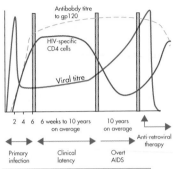

Antibobdy titre to gp120
HIV-specific CD4 cells
Viral titre

2 4 6   6 weeks to 10 years   10 years
              on average   on average

Anti-retroviral therapy

Primary infection   Clinical latency   Overt AIDS

Adapted from Ballingr A, Patchett S. Clinical Medicine, 3rd edn. 2003 Elsevier Ltd, London

D. NRTIs
Abacavir
Didanosine
Emtricitabine
Lamivudine
Stavudine
Tenofor disoproxil
Zalcitabine
Zidovudine

B. Some opportunistic complications of AIDS*

Candidiasis
Invasive cervical carcinoma
Cryptosporidiosis
Cytomegalovirus
HIV-related encephalopathy
Herpes simples
Histoplasmosis
Karposi's sarcoma
Mycobacterium avium
Primary lymphoma of brain
Mycobacterium tuberculosis
Recurrent pneumonia
Toxoplasmosis of brain

*Not comprehensive

HN
CH_3
O
HOH_2C
O

Thymidine

HN
CH_3
O
HO
O
N_3

Zidovudine

E. Liver-related precautions with NRTIs

- Life-threatening lactic acidosis associated with hepatic steatosis and hepatomegaly
- Alcohol abuse
- Hepatitis C treated with interferon-α and ribavirin
- Female patients, especially. obese, with hepatomegaly
- Discontinue treatment with NRTI for lactic acidosis, symptomatic hyperlactinaemia, progressive hepatomegaly, rapid deterioration of hepatic function

Some special precautions*

*Not comprehensive; see also BNF

Abacavir: life-threatening hypersensitivity reactionsl

Didanosine: pancreatitis

Lamivudine: chronic hepatitis

*Stavudine: peripheral neuropathy

*Tenofovir: renal function

Zalcitabine: pancreatitis, peripheral neuropathy

Zidovudine: haematological toxicity

*The only nucleotide NTRI

Non-nucleoside reverse transcriptase inhibitors block reverse transcriptase. Drugs used include **efavirenz** and **nevirapine**. Both are indicated for use in HIV in combination with at least two other anti-retroviral agents. Nevirapine is generally used in more advanced cases. **Adverse effects** of both drugs include Stevens–Johnson syndrome.[49] Efavirenz may cause psychotic episodes, anxiety, nightmares and convulsions, GIT disturbances, photosensitivity and gynaecomastia. Nevirapine is associated with hepatitis, GIT upsets, hypersensitivity reactions, pruritis (common), granulocytopenia and anaemia. **Precautions** with both drugs include hepatitis B or C and renal impairment, especially with efavirenz, which is **contraindicated** while breastfeeding. Nevirapine is contra-indicated in, for example, severe liver impairment and while breastfeeding.

Protease inhibitors block the enzymes that degrade protein. HIV uses a protease to digest host protein, before incorporating it into new copies of the virus. Drugs used include **amprenavir**, atazanavir, **fosamprenavir**, **indinavir**, **lopinavir** together with **ritonavir**, or ritonavir alone, **nelfinavir** and **saquinavir**. Ritonavir in sub-therapeutic doses increases the plasma half-lives of several other agents. **Administration** is oral. **Adverse effects** of protease inhibitors include potential for drug interactions because they are metabolised by the liver cytochrome P450 enzymes, which metabolise many other drugs. Most are associated with dyslipidaemia, lipodystrophy, which is disturbance of fat distribution or metabolism, and insulin resistance, and patients should be monitored for blood glucose and plasma lipids while on protease inhibitors, because these are associated with atherosclerosis. They may cause CNS, GIT and renal problems, skin rashes, electrolyte disturbances, endocrine symptoms including Cushing's syndrome, gynaecomastia and sexual dysfunction. **Precautions** include use with diabetics, haemophiliacs, hepatitis B or C, renal impairment (except with atazanavir and fosamprenavir, which can be used at recommended doses in patients who have renal impairment). **Atazanavir** may exacerbate cardiac conduction problems; there is a risk of nephrolithiasis (kidney stones) with indinavir, which, as with ritonavir, should be avoided in patients with porphyria. Patients on saquinavir should avoid garlic, which reduces plasma concentrations of the drug. **Contraindications** for all protease inhibitors include breastfeeding.

Fusion (entry) inhibitors block HIV's ability to penetrate the host cell. **Enfuvirtide** is licensed for use in the UK in combination with other drugs in cases where patients do not respond to other combinations. It fuses with HIV cell surface glycoprotein gp41, thus blocking its fusion to host cell surface proteins. **Administration** is by injection. **Adverse effects** include injection site reactions, symptoms of systemic hypersensitivity reactions (the drug must be stopped at once), gastro-oesophageal reflux and CNS disturbances, including decreased concentration ability, vertigo, tremor, anxiety and nightmares, lipid disorders, including hypertriglyceridaemia, endocrine disturbances, including diabetes mellitus, skin pupilloma and renal calculi. **Precautions** with enfuvirtide include hepatic disease, chronic hepatitis B or C, and renal impairment. **Contraindications** include breastfeeding.

Treatment strategies include: (i) when to initiate therapy; (ii) special patient needs, e.g. pregnancy, breastfeeding, age, concomitant endocrine, hepatic and renal status of the patient; (iii) decisions about switching treatments; and (iv) post-exposure prophylaxis. Treatment initiation depends on the CD4 count, the viral load and the patient's symptoms. HIV infection is treated with combinations of two or three drugs, mainly to minimise resistance development.

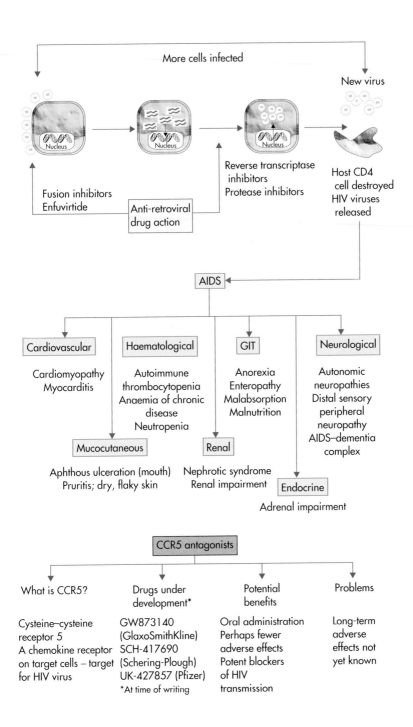

More cells infected

New virus

Nucleus

Nucleus

Nucleus

Fusion inhibitors
Enfuvirtide

Anti-retroviral
drug action

Reverse transcriptase
inhibitors
Protease inhibitors

Host CD4
cell destroyed
HIV viruses
released

AIDS

Cardiovascular

Cardiomyopathy
Myocarditis

Haematological

Autoimmune
thrombocytopenia
Anaemia of chronic
disease
Neutropenia

GIT

Anorexia
Enteropathy
Malabsorption
Malnutrition

Neurological

Autonomic
neuropathies
Distal sensory
peripheral
neuropathy
AIDS–dementia
complex

Mucocutaneous

Aphthous ulceration (mouth)
Pruritis; dry, flaky skin

Renal

Nephrotic syndrome
Renal impairment

Endocrine

Adrenal impairment

CCR5 antagonists

What is CCR5?

Cysteine–cysteine
receptor 5
A chemokine receptor
on target cells – target
for HIV virus

Drugs under
development*

GW873140
(GlaxoSmithKline)
SCH-417690
(Schering-Plough)
UK-427857 (Pfizer)
*At time of writing

Potential
benefits

Oral administration
Perhaps fewer
adverse effects
Potent blockers
of HIV
transmission

Problems

Long-term
adverse
effects not
yet known

Glossary of terms

ACE inhibitors Drugs that inhibit angiotensin-converting enzyme

Acetylsalicylic acid Aspirin

ACh Acetylcholine

Acidosis Abnormally high acidity of body fluids and tissues

Acromegaly Excessive production of growth hormone in adults by a tumour of the pituitary gland

Activated partial thromboplastin time (APTT) Clotting produced by addition to plasma of a mixture of negatively charged phospholipids (PLs), kaolin and Ca^{2+}

Active immunisation Promotion of the production of antibodies or sensitised lymphocytes to bacteria or toxins that are produced by bacteria before infection occurs (see also **Passive immunisation**)

Addison's disease Disease caused by deficiency of **corticosteroid** production and release from the adrenal cortex; the main symptoms are loss of energy, muscle weakness, **hypotension**; low corticosteroids lower the body's defences against stress and infectious diseases

Adipose tissue Connective tissue packed with adipocytes (fat cells)

Adjuvant therapy In cancer treatment, refers to the use of **cytotoxic** drugs to kill remaining cancer cells after surgery or **radiotherapy**, particularly if there is a high risk of recurrence of the tumour

Adrenal medulla

Adrenaline Alternative name for epinephrine

Adrenergic Describes nerves of the sympathetic nervous system that release **norepinephrine**, or receptors that respond to norepinephrine and sympathomimetic drugs (see also **Noradrenergic**)

Adrenocorticotrophic hormone (ACTH) Hormone released by the anterior pituitary gland; releases adrenal cortical hormones

Adverse effects Unwanted effects; also termed side-effects

Aetiology Cause of a disease; the study of disease causation

Affinity Tightness of the binding reaction between two molecules, e.g. between drug and receptor, or between substrate and enzyme

Afterload The arterial pressure against which the heart must pump

Agonist Drug that reacts with a receptor resulting in a cellular response similar to the physiological response of the cell to **endogenous** activation

Ague Rheumatism (historic)

AIDS Acquired immune deficiency syndrome

Allele Alternative forms of a gene

Alopecia Scalp hair loss

Alzheimer's disease Progressive development of **dementia** characterised by short-term memory loss, and progressive loss of cognitive ability; may be caused by loss of certain **cholinergic** neurons in the brain

Amoebiasis Dysentery (severe **diarrhoea** with mucus and blood) caused by infection of the gut with *Entamoeba histolytica*, a protozoan parasite

Anabolic Promoting tissue growth; forming complex substances such as proteins and laying down glucose as **glycogen**

Anaemia Clinically significant reduction in **haemoglobin** in blood

Analgesic Drug that relieves pain

Analogue Drug that is chemically related to a parent substance, e.g. ethinylestradiol is an analogue of the hormone estradiol, and has similar oestrogenic properties, but, unlike estradiol, can be taken by mouth

Anaphylactic reaction Widespread release of histamine as part of an allergic response; can be fatal unless dealt with immediately

Androgen One of a group of compounds, including testosterone, which develops and maintains male sexual function and secondary male characteristics, e.g. hirsutism (hair growth)

Angina A suffocating pain, usually originating in the heart

Anorexia Loss of appetite

Antagonist Drug that blocks the action of an agonist

Anthelmintic Chemical used to destroy parasitic worms

Anti-arrhythmic Any drug used to treat heartbeat irregularities

Antibiotic Any substance produced by or derived from an organism that inhibits the growth of or destroys another organism, usually a bacterial or fungal infection

Antibody Protein produced by a white blood cell, which binds to and renders harmless a specific **antigen** such as a bacterium, a foreign blood cell, a virus or pollen

Anticholinesterase A drug that blocks the enzyme acetylcholinesterase, which breaks down the neurotransmitter **acetylcholine**

Anticoagulant Agent that prevents or slows down the clotting of blood

Anticonvulsant Drug that prevents or reduces the severity of epileptic **seizures**

Antidepressant Drug that alleviates the symptoms of depression

Anti-emetic Agent that inhibits or reduces vomiting

Antigen Substance seen by the body as foreign, and against which the body makes a specific **antibody**

Antihistamine Agent that blocks the action of histamine, usually by blocking histamine receptors

Anti-inflammatory Reducing or blocking inflammation reactions

Antimuscarinic Drug that blocks **muscarinic** receptors

Antipsychotic (neuroleptic) Drug used to treat **psychosis**

Antipyretic Lowering of body temperature (e.g. aspirin is antipyretic)

Antiserum Serum containing antibodies directed against specific antigens; used clinically for **passive immunisation**

Antithrombin III A protein that is part of the system that regulates clotting. It binds to certain **clotting factors** and renders them inactive

Anxiety A term used to describe a condition of generalised, all-pervasive fear

Anxiolytic Drug that reduces **anxiety**

Aqueous humour Fluid that fills the chamber of the eye behind the cornea and in front of the lens (see also **Vitreous humour**)

Aromatase inhibitor Drug that blocks the biosynthesis of oestrogens by inhibiting the aromatase enzyme

Arrhythmia Deviation from the normal sinus rhythm of the heart

Arteriole Small branch of an artery, important in the control of blood flow and blood pressure, because it is innervated by nerves and responds to drugs that may either dilate or constrict it

Arthritis Inflammation of the joints (see also **Osteoarthritis, Rheumatoid arthritis**

Ascites Accumulation of fluid in the peritoneal cavity, which causes the abdomen to swell

Asthma Condition of unknown **aetiology** causing paroxysmal **dyspnoea** because of narrowing of **bronchioles**

Atheroma Degeneration of the inner arterial wall (intima) caused by the deposition of fatty plaques and scarring

Atonic (*n.* atony) Muscles are relaxed and 'floppy' without their usual elasticity, e.g. 'atonic' **seizures** in epilepsy

Atopy Constitutional or hereditary tendency to development of hypersensitivity, e.g. asthma, atopic **eczema**

Atrial fibrillation (AF) Atrial arrhythmia marked by rapid, randomised contraction of small areas of the atrial **myocardium**, causing an irregular and often rapid ventricular rate

Atrioventricular (AV) node Body of modified heart muscle in the lower part of the right ventricle that receives contractile impulses from and transmits these to the ventricles through the **bundle of His**

Atrium Either of the two upper chambers of the heart

Atrophy Wasting away of tissues or organs because of cellular degeneration

Auscultation Listening to sounds made by fluids or gas in the body, usually with a stethoscope

Autonomic nervous system (ANS) Part of the nervous system that controls functions over which there is little or no conscious control; consists of sympathetic and parasympathetic divisions

Autosomal Describes any gene carried on any chromosome other than a sex chromosome

B cell See **B lymphocyte**

B lymphocyte White blood cell made in the bone marrow that matures in the lymph nodes and spleen before entering the bloodstream. B lymphocytes make antibodies (see also **T lymphocyte**)

Bactericidal Able to kill bacteria, usually rapidly

Bacteriostatic Able to stop bacteria from replicating, but not killing them

Basal ganglia Large masses of grey matter embedded within the white matter of the cerebral hemispheres; they are concerned mainly with control of voluntary movements at a subconscious level

BPH Benign prostatic hyperplasia

β-receptor Subclass of adrenergic receptors that mediates, e.g. vasodilatation (β_2-receptor) or cardiac **contractility** and speed (β_1-receptor)

Bioassay Measurement of drug activity or potency *in vivo* or *in vitro*, usually by comparison with standard drugs of known strength

Bioavailability The drug has reached the circulation and is therefore available to all the tissues

'Biologic' drugs Therapeutic agents, including vaccines or genetically engineered proteins, that interact with proteins of viruses or bacteria, bacteria or proteins of the body that mediate, for example, immune reactions

Biopsy Excision of a small sample of living tissue for microscopic or biochemical investigation, usually for diagnostic purposes

Bradycardia Slowing of the heart rate; pulse rate falls below 60

Bradykinesia Symptom of Parkinson's disease – difficulty in maintaining body posture

Bronchiole A subdivision of the bronchial tree

Bronchospasm Narrowing of the bronchial tubes through contraction of bronchial smooth muscle

Bruit Murmur caused by blood flow turbulence in the heart or blood vessels heard through a stethoscope; causes include damaged valves, narrowed arteries, septal defects and arteriovenous communication

Bundle of His Bundle of modified heart muscle fibres called Purkinje fibres that conduct waves of contraction from the atria to the ventricles (also called atrioventricular bundle)

Calcium antagonist Drug that blocks calcium channels; used in hypertension and cardiac arrhythmias

Carcinogen Anything that causes cancer (see also **Oncogen**)

Carcinoid tumour Tumour of argentaffin cells in intestinal glands, often on the tip of the appendix; the tumours produce pharmacologically active amounts of 5-HT, prostaglandins and other chemicals that cause carcinoid syndrome if they escape into the circulation

Cardiac Pertaining to the heart; also used to describe the upper end of the stomach

Cardiomyopathy Chronic disease of heart muscle

Cardioversion Restoring the normal rhythm of the heart by applying a controlled direct current shock to the heart of an anaesthetised patient using electrodes placed on the chest wall; the apparatus used is called a cardiovertor

Catabolic Breakdown of complex substances such as proteins and **glycogen** to glucose to release energy

Catechol-O-methyltransferase (COMT) An enzyme that breaks down catecholamines

Catecholamine An amine that contains the catechol ring; examples are **norepinephrine** and **epinephrine**

CD4 A protein on the surface of **helper T cells** that is important in the development of immunity to viral infections

Cerebral palsy Movement disorder caused by brain damage before, during or soon after birth; brain damage is permanent, but the disorder is non-progressive

Chelating agents Chemicals that form complexes with some metal ions, thus rendering them harmless so that they can be safely excreted; useful agents in cases of, for example, copper poisoning

Chemoreceptor trigger zone (CTZ) Nerve centre in the **medulla** of the brain that, when stimulated by drugs such as apomorphine, triggers the **vomiting centre**

Chemotherapy Treatment or prevention of disease with chemicals; usually refers to treatment of cancer and infectious diseases with drugs

Cholecalciferol Vitamin D

Cholinergic Usually refers to any function or nerve where acetylcholine is the mediator

Chronic obstructive pulmonary (airway) disease (COPD) Group of pulmonary disorders marked by a progressive and irreversible reduction in lung airflow

Cirrhosis Formation of a network of fibrous tissue and regenerating cells in the liver in response to, for example, alcohol, hepatitis, chronic heart failure

Clinical trial Controlled assessment of a new drug or procedure in patients and/or healthy volunteers

Clotting factors (coagulation factors) Components of blood that are part of a cascade of reactions resulting in coagulation

Clotting time (coagulation time) The time taken for blood or plasma to coagulate under controlled laboratory conditions

CNS Central nervous system

Coagulation In the case of blood, the conversion of liquid blood to a solid fibrous mass

Coeliac disease Disease in which the small intestine is unable to digest and absorb food; successfully treated by adopting a strictly gluten-free diet

Compliance A patient's adherence to a prescribed drug or other programme of treatment

COMT Catechol-O-methyltransferase

Congenital Any disorder recognised at birth, whether caused genetically or by environmental factors

Conjugation In pharmacokinetics, refers to the metabolic conversion of a drug to a more soluble form, as either a sulphate or a glucuronide, for excretion via the kidneys

Constipation Difficult, infrequent or painful evacuation of bowel contents

Contractility Degree of power of the muscle to contract

Contraindications Conditions that mean that a drug should not be used

Coronary angioplasty Inflation of part of the coronary artery with a balloon

Coronary thrombosis Thrombus (blood clot) formation in the coronary artery, causing death of some cardiac tissue through a reduction in blood supply

Coronary Relating to the heart

Corpus striatum Part of the **basal ganglia** in the cerebral hemispheres of the brain

Corticosteroid (corticoid) Any steroid hormone synthesised in the adrenal cortex, the two main types being glucocorticoids, e.g. cortisol, and mineralocorticoids, principally aldosterone

COX Cyclo-oxygenase

Cranial nerves Twelve pairs of nerves arising directly from the brain, e.g. vagus (XI)

Crohn's disease (regional enteritis, regional ileitis) Inflammation of segments of the alimentary tract, which become ulcerated, thickened and inflamed. The cause is unknown

CSM Committee on Safety of Medicines

CT Computer tomography

Cushing's disease Disease caused by excessive production and release of corticosteroid hormones due to an ACTH-secreting tumour in the pituitary or elsewhere in the body; Cushing's *syndrome* is a condition where the patient has the symptoms of Cushing's disease, but caused, for example, by large amounts of steroid medication

Cyanosis Skin and mucous membranes turn blue as a result of inadequate oxygen supply to the tissues

Cyclo-oxygenases (COXs) Enzymes in pathway to biosynthesis of, for example, prostaglandins; aspirin reduces inflammation by inhibiting cyclo-oxygenase

Cytokines Proteins released by cells when they are challenged by antigens, e.g. interleukins; part of the body's protective mechanisms

Cytotoxic Destroys cells by blocking cell division

Dementia Chronic mental disorder of intellectual function and behaviour caused by brain degenerative disease or destruction of brain tissue through physical trauma such as stroke; dementia should not be confused with psychological disorders that produce similar symptoms

Depolarising non-competitive drugs Neuromuscular blockers that actually excite the muscle fibre by depolarising the membrane before they block any further membrane depolarisation by acetylcholine released from nerve endings at the neuromuscular junction (e.g. suxamethonium)

Diabetes A term to describe a metabolic disorder characterised by production of abnormally large volumes of dilute urine. When used alone, it usually refers to diabetes mellitus

Diabetes insipidus A rare disease in which the patient produces large amounts of dilute urine due to a deficiency of vasopressin

Diabetes mellitus Raised blood sugar caused by a deficiency of insulin. There are two types: type 1 (juvenile onset, insulin-dependent), which is an autoimmune disease involving destruction of the pancreatic β cells, and type 2 (non-insulin dependent), which is a reduced ability of the islets to produce sufficient insulin

Diarrhoea Abnormally high frequency of bowel evacuation, often with soft or liquid stools; can cause serious loss of water, salts and nutrients

Diastolic blood pressure The pressure recorded at diastole when the heart is filling; the value obtained reflects predominantly the **total peripheral resistance** in the vascular beds

Discoid rash SLE affecting the skin only

Doppler ultrasound Use of ultrasound to study flow direction and velocity in blood vessels, and the movement of heart valves

Dyspnoea Difficult or laboured breathing, apparent to the health professional

Diuretic Drug that increases urine flow

DMARD Disease-modifying anti-rheumatic drug

DNA Deoxyribonucleic acid

Dopaminergic Refers to nerve cells that use dopamine as a **neurotransmitter**

Dose–response relationship Relationship between the dose of a drug used and the magnitude of the response

Drug absorption Movement of a drug into the internal environment

Drug dependence Patient either craves a drug (psychological dependence) or suffers physical symptoms of withdrawal without the drug (physical dependence)

Drug distribution The tissues to which a drug gains access

Drug elimination Movement of the drug out of the body into the external environment (see also **Excretion**)

Drug metabolism How the body transforms the drug chemically

Drug tolerance More of a dose of a drug is required in order to achieve the same effect

Dysmenorrhoea Painful menstruation

Dyspepsia (indigestion) Disorder of digestion during which there may be pain and discomfort in the abdomen or lower chest, and perhaps nausea and vomiting

Dysphasia (aphasia) Language disorder arising in the left hemisphere affecting speech generation and content (not a disorder of speech articulation)

Dyspnoea Shortness of breath

Dystonia Uncontrolled movements

ECG See **Electrocardiogram**

Echocardiogram Visual display of the beating heart action using non-invasive ultrasound

Eczema Itchy skin disorder; there are several types

EEG See **Electroencephalogram**

Efficacy How effective a drug is (see also **Potency**)

Electrocardiogram (ECG) Recording of the heart's electrical activity using surface electrodes

Electroencephalogram (EEG) Tracing produced by recording electrical activity in various parts of the brain using surface electrodes

Embolism Condition when an **embolus** becomes lodged in an artery and blocks blood flow

Embolus Material such as air, fat, blood clot, amniotic fluid or a foreign body that is carried in the blood to lodge elsewhere, e.g. a lung embolism

Embryo In humans, the product of conception up to week 8

EMEA European Agency for the Evaluation of Medicinal Products

Emetic Substance that causes vomiting

Emphysema (pulmonary emphysema) Difficulty with breathing caused by damaged alveoli of the lungs; cause unknown but smokers may be more prone to emphysema

Emulsion A mixture of two immiscible liquids (e.g. oil and water) in which one is dispersed through the other in a finely divided state, e.g. milk of magnesia

Endocarditis Inflammation of the lining of the heart cavity (the endocardium)

Endocrine gland Ductless gland

Endogenous Derived from or arising in the body, e.g. endorphins are endogenous whereas morphine is **exogenous**

Endometrium Mucous membrane that lines the lumen of the uterus

Endoscopic retrograde cholangiopancreatography (ERCP) Technique used to outline the bile ducts and pancreatic duct radiographically

Endoscopy Viewing interior organs, usually with fibreoptics

Enema Fluid infused into the rectum through a tube that has been passed through the anus

Enzyme induction Increasing the activity of an enzyme, usually by stimulating enzyme production. This can have serious implications for the patient, e.g. barbiturates induce enzymes that metabolise warfarin

Enzyme Protein that catalyses biochemical reactions

Epidural injection The injection of a local anaesthetic into the epidural space in the lumbar region of the spinal cord

Epinephrine (adrenaline) Hormone released from the **adrenal medulla**; one of the **catecholamines**

ERCP Endoscopic retrograde cholangiopancreatography

Erythema Skin flushing caused by capillary dilatation in the dermis; **erythematous**: producing erythema

Erythropoietin Hormone secreted by some kidney cells in response to reduced oxygen tension in blood; erythropoietin increases the rate of red blood cell production

Essential hypertension Clinically high blood pressure of unknown cause

Euphoria Elation and optimism for no apparent reason; in extreme form is called **mania**

Exacerbation Worsening

Excretion Ejection of anything from the body

Exfoliation Flaking off of the upper layers of the skin; separation of the surface epithelium from underlying tissue

Exocrine gland Refers to gland that secretes its hormone via ducts

Exogenous Derived from or originating outside the body, e.g. diethyl-stilbestrol is an exogenous oestrogen whereas estradiol is an **endogenous** oestrogen

Extrasystole Also called an **ectopic beat**, it is a heartbeat that originates in the heart away from the sinoatrial node; may be ventricular or supraventricular

Extravasation Escape from blood vessels into other tissues

Febrile Relating to fever

Ferritin A complex of iron and a protein; one of the ways in which iron is stored in the tissues

Fetus (foetus) Unborn child from week 8 of development

Fibrates Drugs that alter the metabolism of **lipoproteins,** and so lower blood cholesterol and triglycerides

Fibrillation Rapid, chaotic beating of individual cardiac muscle fibres

Fibrin Fibrous insoluble protein of the blood clot

Fibrinogen Soluble protein converted to insoluble **fibrin** by **thrombin**

First-pass metabolism Metabolism of a drug in the liver after its absorption from the **GIT**

Flatulence Sensation of distension of the abdomen and expulsion of stomach gases through the mouth

Follicle-stimulating hormone (FSH) Hormone released by the anterior pituitary; promotes spermatogenesis and development of the ovarian follicle

GAD General anxiety disorder

Gallstone (cholelithiasis) A hard body made of cholesterol, bile pigments and calcium that forms in the gallbladder

Gastric Relating to or affecting the stomach

General anaesthetic Drug that produces total unconsciousness for surgical purposes

General anxiety disorder (GAD) The patient feels apprehensive and tense for no particular reason, or as a result of some minor problem

GIT Gastrointestinal tract

Glabellar tap Persistent reflex blinking when tapping the glabellar bone between the eyebrows

Glaucoma Loss of vision caused by abnormally raised intraocular pressure

Globus pallidus Globe-shaped mass within the **basal ganglia** of the brain

Glomerulus Usually refers to the network of blood capillaries in Bowman's capsule of the kidney; an important function is to filter substances out of the blood into the urine

Glucocorticoid See **Corticosteroid**

Glycogen Principal storage form of glucose in the body, consisting of branched chains of glucose

Gonadotrophins Proteinaceous hormones released from the anterior pituitary gland and the placenta; they are concerned with the growth and structural maintenance of the male and female gonads, and with the synthesis and release of the gonadal sex hormones

Gonads Male or female reproductive organs (testis and ovary, respectively)

Gout Disease in which uric acid metabolism and excretion are impaired, resulting in deposition of uric acid in joints and cartilage, especially in the ears

Haemoglobin Oxygen-carrying protein in the red blood cells

Haemoptysis Coughing up blood

Haemorrhage Serious leakage of blood from blood vessels

Haemostasis The balance between **coagulation** and clot dissolution; also used to describe stopping bleeding either naturally through coagulation or as a surgical procedure, e.g. ligation

Haptens Small molecules that combine with larger molecules such as proteins and turn them 'foreign', e.g. aspirin

HDL High-density **lipoprotein**

Heart block When the bundle of His fails to transmit impulses from the atria to the ventricles

Heart failure Inadequate pumping power of the ventricles of the heart

Helper T cells Lymphocytes that stimulate the production of **killer T cells**, which attack and destroy target cells

Hepatic Pertaining to the liver

Hepatosplenomegaly Enlargement of the liver and spleen that can be felt below the rib margin

Hepatotoxic Toxic to the liver

Heroin Diacetylmorphine

Herpes Inflammation of mucous membranes or skin caused by the herpes virus; herpes simplex virus type I causes the cold sore and type II causes genital herpes; herpes zoster causes shingles

Hirsutism Inappropriate and unwanted growth of body hair

HMG-CoA Hydroxymethyl glucoyl-coenzyme A

HRT Hormone replacement therapy

Human immunodeficiency virus (HIV) Retrovirus responsible for AIDS

Hypercalcaemia High blood calcium

Hyperglycaemia Clinically high blood glucose

Hyperkalaemia High blood potassium

Hyperlipidaemia Abnormally high concentration of fats in the bloodstream

Hyperparathyroidism Over-activity of the parathyroid glands

Hyperplasia The increased production and growth of more normal cells in any organ or tissue, e.g. benign prostatic hyperplasia (BPH) in older men

Hypertension Clinically raised blood pressure that could damage perfused tissues; see also **Essential hypertension**

Hyperthyroidism Over-secretion of thyroid hormone

Hypertrophy The enlargement of the cells themselves without necessarily an increase in cell number; the increase in muscle size following exercise or 'pumping iron' is an example of hypertrophy

Hyperuricaemia (lithaemia) Abnormally high uric acid concentrations in blood

Hypnotic Drug that induces sleep

Hypoglycaemia Clinically low blood glucose

Hypokalaemia Low blood potassium

Hypokinesia Inhibition of voluntary movements

Hyponatraemia Low blood sodium

Hypotension Clinically low blood pressure

Hypothyroidism Under-secretion of thyroid hormone

Idiopathic A condition with an unknown cause and that appears to arise spontaneously

In vitro Refers to events, e.g. heart rate, or chemical reactions, e.g. glycolysis, outside living systems, e.g. in a test tube

In vivo Refers to events, e.g. blood pressure, or chemical reactions, e.g. insulin biosynthesis, within whole, living systems

Incontinence Involuntary passage of urine

Infarct Localised area of dead tissue caused by failure of blood supply

Infarction Tissue death caused by interruption of blood supply, e.g. **myocardial infarction** after a coronary thrombosis

Infective endocarditis Infection of the mural surface of the endocardium or of the cardiac valves

Inflammatory bowel disease Any of a group of intestinal inflammatory disorders including **Crohn's disease** and **ulcerative colitis**

Infusion Slow injection of a volume into the body, usually into a vein

Insomnia Inability to fall asleep or remain asleep for an adequate time

Intercurrent illness The occurrence of an illness that may modify the course and treatment of another illness that is present at the same time

Interferons Peptides that are produced by cells infected with viruses

Intrathecal injection Administration of a drug directly into the central nervous system (CNS), thus bypassing the blood–brain barrier

Ionisation Conversion of an electrically neutral chemical into a charged one by either gaining or losing electrons

Ischaemia Inadequate blood flow to a part of the body (adj. ischaemic)

Kaolin cephalin time A method of measuring the clotting time

Ketone Member of a group of organic compounds containing a carbonyl group (C=O) that has two alkyl groups attached, e.g. acetone and β-hydroxy-butyric acid

Killer T cells Lymphocytes that target and destroy other cells

Kinase Intracellular enzyme that can convert an inactive enzyme into an active one; kinases themselves can exist in either inactive or activated states

LDL Low-density **lipoprotein** that carries cholesterol in the bloodstream

Lennox–Gastaut syndrome Very severe form of childhood epilepsy

Lewy body dementia Dementia with symptoms overlapping those of **Alzheimer's disease**, with loss of cognition, hallucinations and symptoms of **Parkinson's disease**; Lewy bodies are abnormal lumps seen in degenerating cells of the cortex and substantia nigra

Libido Sexual drive

Ligand Any chemical that binds to another (in pharmacology, almost always refers to drugs that bind to macromolecular receptors)

Lipid Fat (see also **Adipose tissue**)

Lipophilic Literally 'fat loving'; in pharmacy usually describes solubility of a solute or solvent in a lipid medium; in physiological, pharmacological and chemical terms lipophilic often describes an uncharged molecule, e.g. a steroid

Lipophobic Literally 'fat hating'; the inability of charged molecules such as ions to diffuse freely across the fatty plasma membrane

Lipoproteins Molecules in the blood and lymph consisting of protein and lipids; important in the transport of cholesterol and the uptake of cholesterol into cells

Local anaesthetic Drug that reduces or abolishes pain in a limited body area, e.g. the gums in dentistry

Loop diuretic **Diuretic** that acts in the ascending limb of the loop of Henle

Malar rash Red 'butterfly' rash on cheeks, a symptom of **SLE**

Malaria Infectious disease caused by parasitic protozoa of genus *Plasmodium*

Malnutrition Condition arising from improper balance between an individual's diet and what is required in a diet for maintenance of health

Mania Wild, extravagant and incoherent speech and behaviour

MAOI See **Monoamine oxidase inhibitor**

Medulla The inner part or region of a tissue, which can be anatomically distinguished from an outer region called the cortex; examples include the kidney, **adrenal medulla**, lymph nodes and brain

Meningitis Inflammation of the meninges, the three membranes that enclose the brain and spinal cord; symptoms include severe headache, photosensitivity, fever, loss of appetite, muscle rigidity, especially in the neck, and in severe cases delirium, convulsions and death

Menopause When cessation of ovulation and menstruation starts to occur

Metastasis Spread of a malignant tumour to distant sites in the body

MI See **Myocardial infarction**

Microsomal Refers to particles of endoplasmic reticulum to which ribosomes become attached. Several metabolic enzymes are associated with the microsomal fraction of cells

MMR vaccine Combined vaccine against measles, mumps and German measles (rubella)

Monoamine oxidase inhibitor (MAOI) Drug that inhibits the enzyme monoamine oxidase, which breaks down **catecholamines** such as **norepinephrine** and **epinephrine**; used chiefly to treat depressive illness

Monoclonal antibody Antibody produced from an artifical cell made by fusing a mouse spleen lymphocyte that produces the antibody to a mouse myeloma cell; the resulting artificial cell makes only the one antibody that the lymphocyte originally made

Monocyte Type of white blood cell with kidney-shaped nucleus, with the function of taking in foreign particles, e.g. bacteria and debris

Morbidity Condition or state of being diseased

Mortality Death, e.g. mortality rate = death rate

MRSA Meticillin-resistant *Staphylococcus aureus*

Muscarinic Describes drugs that bind to and activate muscarinic acetylcholine receptors of the parasympathetic division of the autonomic nervous system, or to drugs that mimic the effects produced by stimulation of muscarinic receptors

Myocardial infarction (MI) Death of part of the heart muscle, usually in the left ventricle, following interruption of the blood supply

Myocardium Middle layer of heart wall tissue, composed of muscle

Myoclonic jerks Sudden jerking of the limbs that occurs in patients with epilepsy and in those with degenerative neurological disease

Myopathy Any disease of muscle (e.g. **cardiomyopathy**)

NADPH Reduced nicotinamide adenine dinucleotide phosphate; a coenzyme that acts as a hydrogen acceptor in oxidation–reduction reactions

Necrosis Death of cells within a tissue or organ

Negative feedback A regulatory system whereby the end-product (e.g. testosterone) controls its own synthesis and/or release by inhibiting the system that stimulates its production

Negative inotropic Decreased heart contractility

Nephrotic syndrome Protein loss in the urine and cirrhosis of the liver where there is a failure to make protein

Nephrotoxic Toxic to the kidneys

Neural transplantation Transplanting human fetal tissue, e.g. containing dopaminergic neurons into the brains of patients with Parkinson's disease

Neuroleptic Antipsychotic drug

Neurotransmitter Chemical, e.g. ACh, norepinephrine or 5-HT, released from nerve terminals by arrival of a nerve impulse, and which binds to specific receptors on pre- and/or post-synaptic membranes

Neutropenia Clinically significant reduction in the numbers of neutrophils in the blood

NHS National Health Service

NICE National Institute for Health and Clinical Excellence

Nicotinic Describes drugs that bind to and activate nicotinic acetylcholine receptors of the parasympathetic division of the autonomic nervous system, or to drugs that mimic the effects produced by stimulation of nicotinic receptors

Noradrenergic Describes nerves that release **norepinephrine** as **neurotransmitter,** or receptors that respond to norepinephrine

Norepinephrine (also called noradrenaline) A **catecholamine** neurotransmitter released from **noradrenergic** nerve terminals; small amounts are also released from the **adrenal medulla**

NSAID Non-steroidal anti-inflammatory drug

Nucleoside A chemical consisting of a pyrimidine or purine base attached to a sugar, e.g. adenosine

Nucleotide A pyrimidine or purine base attached to a sugar to which is attached a phosphate group; the building blocks of **RNA** and **DNA**

Obese Possessing excess fat; an individual who weighs 20% or more than the recommended weight for his or her age, build and height is usually considered obese

Obsessive–compulsive disorder Characterised by repetitive, anxiety-driven behaviour such as the repeated washing of hands or obsessive thoughts and doubts

Oedema Accumulation of excess fluid in body tissues (called dropsy in the past)

Oestrogen One of a group of chemicals, including estradiol, that develops and maintains female sexual function and secondary female characteristics such as breast development

Oliguria Abnormally low urine production

Oncogen Anything that causes a tumour

Opiates Strictly speaking, *synthetic* morphine analogues such as diacetyl-morphine (heroin), but in many texts the term is used to describe both natural and synthetic morphine analogues

Opioid Natural substances that produce morphine-like effects such as analgesia, euphoria and sedation. Examples include morphine, codeine, enkephalins and endorphins. Strictly speaking, these are *natural* morphine analogues but in many texts the term is used to describe both natural and synthetic morphine analogues

Optic chiasma Crossing over of the two optic nerves near the pituitary gland

Oral anticoagulants Anticoagulants that can be taken by mouth, e.g. warfarin

Oral contraceptive (OC) Tablet taken orally that blocks conception

Osteoarthritis (osteoarthrosis) Degenerative joint disease, involving wear of articular cartilage, which may cause secondary changes in underlying bone; can be primary, or secondary to abnormal loads to joints or damage to cartilage caused by trauma or inflammation

Osteoporosis Loss of bony tissue, resulting in fracture-prone brittle bones

Ototoxic Toxic to the organs of hearing or balance in the inner ear or on the vestibulocochlear nerve

PABA Para-Aminobenzoic acid, a precursor of folic acid, which is essential in cell division

Palliative therapy Drug treatment to relieve symptoms, without actually curing a disease; commonly used in cancer

Pallidotomy (pallidectomy) Introduction of electrodes into the brain to destroy a particular part of the brain in an area called the **globus pallidus**

Pancreatitis Inflammation of the pancreas

Panic attacks Unexpected attacks of anxiety, often with marked physical symptoms such as tremor, palpitation and dry mouth, caused by over-activity of the sympathetic nervous system

Parasympathomimetic Drug that mimics the stimulation of the parasympathetic division of the autonomic nervous system

Parenteral Administration of a drug by any route other than orally, e.g. by injection

Parkinson's disease Degenerative brain disorder in the **basal ganglia** with the loss of dopaminergic neurons, resulting in rigidity, tremor and progressive difficulty in initiating and stopping movement

Partial agonist A drug that is both **agonist** and **antagonist** under different conditions (often dose dependent)

Parturition Childbirth

Passive immunisation The appropriate antibody against the invading organism or toxin is injected (see also **Active immunisation**)

Patch Adhesive impregnated with medicine and applied to the skin for slow, continuous release of active agent

Pepsin Stomach enzyme that breaks down proteins

Peptic Relating to **pepsin** or digestion

Peptide Molecule consisting of two or more amino acids, e.g. oxytocin

Peripheral neuropathy Damage to peripheral nerves, notably in the extremities such as fingers or toes, and caused by, for example, diabetes

Peristalsis Wave of involuntary contractions of tubular tissue, e.g. intestine

Peritonitis Inflammation of the peritoneum

Petit mal (absence **seizure**) Brief interference with consciousness

pH Measure of acidity or alkalinity in units from 1 to 14; 'pH' means −log of the hydrogen ion concentration

Phaeochromocytoma A **catecholamine**-secreting tumour of the adrenal gland

Pharmacodynamics Study of how the body recognises the drug; how the drug exerts its effect

Pharmacoeconomics The economic implications of prescribing and dispensing increasingly more expensive treatments

Pharmacokinetics Study of how the body processes the drug

Pharmacology Science of drug properties and actions on living systems

Pharmacovigilance The follow-up of drug use in patients, including safety and effectiveness monitoring

Pharynx Muscular tube lined with mucous membranes that extends from the base of the skull down to the beginning of the oesophagus; its functions are to carry air from the nose and mouth to the larynx, to act as a resonating chamber for the larynx, and to carry food from the mouth to the oesophagus

Phobic states The patient fears certain situations; the commonest is agoraphobia in which the subject is frightened to go out

Phosphodiesterase Enzyme that breaks down cyclic AMP

Pituitary fossa Hollow in the sphenoid bone that houses the pituitary gland

pK_a pH at which a solute is 50% ionised, usually in aqueous solution

Placebo effect Therapeutic effect of a **placebo**

Placebo A treatment that is pharmacologically inert, e.g. a lactose tablet; placebos are often used in **clinical trials**

Plasma half-life The time taken for the plasma concentration of a drug to decline to one-half its original value

Plasma Straw-coloured fluid in which the blood cells are suspended

Plasmodium Genus of **protozoans** that live in human red blood and liver cells; they cause, for example, malaria

Platelets (thrombocytes) Disc-shaped bodies in blood, 1–2 μm in diameter, with functions related to stopping bleeding

Platelet aggregation Sticking together of **platelets** in the blood

PMS See **Premenstrual syndrome**

Pneumocystis A protozoan that can cause pneumonia in immunosuppressed patients

Polyarteritis nodosa (periarteritis nodosa) Potentially dangerous inflammation of the walls of arteries, producing symptoms of, for example, arthritis, asthma, fever, hypertension, kidney failure and neuritis; treated with prednisolone or other corticosteroids

Positive inotropic Increased heart contractility (see **Negative inotropic**)

Post-ictal After a stroke or (more usually) a **seizure**

Post-thrombotic syndrome Long-term adverse effects in legs after a venous thrombosis; effects include valvular damage, pain, swelling, leg ulcers

Post-traumatic stress disorder The anxiety that follows traumatic experiences such as rape or warfare

Potency How powerful the drug is; the lower the dose, the more powerful the drug

Pre-eclampsia Sudden rise in blood pressure in a pregnant woman (> 140/90), in whom blood pressure was previously normal

Pre-ganglionic Refers usually to nerve fibres leaving the CNS before making their synapses in the ganglia

Pre-load The pressure in the venous system filling the heart and stretching the heart muscle

Premenstrual syndrome (PMS; premenstrual tension) Irritability, nervousness and depression before menstruation, associated with accumulation of water and salts in the tissues; usually disappears when menstruation begins

Prodrug A drug that is metabolised to the therapeutically active form, e.g. the antidepressant imipramine loses a methyl group to become desipramine

Prolactin Hormone released by the anterior pituitary; promotes milk production

Prolapse Downward displacement of an organ

Prosthesis Any artificial aid attached to the body, e.g. prosthetic heart valve

Protease Enzyme that catalyses the splitting of proteins

Proteinuria Protein in the urine

Prothrombin time (PT) The time taken for clotting to occur in a sample of blood to which thromboplastin and calcium have been added

Prothrombin Protein that is converted to **thrombin** by **thromboplastin**

Protozoa Group of microscopic, single-celled organisms, e.g. *Trypanosoma*

Psoriasis Relatively common chronic skin disease, often in families, in which scaly, pink patches occur on the scalp, elbows, knees and other parts of the body

Psoriatic arthritis Arthritis that is associated with psoriasis

Psychosis One of a group of psychiatric disorders in which the patient loses contact with reality

Pulmonary embolism Blood clot lodged in a lung blood vessel, obstructing blood flow

Purgatives Drugs that loosen the bowel

Pyridoxine Vitamin B_6

RA Rheumatoid arthritis

Radiotherapy Therapy with any penetrating radiation, e.g. X-rays, β-rays or γ-rays to treat, for example, malignant growths or other tumours

Receptor Protein that recognises another chemical and binds it, usually transducing the binding reaction into a message to the cell

Recessive Describes a gene or its corresponding characteristic that will appear in an individual only when two identical **alleles** of a gene occur in that individual. Defective genes that occur as a double autosomal recessive may cause inherited diseases, e.g. cystic fibrosis

Refractory period Period between muscle contraction or nerve impulse generation when muscle or nerve recovers and is unable to respond to an incoming impulse

Renin Enzyme released into the circulation by the kidney in response to stresses such as haemorrhage or other causes of low blood pressure

Response element Deoxynucleotide sequence in the genomic DNA involved in the switching on and off of transcription

Retinoids Group of drugs derived from vitamin A

Retrovirus RNA-containing virus that converts its RNA into DNA using an enzyme called reverse transcriptase

Reye's syndrome Childhood symptoms of encephalitis with symptoms of liver failure; aspirin is implicated and contraindicated in children below 12 (named after R.D.K. Reye, Australian histopathologist, 1912–1977)

Rheumatic fever Acute rheumatism; disease affecting mainly children and young adults as a delayed complication of haemolytic streptococcal infection of the upper respiratory tract; may progress to chronic rheumatic heart disease

Rheumatoid arthritis (RA) An autoimmune disease; very common form of progressive arthritis, second only to osteoarthritis, affecting soft tissue of joints of fingers, wrists, ankles and feet, and eventually knees, hips, shoulders and neck. Ligaments and bone become damaged; more prevalent in women (women:men = 3:1)

RNA Ribonucleic acid

SBP Systolic blood pressure

Schizophrenia Change of personality with disordered thought processes, which may be associated with hallucinations, delusions and withdrawal

Scleroderma Possibly an autoimmune disorder, with skin thickening and sometimes becoming systemic to lungs and other tissues

Scurvy Disease caused by vitamin C deficiency

Second messenger Intracellular chemical that carries the message that a hormone, neurotransmitter, etc. has bound to its receptor on the cell membrane; examples include cyclic AMP and inositol trisphosphate

Seizure Convulsion or fit

Serotonin (5-hydroxytryptamine, 5-HT) Neurotransmitter widely found in the body, especially platelets, the **CNS** and the **GIT**

Serum Fluid that separates from clotted blood; it is essentially plasma without fibrinogen and other factors involved in coagulation

Sinoatrial (SA) node Tiny modified body of heart muscle in the upper right ventricle near the entry point of the vena cava; called the pacemaker because it has an independent rhythmic beat of about 70 per minute

Sinus rhythm The normal heart rhythm that originates in the **sinoatrial node**

Skeletal (striated) muscle Muscles attached to the skeletal frame, which are under voluntary control

SLE See **Systemic lupus erythematosus**

Smooth muscle Muscle of the autonomic nervous system that mediates involuntary contractions, e.g. of arterioles and bronchi

Splanchnic Refers to the **viscera**, which in turn means the organs within the body cavities, especially those in the abdominal cavities

Specificity Describes the selectivity of a receptor for drugs

Spirometry Measurement of air volume inhaled and exhaled; used in ventilation tests

Statins (HMG-CoA reductase inhibitors) Drugs that block the synthesis of cholesterol in the liver

Steatorrhoea Fatty, pale stools

Stenosis Abnormal narrowing of, for example, blood vessels or heart valves

Stent Device inserted into blood vessel to keep the lumen open in, for example, bile ducts, urethra, ureter, oesophagus or an artery

Stricture Narrowing of any tubular structure, e.g. bowel, oesophagus, ureter

Stroke Weakness or paralysis on one side of the body caused by interruption of blood flow to the brain; in the past was called apoplexy

Sublingual Under the tongue

Suppository Formulation for administration of medicine into the rectum

Supraventricular rhythm Any cardiac rhythm originating above the ventricles

Sustained release Refers to a medicinal formulation that continuously releases the active agent from, for example, the GIT (also called 'retard' preparations)

Sympathomimetic Drug that mimics the stimulation of the sympathetic division of the autonomic nervous system

Synovitis Inflammation of the membrane (synovium) that lines the joint capsule

Systemic lupus erythematosus (SLE) Chronic autoimmune inflammatory disorder affecting the connective tissue; many different organs, including joints, brain and kidney, may be affected; treatment is currently with corticosteroids, antimalarials and immunosuppressive drugs

Systole Period of the cardiac cycle when the heart is contracting

Systolic blood pressure The blood pressure at systole, when the ventricles contract and pump blood into the arterial circulation

T lymphocytes White blood cells that mature in the thymus gland before they enter the general circulation

Tachycardia Very rapid heart rate (> 100 beats/minute)

TED stockings Graduated compression stockings (also called thromboembolic deterrent stockings)

Tendinitis Inflammation of a tendon

TENS Transcutaneous electrical neural stimulation

Teratogenic Causes birth defects

Therapeutic index Ratio of a therapeutic dose to a toxic dose. The higher the therapeutic index, the safer the drug

Thiamine Vitamin B_1

Thrombin Enzyme that converts soluble **fibrinogen** to insoluble **fibrin** in the clotting process

Thrombocytopenia Reduction in blood **platelets**, resulting in bruising of the skin and prolonged wound bleeding

Thrombocytopenic purpura Bleeding into the skin

Thrombolytic A drug that dissolves a thrombus

Thromboplastin (thrombokinase) Enzyme that converts prothrombin to **thrombin**

Thrombosis Blood solidification in a blood vessel through formation of a blood clot

Thrombus Blood clot

Thyrotoxicosis Syndrome caused by excessive circulating thyroid hormones

Thyroxine (T_4) Hormone produced by and secreted from the thyroid gland

TIA See **Transient ischaemic attack**

Tinnitus Sensory experience of sound (e.g. hissing, bells) without any external stimulus

Tissue factor Protein released from damaged tissue, which accelerates the clotting cascade through binding to factor VIIa

TNF Tumour necrosis factor

Tocolytic agents Drugs that inhibit uterine contractions

Tonic–clonic (grand mal) seizure A generalised focal discharge causes the patient to fall unconscious and pass through typical tonic and clonic phases; the patient regains consciousness after a varying interval

Total peripheral resistance (TPR) Resistance to blood flow in diastole, i.e. caused by resistance in the peripheral vascular beds only

Transdermal Literally 'across skin'; refers mainly to skin patches containing medication for direct absorption through the skin

Transient ischaemic attack (TIA) A set of neurological symptoms that clear up completely within 24 hours, caused by a temporary stoppage of blood to a part of the brain by a tiny blood clot

Triiodothyronine (T_3) Released together with thyroxine from the thyroid gland, and the active form of thyroxine in the tissues

Trophic Causing growth

Tubocurarine A non-depolarising neuromuscular blocker extracted from curare bark

Tumour Abnormal swelling in or on the body; may be benign or malignant

Ulcer Break in the skin through all its layers or a break in any mucous membrane

Ulcerative colitis (UC) Inflammatory, ulcerative disease of the colon and rectum

Ultrasound Sound waves usually in excess of 1 MHz, used to generate images of organs and the fetus

Uric acid Chemical excreted in the urine; an end-product of nucleic acid metabolism, which causes gout if deposited in joints

Uricosuric drugs Drugs that increase uric acid excretion in the urine

Urinary retention Difficulty with micturition, e.g. in BPH

Vaccine Preparation of material from deactivated bacteria or viruses, containing antigens against which the body produces antibodies

Varices Distended veins

Vasoconstriction Decrease in diameter of blood vessels, especially arterioles

Vegetation Abnormal outgrowth from membranes; in cardiology refers to outgrowths of fibrin with enmeshed blood cells in ulcerative endocarditis associated with bacterial infection

Ventricle Either of the two lower chambers of the heart; also refers to fluid-filled chambers of the brain

Ventricular fibrillation Cardiac arrhythmia marked by fibrillary contractions of the ventricular muscle due to rapid, repetitive excitation of myocardial fibres without coordinated ventricular contraction and by absence of atrial activity. It is usually fatal unless treated immediately with a **defibrillator**

Virus Particle visible with the electron microscope that survives only within living cells; can infect other micro-organisms such as bacteria, plants and animals

Viscera The organs within the body cavities, especially those in the abdominal cavities (see also **Splanchnic**)

Vitamin One of a group of chemicals not synthesised in the body but taken in the diet; they are required in tiny amounts for normal development and cellular function

Vitreous humour Jelly-like transparent substance that fills the chamber of the eye behind the lens (see also **Aqueous humour**)

Vomiting centre Nerve centre in the medulla of the brain that, when stimulated electrically, causes vomiting (see also **Chemoreceptor trigger zone**)

Wernicke's encephalopathy Brain disorder with delirium or mental confusion caused by vitamin B_1 deficiency, usually associated with alcoholism; treated with vitamin B_1

Whipple's disease Rare disease occurring only in men, when food absorption of the gut is reduced, resulting in malabsorption and often skin pigmentation and arthritis

Zymogen (pro-enzyme) Inactive precursor of an enzyme

Sources

Dorland's Pocket Medical Dictionary, 25th edn. Philadelphia: W. B. Saunders Company, 1995.

Oxford Concise Colour Medical Dictionary, 2nd edn. Oxford: Oxford University Press, 1998.

Ballinger A, Pratchett S. *Saunders' Pocket Essential of Clinical Medicine*, 3rd edn. Edinburgh: Elsevier Ltd, 2004

Trounce's Clinical Pharmacology for Nurses, 17th edn. Edinburgh: Churchill Livingstone, 2004.

Notes

1. There is controversy over whether viruses are 'alive'.
2. False positive: a trial demonstrates a significant, desired effect of the drug compared with placebo when such an effect does not exist.
3. In the *Oxford Concise Medical Dictionary, parenteral* is defined as 'by any way other than through the mouth' (Oxford University Press, 1998, 2nd edn, p. 487).
4. This is an average estimate; total body water per kilogram would be lower in an obese individual.
5. Reminder: the V_D is the theoretical volume of water that the body would need to possess in order to ensure a uniform distribution of a dissolved drug in the body.
6. Treadmill exercise or radionuclide use.
7. SBP: systolic blood pressure; DBP: diastolic blood pressure.
8. Wall PD, Melzack R (eds). *Textbook of Pain*. Edinburgh: Churchill Livingstone, 1994.
9. Olanow CW *et al*. *Neurology* 2001; **56**: 11 (Suppl. 5).
10. Moryama E *et al*. *Neurol Med Chir* 1999; **39**: 350–356.
11. Schuurman PR *et al*. *N Engl J Med* 2000; **342**: 461–468.
12. *Hospital Medicine* 2001 **62**: No. 8.
13. Katzung BG (ed.). *Basic and Clinical Pharmacology*. Stamford, CT: Appleton & Lange, 1998: p. 386
14. Newer drugs for epilepsy in children. *NICE Technology Appraisal 79*, April 2004.
15. *Drugs and Aging* 2003; 20(2): 141-152.
16. This classification based on Dowson AJ. *Pharm J* 2002; **268**: 176.
17. Dowson AJ. *Pharm J* 2002; **268**: 141–143.
18. *Cephalalgia* 1988; **88**: 1–96.
19. NICE. *Anxiety Clinical Guideline 22*, December 2004.
20. Allen S. *Pharm J* 2005; **274**: 243–246.
21. NICE TAO77, Newer hypnotics for insomnia. 28 April 2004.
22. The terms 'neuroleptic' and 'major tranquilliser' are obsolete.
23. NICE. Press release 2002/030.
24. NICE. Appraisal Committee's preliminary recommendations, March 2005.
25. Dada MA, Kaplan AA. *Ther Apher Dial* 2004; **8**: 409–412.
26. Beral V *et al*. *Lancet* 2002; **360**: 942–944.
27. MeReC Bulletin 15, Number 4, 2005.

28. Schneider LS *et al. JAMA* 2004; **291**: 3005–3007.
29. Shumaker SA *et al. JAMA* 2004; **291**: 2947–2958.
30. Human epidermal growth factor receptor detected using immuno-histochemistry; over-expression is associated with a poor prognosis.
31. NICE. *Technology Appraisal Guidance No. 34*, March 2002.
32. Doxorubicin encapsulated in a liposome, with the surface covered with methoxypolyethylene glycol, which renders the liposome invisible to the immune system (pegylation).
32. Alendronate may also be prescribed once monthly for postmenopausal patients.
34. Endomysium: fine connective tissue sheath surrounding a single muscle fibre.
35. **Dermatitis herpetiformis**: a symmetrical itchy, blistering rash on knees, buttocks, elbows and shoulders that responds well to dapsone.
36. Smoking as a prophylactic measure against ulcerative colitis is *not* recommended.
37. Although labelled here as a large bowel condition, Crohn's disease can affect all of the GIT from mouth to anus.
38. NICE CG12. Chronic obstructive pulmonary disease. Full guideline. 3 March 2004.
39. Fabbri LM, Hurd SS. Global strategy for the diagnosis, management and prevention of COPD: 2003 update. *Eur Respir J* 2004; **23**: 932–946.
40. For serious staphylococcal infections, Legionnaire's disease, brucellosis and endocarditis, rifampicin may be given intravenously or orally.
41. Avoid pyrazinamide during an acute attack of gout.
42. *Thorax* 2001; **56**(suppl IV).
43. Patients should be warned that copious urination may occur, as this may frighten some patients.
44. Patients should be stabilised before using thiazides for this purpose.
45. See BNF for more information on the preparations, use and administration of erythropoietin.
46. Bladder retraining is the conscious attempt to increase gradually the time interval between voiding urine.
47. Abscess formation in Bartholin's glands, a pair of glands that open at the juncture of the vagina and vulva.
48. HAART is highly active antiretroviral therapy.
49. An exfoliative skin condition resulting mainly from a toxic reaction to drugs.

Index

liver disease, 26, 80, 220, 222, 228
loading dose, 32
lobar pneumonia, 234
local anaestheics, 110, 112, 168–9
lofepramine, 156
lofexidine, 166
loop diuretics, 240, 241, 242, 243, 246
loperamide, 206, 207
lopinavir, 256
lorazepam, 134, 138, 139, 148, 149,
    158, 160, 161
lornoxicam, 88
losartan, 74
low density lipoprotein receptor, 80, 82,
    186
  mutations, 80
low density lipoproteins, 80, 81, 82, 186
low molecular weight heparin, 52, 53,
    62, 63
luteinising hormone, 175, 182
Lyme disease, 220, 221

macrogols, 212, 213
magnesium sulphate, 212, 213
magnesium-based antacids, 198, 199
maintenance dose, 32
malabsorption, 204, 206–7, 236
mania, 162
mannitol, 240
Mantoux (tuberculin) test, 230, 231
maprotilene, 156, 157
mebendazole, 218, 219
medroxyprogesterone acetate, 184
melatonin, 160
memantine, 164, 165
membrane channel-linked receptors
    (ionotropic), 10, 11
membrane penetration, 20, 21
Mendelson's syndrome, 148
meninges, 147
meningitis, 146–7, 232, 244
  meningococcal, 146, 147
menopause, 186, 187, 196
menstural cycle, 182, 183
mepacrine hydrochloride (quinacrine),
    216, 219
meptazinol, 114, 115, 116
mercaptopurine, 208
mesalazine, 208, 209, 210
met-enkephalin, 110, 114, 115
meta-analysis, 16
metabolism, 24–5
  elderly patients, 136

metabotropic (G-protein-coupled)
    receptors, 10, 11
metapyrone, 180
metformin, 176, 194, 195
methacholine, 40, 41
methadone, 4, 114, 115, 116, 166
methimazole, 178
methotrexate, 98, 99, 100, 101, 104,
    105, 106, 188, 189, 210, 220, 244
methylcellulose, 212, 213
methyldopa, 30, 74
methylnorepinephrine, 41
methylprednisolone, 92, 99
methysergide, 142, 143, 204, 205
metoclopramide, 61, 63, 142, 148, 149,
    198, 199
metolazone, 76, 242
metoprolol, 62
metrimazide, 129
metronidazole, 42, 55, 200, 208, 210,
    214, 216, 217, 235
  adverse effects/contraindications,
    216
    mechanism of action, 217
    pharmacokinetics, 217
mianserin, 156, 157
microconazole, 221
microscopic polyangiitis, 244
midazolam, 113
mifeprostone (RU486), 182
migraine, 91, 140, 142–3
mineralocorticoid replacement, 180
misoprostol, 200
mitomycin, 189
mitoxanthrone, 188, 189, 190
mivacurium, 155
moclobemide, 156, 157
monoamine oxidase B inhibitors, 120,
    121, 122
monoamine oxidase inhibitors (MAOIs),
    4, 148, 149, 156, 157
  drug/food interactions, 156
  sites of action, 157
montelukast, 224, 226, 227
morphine, 24, 30, 60, 110, 113, 114,
    115, 116, 117
  administration routes, 116, 117
  dependence, 166
  renal excretion, 28
  synthetic analogues, 4, 5
morphoea, 106
motility stimulants, 198, 199
muscarine, 41